Frontline Operational Resuscitation and Combat Emergencies (FORCE) Manual

Neha Thakur Rai • Samir Misra
Editors

Dr. Aaditya Katyal
Associate Editor

Frontline Operational Resuscitation and Combat Emergencies (FORCE) Manual

Springer

Editors
Neha Thakur Rai
Department of Paediatrics
Dr. Ram Manohar Lohia Institute of Medical Sciences
Lucknow, Uttar Pradesh, India

Samir Misra
Department of Traumatology & Surgery
King George's Medical University
Lucknow, Uttar Pradesh, India

ISBN 978-981-92-1621-5 ISBN 978-981-92-1622-2 (eBook)
https://doi.org/10.1007/978-981-92-1622-2

This Springer imprint is published by the registered company Springer Nature Singapore Pte Ltd.
The registered company address is: 152 Beach Road, #21-01/04 Gateway East, Singapore 189721, Singapore

Foreword

The future of our national security needs a comprehensive strategy by our uniformed forces, modern weaponry, and technology, including Artificial General Intelligence. However, our ability to save the lives of our uniformed personnel in the moments of terrorist operations and combat matters most and of paramount importance. Toward achieving this objective, we need different protocols and their implementation for and by the medical, paramedical, and nonmedical uniformed personnel.

The creation of Frontline Operational Resuscitation and Combat (Traumatic) Emergencies (FORCE) Manual is a visionary and significant step toward the future—a trauma doctrine rooted in Indian soil, forged by operational realities, and driven by the utmost commitment to protect every precious life possible.

India's defense and disaster forces operate in environments unmatched in complexity—from sub-zero Himalayan passes and borders to riot-torn metros and insurgency zones where evacuation is measured in days, not minutes. In such terrain, conventional trauma care frameworks fall short. FORCE rises to meet this challenge.

By integrating global gold standards like TCCC and ATLS with indigenous improvisation, FORCE delivers a modular, field-adaptable model that empowers all levels of personnel—from combat buddy to commanding officer. It recognizes that in asymmetric warfare, mass casualty events, and remote deployments, care must begin at the point of injury—and continue through prolonged field care and during transfer for definitive care.

This manual is more than a protocol—it is a comprehensive systems-level shift. It emphasizes interoperability, scalable training, and an ingrained culture of preparedness. It bridges medical care and mission planning, leadership and survival, knowledge and action.

FORCE defines India's vision and determination for combat trauma leadership in the decades to come—a doctrine where bravery meets preparedness, and readiness is no longer an aspiration but a discipline instilled through training, trust, and tactical excellence.

We are proud to see this contribution emerge from our frontline experiences as well as mass casualty events affecting civil society—ready to serve the most precious resource by creating a strong system.

We envision that capacity building toward protocolized trauma care must become an integral part of induction training of all viz. Medical, Paramedical, as well as the uniformed personnel engaged in dealing with national security in basic lifesaving skills and safe transfer for definitive care.

I compliment and congratulate the team of experts who have worked overtime to develop this much needed "Manual" which must become the Bhagavad-Gita for all.

Jai Hind

ATLS Chair, India
New Delhi, India

M. C. Misra

Former Director, JPNATC, AIIMS Delhi
New Delhi, India

Preface

In the high-stakes theater of modern conflict and disaster response, the interval between injury and definitive care is often measured not just in miles but in the unforgiving realities of terrain, climate, and tactical isolation. While clinical excellence is the goal, the battlefield demands more than just medical knowledge—it requires an *operational mindset.*

The *Frontline Operational Resuscitation and Combat Emergencies (FORCE) Manual* stands as India's inaugural trauma care doctrine, specifically forged for the unique challenges faced by our military, paramilitary, and first responders. It acknowledges a hard truth: in the "Golden Hour," the luxury of a sterile hospital environment is often replaced by the grit of a mountain pass, the density of a jungle, or the chaos of an urban blast site.

Bridging the Gap

Traditional trauma models often assume rapid evacuation and infinite resources. *FORCE* reimagines this paradigm. By integrating international gold standards—such as Tactical Combat Casualty Care (TCCC) and Advanced Trauma Life Support (ATLS)—with the pragmatic necessity of *prolonged field care*, this manual provides a framework that is both evidence-based and improvisation-ready.

This doctrine is structured to be modular and role-based, ensuring clarity whether you are a first-responder medic or a specialized physician. Key highlights include:

- *Operational Integration*: Protocols tailored for gunshot wounds, blast injuries, and hand trauma—the hallmarks of asymmetric warfare
- *Tactical Decision-Making*: Simple, field-tested algorithms designed for high-stress environments where clarity is as vital as the kit in your bag
- *Resilience and Leadership*: A dedicated focus on the psychological readiness and mission planning required to maintain a "chain of survival" under fire

A Call to Action

FORCE is more than a collection of protocols; it is a commitment to the life of the individual soldier and citizen. It empowers every provider to act with decisive courage, transforming resource constraints into opportunities for innovation.

As you navigate through the pages of this book, let them instill in you the "FORCE mindset"—the unwavering resolve to lead, to adapt, and to save lives when the stakes are at their highest.

Lucknow, Uttar Pradesh, India Neha Thakur Rai
Lucknow, Uttar Pradesh, India Samir Misra

Acknowledgments The *Frontline Operational Resuscitation and Combat Emergencies (FORCE) Manual* is more than a clinical guide; it is a labor of deep respect for those who serve in the shadow of risk. This doctrine was born from the realization that in the most remote corners of our nation, the "Golden Hour" is not a medical guarantee, but a tactical challenge to be conquered through skill, grit, and unwavering resolve.

Operation Sindoor serves as the primary inspiration for this work. As a milestone of Indian operational excellence, it underscored the vital necessity for a trauma doctrine that thrives in austerity. It proved that when evacuation is delayed and resources are scarce, medical ingenuity becomes the ultimate lifeline.

I owe a profound debt of gratitude to my husband, *Major (Retd) Dr. Narendra Rai*. His distinguished service in the elite *9 Para (Special Forces)* and the *20 Punjab Regiment* provided the "boots on the ground" perspective essential to this manual. His firsthand dedication to his men in the world's harshest environments inspired every protocol within these pages, ensuring they are practical for those who carry the weight of a life in their hands.

I also extend my sincere gratitude to *Prof. M. C. Misra*, the pioneer who ignited the flame of trauma education in India. His visionary leadership laid the groundwork for modern emergency care in our country. Furthermore, I am highly indebted to *Dr. Aaditya Katyal* for his invaluable assistance and tireless effort in preparing and refining this manual.

Finally, I am deeply grateful to the leadership of *all Indian Combat Forces*. This manual is a tribute to your collective bravery. Your resilience in the face of asymmetric threats is the heartbeat of this doctrine. You are the silent guardians of our sovereignty; may this manual empower our first responders to act with clarity and courage, ensuring the chain of survival remains unbroken—no matter the terrain or the region.

Lead with courage. Act with clarity.

Neha Thakur Rai
Samir Misra

Contents

Introduction to FORCE: Frontline Operational Resuscitation and Combat Emergencies

1

Neha Thakur Rai, Vimal Krishnan S, and Aaditya Katyal

Learning Objectives

By the end of this chapter, the reader will be able to:

- Understand the rationale and relevance behind the FORCE model.
- Define the operational challenges that differentiate FORCE from conventional trauma systems.
- Identify the influence of models such as TCCC, ATLS, and PHTLS in shaping FORCE.
- Recognize the FORCE framework as an evolution of role-specific resuscitation strategies.
- Appreciate its evolution, core principles, and real-world applicability in Indian military, paramilitary, and humanitarian response settings.

Introduction

The nature of conflict and crisis in India has evolved—stretching far beyond traditional battlefields into insurgency zones, high-altitude patrols, riot-stricken cities, and disaster-hit rural expanses. In these diverse and demanding environments,

N. T. Rai
Department of Paediatrics, Dr. Ram Manohar Lohia Institute of Medical Sciences, Lucknow, Uttar Pradesh, India

V. K. S. · A. Katyal (✉)
Department of Emergency Medicine, Kasturba Medical College, Manipal, Karnataka, India
e-mail: vimal.krishnan@manipal.edu

N. T. Rai, S. Misra (eds.), *Frontline Operational Resuscitation and Combat Emergencies (FORCE) Manual*, https://doi.org/10.1007/978-981-92-1622-2_1

medical response must be immediate, adaptive, and resilient. Whether the provider is a military medic in Kupwara, a paramilitary jawan in Bastar, or a border unit handling high-altitude trauma in Arunachal Pradesh, the one constant is this: *chaos, limited resources, and lives hanging by seconds.* Yet, conventional trauma systems often fall short in the face of delayed evacuation, limited resources, and operational unpredictability.

FORCE (Frontline Operational Resuscitation and Combat Emergencies) was developed as a direct response to this reality. It is a tactical trauma care framework built specifically for the Indian military and paramilitary ecosystem—where lives depend not only on advanced care but on timely, improvised interventions in the field. It presents a practical, modular framework to manage life-threatening injuries in operational environments where time is short, evacuation is delayed, and improvisation is often the only available tool. Whether it's a buddy applying a tourniquet under fire or a medic managing a chest wound in sub-zero temperatures, FORCE emphasizes that survival begins not at the hospital, but at the point of injury.

Unlike traditional trauma manuals that assume access to a hospital within the golden hour, FORCE empowers ground-level providers to resuscitate, stabilize, and prepare casualties for delayed or staggered evacuation. It blends evidence-based trauma care with battlefield adaptability, enabling first responders to make life-saving interventions in the most hostile of settings.

Drawing from global best practices like TCCC, ATLS, and PHTLS—but redesigned for India's terrain, gear limitations, and manpower structure—*FORCE is as much a mindset as a model!*

Case Scenario

A four Indian Army personnel troop, returning from a night reconnaissance patrol near the Line of Control (LoC), is ambushed by insurgents. Amid the exchange of fire, a jawan sustains a gunshot wound to the left chest and collapses, gasping (Fig. 1.1). The team has no radio contact with base, and the nearest road is 7 km of treacherous terrain away. The temperature is –8 °C.

The unit medic, armed with a limited trauma kit, identifies a suspected tension pneumothorax. There is no portable suction, no monitors—just training, torchlight, and grit. Using a decompression needle and makeshift seal, he creates an occlusive dressing, stabilizes the airway, and provides thermal insulation. Over the next two hours, the team shelters in silence as the jawan's condition stabilizes enough for staggered evacuation at first light.

This scenario is not fiction. It reflects the daily reality of forward-deployed troops in India's highest-threat zones. It also reflects why FORCE was created.

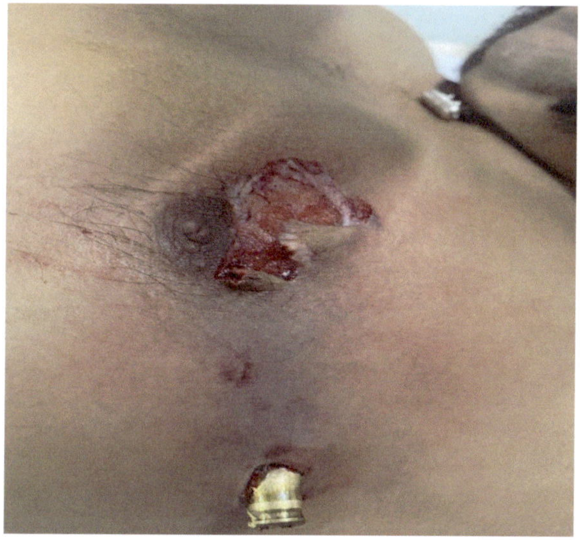

Fig. 1.1 Soldier with a gunshot wound to the left chest with impaled bullet

Historical Context and Evolution of FORCE

The story of FORCE is rooted in the enduring challenge of saving lives in battle—not in idealized, sterile conditions, but in the gritty, unpredictable reality of the field. Historically, trauma care in combat has evolved through hard-earned lessons from every major conflict. In the early twentieth century, World Wars I and II gave rise to the concept of tiered evacuation, battlefield triage, and the need for rapid surgical intervention. Yet despite a century of innovation, a central truth remains: *when bullets fly, time bleeds.*

The evolution of modern battlefield trauma care has largely been shaped by Western doctrines. ATLS (Advanced Trauma Life Support), developed by the American College of Surgeons in the late 1970s, provided a structured approach for hospital-based resuscitation. Later, in the 1990s, Tactical Combat Casualty Care (TCCC) was developed by the U.S. Special Operations Command to adapt trauma principles to combat environments. These doctrines revolutionized outcomes, especially in Afghanistan and Iraq, where structured care pathways, rapid air evacuation, and tiered trauma centers were accessible. The model emphasized early hemorrhage control, airway management, and rapid MEDEVAC—a concept often supported by robust air mobility and trauma team activation within the "Golden Hour."

However, as effective as these frameworks were in their respective theaters, they emerged from specific operational ecosystems—well-resourced, highly mobile, and technologically integrated. They assumed access to helicopters within minutes, medical evacuation corridors, and forward surgical teams within range. However, India's operational environments tell a different story.

Indian forces operate across some of the most logistically and geographically diverse environments on earth. From the dizzying altitudes of the Siachen

Glacier to the heat-blasted deserts of Rajasthan, the swampy jungles of the northeast to dense urban riots—each operational context presents unique barriers to traditional trauma protocols. Most notably, the assumption of timely evacuation often fails.

Indian counterinsurgency zones (e.g., Jammu & Kashmir, Chhattisgarh, Manipur) present operational constraints that are distinct from conventional battlefield engagements. Ambushes, IED blasts, sniper fire, and civilian presence often prevent immediate access to casualties. Medical evacuation may be delayed not by hours, but days. Poor weather, lack of airspace clearance, and denied territory further restrict the application of standard trauma doctrine.

What also sets India apart is its scale and distribution of manpower. A large number of personnel operate in small units—often a four-to-six-person patrol—across vast terrains. The reality is that not every unit has a full-time medic. Frequently, the first response comes from a fellow jawan, who must act with whatever is at hand*: a rifle sling, a torch, a pouch of ORS!* While TCCC assumes a level of medic proficiency and gear availability, Indian field scenarios demand resilience through improvisation.

It is in these gaps—between doctrine and field, theory and practice—that the FORCE model was born.

FORCE stands for Frontline Operational Resuscitation and Combat Emergencies. It is not a reinvention of trauma science—*it is a recalibration*. The model emerged not from conference halls but from field feedback—from combat medics stationed in Kupwara, from CRPF teams patrolling Bastar, from border troops navigating the high passes of Ladakh. Each of these personnel contributed to an evolving understanding: that survival in the Indian operational context requires a modular, adaptive, and improvisation-ready system.

FORCE draws upon the strengths of multiple doctrines:

- From TCCC, it inherits the urgency of bleeding control and phased care delivery.
- From ATLS, it borrows the systematic logic of trauma assessment.
- From PHTLS (Prehospital Trauma Life Support), it adopts prehospital decision-making skills.
- And from prolonged field care (PFC) models used in SOF and wilderness medicine, it integrates concepts of delayed evacuation, limited monitoring, and phased resuscitation.

But FORCE adds something more: *indigenous adaptability*.

For example, while TCCC may recommend a commercial chest seal, FORCE acknowledges that a food wrapper, tape, and glove can save a life in the hands of a trained soldier. While ATLS emphasizes airway adjuncts, FORCE emphasizes head tilt-chin lift, thermal protection, and sustained monitoring—because that is what is realistically possible when help is three hours away on foot.

Crucially, FORCE does not aim to supersede these global doctrines. Instead, it operationalizes them for Indian conditions. It integrates terrain, training level, logistics, and role distribution into its matrix. It doesn't teach every provider to perform a cricothyrotomy—*it teaches each one what they can do, given their role, with their gear, in their time window.*

The FORCE evolution is also shaped by Indian military medical traditions. The Indian Army Medical Corps has historically delivered exceptional outcomes in war and peace. However, a gap remained between medical officers and frontline combat units. That gap—of time, of gear, and of geography—needed to be bridged not just with medical support, but with training, doctrine, and mindset.

The emergence of asymmetric warfare and mass-casualty terror events further pushed the need for a system like FORCE. Whether it's a surgical strike, a civilian riot, or a cross-border skirmish, the first responder is no longer always a medic. He could be a buddy, a fireteam member, or even a civilian support volunteer. FORCE was designed for that uncertainty.

It is also a living model. FORCE evolves through feedback. Every deployment, every field case, every debrief adds to its corpus. Thus, FORCE is not just a response to a medical need—it is a doctrinal evolution. It reflects India's geography, India's enemy profile, India's training ecosystem, and India's resource profile**.** *It is battlefield trauma care for India, by India.*

While the world gave us ATLS and TCCC, India now has FORCE—a model forged not in textbooks, but in trenches, outposts, and patrol routes. A model where the doctrine doesn't merely follow the casualty—*it follows the reality!*

Philosophy and Purpose of FORCE

FORCE—Frontline Operational Resuscitation and Combat Emergencies—is more than a tactical medical model. It is a mindset forged in adversity, designed to function where doctrine meets dust, blood, and chaos. While its protocols and phases can be learned, its philosophy must be absorbed—because on the battlefield, survival is not determined solely by what you know, but by how you think under pressure.

At its core, FORCE is built upon *four interdependent pillars: tactical awareness, tiered responsibility, operational improvisation, and mission integration.* These four pillars are not simply teaching modules—they represent a strategic shift in how we perceive prehospital trauma care in military and paramilitary environments.

Tactical Awareness: Medicine That Understands the Battlefield

In traditional trauma care systems, the medical intervention is prioritized above all else. In FORCE, *tactical context always precedes clinical action.* A tourniquet that exposes a provider to enemy fire is not heroic—it is potentially fatal. FORCE teaches that no medical act is worth more than unit survivability. Every intervention is filtered through the lens of operational feasibility.

This emphasis on situational awareness trains providers to assess not only the patient but the environment. Can airway support be provided in a firefight? Should you drag the injured or suppress the threat first? Is lighting a torch worth the sniper's attention? Tactical awareness reframes resuscitation as a dance between clinical urgency and operational prudence.

This is especially relevant in Indian theaters—like Manipur or Rajouri—where operations unfold in narrow alleys, dense forests, or open mountain trails. The doctrine of FORCE demands that a provider be as tuned into the ambush arc as into the injured fellow teammate's breath sounds.

Tiered Responsibility: Everyone Is a Link in the Survival Chain

FORCE does not rely on "medical saviors." It thrives on distributed competence. Recognizing that not every soldier is a medic and not every unit has access to a medical officer, FORCE trains providers according to their role, proximity, and mission criticality.

- The *combat buddy* focuses on immediate hemorrhage control, airway positioning, and calling for help.
- The *trained field medic* delivers needle decompression, fluid resuscitation, and prolonged field care.
- The *team commander* prioritizes extraction planning, triage, and communication.
- The *medical officer* executes advanced trauma procedures, if available.

This role-based scaffolding ensures that trauma care is layered, redundant, and fail-safe. It avoids the unrealistic expectation that a single provider can "do everything." Instead, it distributes capacity across the team—so that no life is lost waiting for expertise to arrive.

Tiered responsibility also builds morale and accountability. When every soldier knows that they are trained to do *something*, no one is helpless, and no injured teammate is alone.

Operational Improvisation: Skills First, Tools Second

Perhaps the most defining trait of FORCE is its relentless emphasis on functional improvisation. In Indian deployments, medics often operate without commercial airway adjuncts, vacuum dressings, or heated IV fluids. Here, survival hinges not on kit, but on creativity.

FORCE teaches its providers that *a lack of tools is not a lack of options*:

- A *glove and tape* can substitute a chest seal.
- A *pen cap and blade* can create an airway.
- A *hydration bag and IV cannula* can act as an infusion setup.
- A *rifle sling and stick* can become a windlass tourniquet.

These techniques are not "alternatives." In FORCE, they are the primary tools taught during training. Every protocol is followed by a "field-ready" variant, preparing the provider for both textbook care and zero-resource improvisation.

This is where FORCE diverges from Western doctrines. While TCCC assumes combat gauze, FORCE assumes pressure, cloth, and knowledge. While ATLS emphasizes imaging and labs, FORCE emphasizes sound, smell, and feel. This not only increases self-reliance but builds clinical confidence under uncertainty.

Mission Integration: Embedding Medicine into Operations

In conventional training, medical considerations begin after a casualty occurs. In FORCE, *medical preparedness begins during mission planning*. This integration transforms medical care from a reactive to a proactive domain.

During the pre-mission briefing, FORCE-trained leaders assess:

- Medic-to-operator ratios
- Likely injury patterns based on past ops
- Evacuation routes and delays
- Availability of resupply or reinforcements

During mission execution, commanders know what level of care can be expected within minutes, who is trauma-trained, and what triage principles apply. Casualty collection points are designated. Communications include casualty codes, expected delays, and alternate extraction routes.

In the postoperation phase, debriefs include medical reviews. "What went wrong clinically?" is discussed alongside "What went wrong tactically?" This reinforces the idea that *trauma outcomes are command responsibilities—not just medical ones!*

This model reflects global best practices but adds Indian realism. In counterinsurgency-counterterrorism ops or riot control duties, planning rarely includes a trauma insert—FORCE changes that. It makes casualty care a shared responsibility, embedded in every operational order.

Psychological Readiness: The Fifth, Invisible Pillar

Though not a formal doctrine pillar, psychological readiness permeates FORCE philosophy. The provider must not only know what to do—*they must be ready to do it, under pressure, under fire, and, often, in moral isolation.*

FORCE training includes:

- *Stress inoculation drills*: Designed to mimic combat chaos
- *Cognitive offloading techniques*: To streamline memory in adrenaline surges
- *Peer-debriefs*: After trauma simulations, to process guilt, errors, and anxiety

This psychological training is critical in Indian ops, where evacuation is slow, support is limited, and emotional decompression may take days. It ensures that our providers remain not just physically trained but mentally equipped to act with courage and clarity.

The philosophy of FORCE redefines battlefield medicine as a team function, a tactical variable, and a survivability doctrine. It empowers providers by acknowledging their limits, maximizing their strengths, and embedding trauma readiness into every phase of the mission.

FORCE does not teach heroism. It teaches preparedness. It replaces panic with purpose. And it ensures that *when life begins to slip away, someone on the team knows what to do—clearly, calmly, and courageously.*

Core Domains and Principles of FORCE

The operational power of FORCE lies in its structured yet flexible foundation of *six core domains*. These domains collectively guide the execution of life-saving interventions in diverse and often austere settings. Each domain represents a pillar of action, but also a mindset shift—moving from hospital-based routines to field-ready responsiveness, adapted for India's multifaceted terrains and combat profiles.

The six core domains of FORCE are not checklists. They are mindsets converted into actions. From rapid hemorrhage control to structured communication, from improvised thermoregulation to mission-phase planning—each domain equips the Indian combat provider to work with clarity, courage, and clinical efficiency.

Together, they form a trauma care model that is not only functional but field-proof—designed for war, disaster, and everything in between.

Role-Based Resuscitation: A Shared Chain of Care

In traditional trauma care models, clinical decisions and interventions are centralized—carried out by physicians or senior medics. FORCE challenges this top-down model by introducing distributed trauma capability through role-based resuscitation.

Each provider—from the buddy to the commanding officer—has a clearly defined scope of practice:

- *Buddy providers* are trained in hemorrhage control, airway positioning, and monitoring vital signs.
- *Unit medics* perform higher-order tasks like decompression, IV/IO insertion, splinting, and fluid resuscitation.
- *Team leaders* oversee triage, casualty movement, and tactical integration of medical actions.
- *Medical officers*, when available, assume definitive control, surgical triage, and advanced interventions.

This layered model creates redundancy and avoids bottlenecks. Most importantly, it fosters confidence without confusion: each person knows *what* they are trained to do, *when* to do it, and *who* is next in the chain of care. In the fog of conflict, this clarity can mean the difference between chaos and coordination.

Phased Trauma Response: Stabilize, Sustain, Transition

The FORCE approach reframes trauma care not as a singular event, but as a timeline of interlinked phases (Fig. 1.2). This longitudinal view is crucial in Indian contexts where *delayed evacuation is the norm, not the exception!*

The Three Key Phases Are:

- *Point-of-injury care (POI)*: Delivered immediately after the casualty is down, usually under fire. The aim is to preserve life using rapid, low-risk interventions—tourniquets, airway opening, hemostatic agents, and patient positioning.
- *Prolonged field care (PFC)*: Encompasses all interventions post-POI when evacuation is delayed for hours. This may include wound dressing, fluid maintenance, monitoring, hypothermia control, and even pain management.

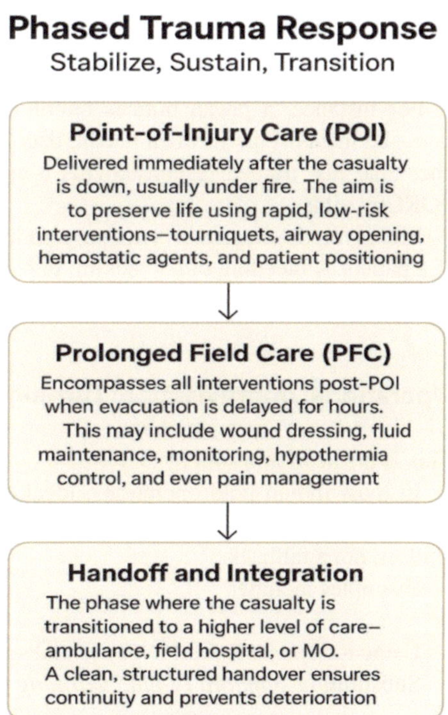

Fig. 1.2 Phased trauma response—the FORCE approach

- *Handoff and integration*: The phase where the casualty is transitioned to a higher level of care—ambulance, field hospital, or MO. A clean, structured handover ensures continuity and prevents deterioration.

This time-based triage model also adapts dynamically to the scenario. In Kupwara or Siachen, a provider might move fluidly between all three phases within a 12-h cycle—something no Western doctrine traditionally prepares them for.

Rapid Recognition of Life-Threatening Injuries

FORCE simplifies clinical triage into an instinctive process. Rather than exhaustive examination, it trains providers to *recognize and act upon five immediately correctable threats:*

- Massive hemorrhage
- Airway obstruction
- Tension pneumothorax
- Shock
- Hypothermia

This rapid assessment model is built around the *MARCH algorithm* (massive bleeding, airway, respiration, circulation, hypothermia/head injury). It needs to be drilled into every provider's mental toolkit to such an extent that even under gunfire, *pattern recognition overrides panic.*

For instance, a jawan notices bubbling chest wounds and decreasing breath rate—he instantly performs a needle decompression, no protocol consultation, no checklist, just trained response. This is not luck—it is the muscle memory that FORCE builds.

Moreover, the emphasis is not only on what to do, but what not to waste time on. If a patient is bleeding out, checking pupils is irrelevant. FORCE prioritizes time-sensitive decision-making above procedural thoroughness.

Operational Improvisation: Turning Limitations into Assets

This is the heart and soul of FORCE.

In most Indian field operations, ideal equipment is unavailable, exhausted, or forgotten. Rather than delay care, FORCE promotes pre-planned improvisation as a skillset, not a fallback.

Examples include:

- Using a *disposable food wrapper* and surgical tape as an occlusive chest seal
- Substituting *standard IV fluid warming* with body heat and insulation

- Adapting a *camelback line* to provide oral rehydration tubing
- *Repurposing vehicle blankets* to prevent hypothermia

What sets FORCE apart is that these *improvisations are taught, rehearsed, and documented.* They are part of SOPs and evaluated during drills. *The goal is to normalize creativity in trauma care—to empower providers not to freeze when protocol fails, but to innovate safely.*

This also makes FORCE uniquely resilient during natural disasters, civilian riots, or border skirmishes, where even the best preloaded kits are rendered useless by chaos.

Tactical Communication as Clinical Intervention

FORCE elevates communication to the level of a clinical skill.

A provider who performs perfect decompression but fails to report patient condition may delay evacuation. A medical officer who receives no SITREP may misprioritize triage.

Hence, FORCE trains all providers to:

- Deliver concise, structured updates ("Chest wound decompressed, HR stable, RR 26, moving to commands")
- Use color-coded urgency codes in the absence of radios
- Transmit MEDEVAC triggers such as blood loss volume, shock index, or airway difficulty

Even during buddy rescue, a simple "Pulse present, bleeding controlled" can change how backup responds.

In many ways, *communication is resuscitation.* It keeps leadership informed, avoids duplication, and prevents loss of information during handover. This is especially vital in dense operational zones like border crossings or urban conflict areas.

Integrated Training and Doctrine

FORCE is not merely a collection of skills—*it is a teaching philosophy.*

Every intervention has to be taught within operational context. A tourniquet is not taught on a bench, but in the rain, under stress, with eyes closed. Simulations mimic true field constraints. Debriefs are mandatory. Role-swaps allow buddies to feel the medic's pressure.

This ensures that FORCE is not a "top-down" model. *Everyone trains. Everyone understands. Everyone plays a role.* The doctrine is also living—built on feedback loops, evolving SOPs, and after-action learning.

Utility in the Combat Field

The Indian subcontinent, with its staggering geographic diversity, sociopolitical volatility, and varied security operations, presents unique challenges in combat trauma care. From avalanche-prone glaciers to jungle insurgencies, riot control in urban slums to humanitarian rescue after cyclones, India's military, paramilitary, and disaster response forces confront trauma scenarios that defy conventional frameworks. The FORCE model—Frontline Operational Resuscitation and Combat Emergencies—was designed to meet this challenge head-on.

It is not just relevant in the Indian context—it is essential. Its principles resonate across the spectrum of operations where the gap between injury and definitive care is not measured in minutes, but in hours, terrain, and ingenuity.

Evacuation Delays and Terrain Constraints

One of the most pressing challenges in Indian trauma response is delayed evacuation, often due to terrain, weather, or tactical exposure. In high-altitude operations like those in Siachen, Kargil, and Arunachal Pradesh, a casualty cannot be evacuated instantly. Snowstorms, avalanches, altitude sickness, and low visibility frequently render airlifting impossible. In some cases, casualties must be stabilized and carried manually for hours through steep ridges or glacial cracks.

Similarly, in jungle warfare scenarios across Chhattisgarh, Jharkhand, and Nagaland, access to injured personnel may be delayed due to active hostilities, IED threats, or lack of secure landing zones. Often, the first golden hour passes with no external support—placing the burden of care squarely on the patrol itself.

FORCE explicitly acknowledges these delays and trains providers for "Care in Place"—a concept rarely emphasized in Western protocols. *It promotes field-prolonged care as a standard, not an exception.* Its modular protocols for airway maintenance, wound dressing, hypothermia prevention, and analgesia allow care to begin and continue long before formal evacuation occurs.

Manpower Constraints and Variable Training

Indian forces are often deployed in small patrol units, with limited medical representation. A 10-person CRPF or Assam Rifles team may carry only one trained medic—if any. Sometimes, the only intervention available comes from a fellow jawan with no more than basic trauma training.

Western models such as TCCC assume a 1:4 medic-to-combatant ratio, often with MEDEVAC or CASEVAC within reach. In India, such ratios are unrealistic in border operations and counterinsurgency duties. FORCE addresses this by emphasizing tiered role-based care, where the buddy, the squad leader, and the medic each perform within their competencies.

For instance, the buddy might apply a tourniquet and move to cover, while the medic begins IV access or decompression. The commanding officer ensures extraction planning and updates to base. This distributed resuscitation model enables maximal utility of limited personnel.

Additionally, training levels vary widely—from highly skilled RMO cadres to young recruits with minimal exposure to real trauma. FORCE embraces this reality by providing scalable training pathways, enabling soldiers, medics, officers, and even civilian volunteers to engage meaningfully in trauma response.

Hybrid Deployments: Combat Meets Civil Support

India's military and paramilitary forces routinely shift between counterterrorism and civil humanitarian assistance. The same team may patrol Maoist-affected areas one month and lead flood relief the next. In these dual-use deployments, trauma scenarios evolve—from gunshot wounds and blast injuries to drowning, crush trauma, burns, and hypothermia.

FORCE is designed to bridge this spectrum. Its protocols address both combat-specific injuries and mass-casualty civil events. During the Chamoli glacier burst (2021) and the Kerala floods (2018), Indian military and NDRF teams executed improvised casualty evacuation, field dressing, and cold-exposure management—actions directly aligned with FORCE principles.

Whether the casualty is a fellow soldier, a civilian child, or a stranded villager, FORCE promotes context-sensitive triage and improvisational treatment with limited resources. It also empowers nonmedical personnel to lead early response efforts during large-scale disasters—crucial in India's vast and often inaccessible hinterlands.

Cross-Agency Interoperability

India's internal security response involves a mosaic of stakeholders: Army, BSF, ITBP, CRPF, SSB, NDRF, state police, and more. However, trauma care protocols often remain compartmentalized, with little standardization across agencies. FORCE offers a common doctrine, enabling interoperability during joint operations.

Imagine an NDRF provider stabilizing a riot-injured civilian using FORCE hemorrhage control, handing over to an Army MO for secondary care during disaster response in Bengal, or a CRPF medic performing PFC under sniper fire in Chhattisgarh, using the same checklist as an ITBP unit in Tawang. Such standardization ensures smoother transitions, fewer errors, and better survivability.

The uniform language of FORCE (e.g., MARCH algorithm, POI-PFC-handoff phases, code-based triage) allows seamless collaboration even when agencies have different chains of command. In a crisis, clarity saves lives—and FORCE provides that clarity.

Inclusion of Civilian and Disaster Responders

While developed for military and paramilitary personnel, FORCE is equally applicable to civilian providers. In regions like Kashmir, Assam, or Uttarakhand, many mass-casualty events involve local volunteers, home guards, or civilian doctors. FORCE's simplicity, field readiness, and improvisation-friendly structure make it a natural fit.

The model can be adapted into:

- Short training modules for schoolteachers, panchayat workers, and community leaders in vulnerable districts
- Urban disaster provider toolkits for firemen and police teams
- Medical college training on prehospital trauma care

In doing so, *FORCE becomes not just a military doctrine, but a national trauma resilience initiative*—one that strengthens India's capacity to respond to both conflict and catastrophe.

Cultural Fit and Practical Realism

FORCE also considers India's cultural and operational nuances:

- The tendency to defer medical decisions to senior officers
- The practice of jury-rigging tools when equipment fails
- The necessity of hiding medical activity during ongoing hostilities
- The language diversity that requires non-verbal or color-coded triage cues

Rather than resisting these realities, FORCE embraces and builds around them. For example, it encourages nonmedical commanders to lead tactical triage; it promotes pictorial training material for low-literacy environments; it builds protocols that do not require verbal confirmation but rely on observable metrics like bleeding control and chest rise.

It is a doctrine born not in air-conditioned simulation labs, but in patrol huts, mountain posts, and after-action debriefs.

Building a Trauma-Ready India

In India's current national security scenario, the role of a first responder is no longer exclusive to doctors or medics. Every patrol member, every rescue volunteer, and every police constable may become the difference between life and death. FORCE equips them for that moment.

By integrating field medical principles into a scalable, modular, Indianized trauma doctrine, FORCE offers:

- A field-tested, feedback-driven approach rooted in Indian soil
- A bridge between doctrine and delivery, even where the golden hour has long passed
- A symbol of tactical compassion, where every provider is a potential lifesaver

India needed a trauma care model that understood its terrain, its tempo, and its people. In FORCE, that model exists. It is as at home in a CI-CT ambush as it is in a flood rescue or a riot intervention. It speaks the language of Indian deployment—practical, adaptable, and field-first.

Its relevance is not confined to manuals. It is proven every time a tourniquet saves a limb in Bastar, every time a chest decompression stabilizes a jawan in Kupwara, and every time a buddy stabilizes a bleeding civilian in Guwahati.

FORCE is not a clinical guide alone—*it is a combat ethos, a tactical doctrine, and a trauma survival mindset.* It recognizes that on the frontlines, *time kills, and training saves.* It prepares providers for a war not only of weapons but of seconds. FORCE teaches that survival is a chain—one built on the strength of each link, from the buddy to the evacuation officer.

In the coming chapters, this manual will explore specific interventions, role-based competencies, decision-making tools, and field-tested protocols. Whether in counterinsurgency, border skirmishes, or humanitarian deployments, FORCE is designed to be India's answer to frontline trauma leadership.

FORCE is not only India's answer to battlefield trauma—it is India's offering to the world.

Case Resolution

Returning to the Kupwara case—by the time the QRT (Quick Reaction Team) reached the injured jawan at dawn, he was alert, perfused, and semi-reclined with sealed wounds. The decompression had worked. The thermal protection had prevented hypothermia. And the improvised airway support bought him critical hours. Evacuation to the RR Hospital was delayed by snowdrift, but by then, the resuscitation was complete.

The medic had not followed a textbook. He had followed training—*and a FORCE mindset.* He was not just a care provider; he was a tactical lifeline.

Key Messages

- FORCE is a trauma care doctrine designed specifically for Indian military, paramilitary, and disaster-response operations.
- It addresses the reality of delayed evacuation, limited resources, and the need for immediate frontline interventions in diverse terrains.
- The model draws from global best practices like TCCC, ATLS, and PHTLS, but adapts them to India's operational and logistical contexts.

(continued)

- FORCE introduces role-based resuscitation, assigning clear responsibilities to buddies, medics, officers, and commanders.
- It structures trauma care across three dynamic phases: point-of-injury care, prolonged field care, and handoff to higher echelons.
- Emphasis is placed on operational improvisation, turning locally available materials into life-saving tools.
- FORCE integrates tactical decision-making and communication as essential components of trauma care.
- The doctrine supports inter-agency interoperability, scalable training modules, and modular instruction across combat and humanitarian scenarios.
- It is a living, feedback-driven system, shaped by real experiences from India's diverse conflict and disaster zones.
- FORCE aims to empower every provider with the skills, mindset, and confidence to act decisively when time and tools are scarce.

Conclusion

FORCE represents a paradigm shift in battlefield trauma care—rooted in Indian terrain, designed for Indian realities, and responsive to Indian needs. It transforms frontline providers into capable lifesavers through modular training, improvisation, and mission integration. Drawing from global best practices but forged in operational adversity, FORCE redefines survival not as luck or logistics, but as preparedness, adaptability, and teamwork. As a living doctrine shaped by field feedback, FORCE is India's contribution to trauma care excellence—bridging doctrine with dust, and skill with courage. In every provider, it instills the power to act when every second—and every life—counts.

Bibliography

1. "Battlefield advanced trauma life support (BATLS)." *Journal of the Royal Army Medical Corps*; 146,3 (2000): 215–27. doi:https://doi.org/10.1136/jramc-146-03-12
2. Agarwal, Divyansh et al. "Reciprocal Learning Between Military and Civilian Surgeons: Past and Future Paths for Medical Innovation." Annals of Surgery; 274,5 (2021): e460–e464. doi:https://doi.org/10.1097/SLA.0000000000003635
3. American College of Surgeons Committee on Trauma. ATLS: Advanced Trauma Life Support. 10th ed. Chicago: American College of Surgeons; 2018. ISBN: 978-0996826235
4. Butler, Frank K Jr. "Tactical Combat Casualty Care: Beginnings." Wilderness & Environmental Medicine; 28,2S (2017): S12–S17. doi:https://doi.org/10.1016/j.wem.2016.12.004
5. Hodgetts, T J, and P F Mahoney. "Military pre-hospital care: why is it different?." Journal of the Royal Army Medical Corps; 155,1 (2009): 4–8. doi:https://doi.org/10.1136/jramc-155-01-01

6. Kotwal, Russ S et al. "The Effect of a Golden Hour Policy on the Morbidity and Mortality of Combat Casualties." JAMA surgery; 151,1 (2016): 15–24. doi:https://doi.org/10.1001/jamasurg.2015.3104
7. Lerner, E Brooke et al. "Comparison of the 1999 and 2006 trauma triage guidelines: where do patients go?." Prehospital emergency care; 15,1 (2011): 12–7. doi:https://doi.org/10.3109/10903127.2010.519819
8. Mabry, Robert L, and Robert DeLorenzo. "Challenges to improving combat casualty survival on the battlefield." *Military medicine*; 179,5 (2014): 477–82. doi:https://doi.org/10.7205/MILMED-D-13-00417
9. Ronald F. Bellamy, The Causes of Death in Conventional Land Warfare: Implications for Combat Casualty Care Research, Military Medicine, Volume 149, Issue 2, February 1984, Pages 55–62, doi:https://doi.org/10.1093/milmed/149.2.55

Soldier's Anatomy and Physiology

2

Bharath Gopinath

Learning Objectives
By the end of this chapter, readers should be able to:

- Recognize the unique anatomical and physiological demands of soldiers
- Apply knowledge of these adaptations in assessing and managing combat trauma
- Understand the impact of physical, psychological, and environmental stressors on soldiers
- Implement strategies to optimize field medical care, taking into account these unique considerations—especially in Indian settings of high altitude and cold weather

Introduction

The anatomy and physiology of a soldier differ considerably from those of civilians due to the extreme physical, psychological, and environmental demands inherent to combat and military training. Physiological adaptations in soldiers enhance resilience, enabling quick response and sustained endurance under stress. Soldiers often operate in extreme environments, including the high-altitude, cold, and hypoxic conditions of regions like the Himalayas and Siachen glacier. This chapter discusses specialized anatomical and physiological adaptations and how they influence trauma response, injury patterns, and treatment needs in combat.

B. Gopinath (✉)
Department of Emergency Medicine, AIIMS, New Delhi, India

N. T. Rai, S. Misra (eds.), *Frontline Operational Resuscitation and Combat Emergencies (FORCE) Manual*, https://doi.org/10.1007/978-981-92-1622-2_2

Case Scenario

A 30-year-old soldier, recently deployed to a forward observation post at an altitude of 15,000 feet in the Northern Himalayas, sustains blunt trauma after slipping on icy terrain during a night patrol. The ambient temperature is well below freezing, and wind chill further accelerates heat loss. He is found conscious but disoriented, with visible bruising on the chest and left flank (Fig. 2.1). His vital signs show tachypnea (RR 28/min), hypoxia (SpO_2 84% on room air), and a core body temperature of 34 °C.

The soldier complains of generalized fatigue, severe headache, and breathlessness. He is shivering and pale, with delayed capillary refill. His GCS is 14/15. Auscultation reveals reduced breath sounds on the left side. No overt bleeding is noted, but his extremities are cold and cyanotic.

- What environmental and physiological factors complicate trauma care at high altitude?
- How does high-altitude physiology affect shock recognition and fluid resuscitation decisions?

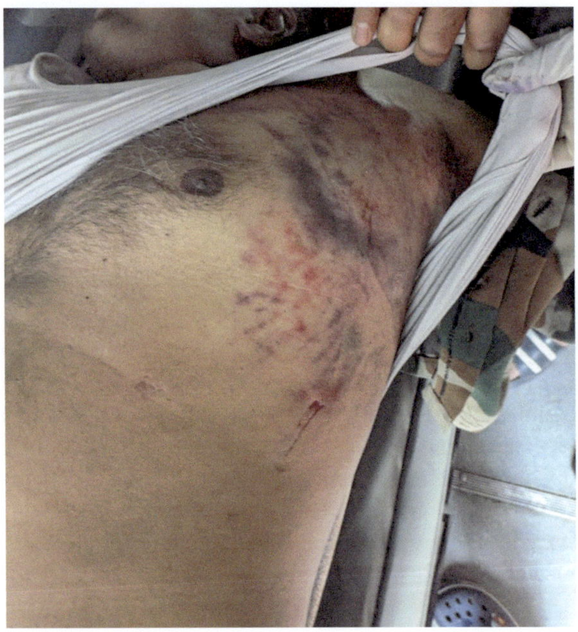

Fig. 2.1 Soldier with blunt trauma with visible bruising on the chest

Approach to Understanding Soldier's Anatomy and Physiology in Combat

The anatomy and physiology of soldiers are adapted to endure the high physical demands, psychological pressures, and environmental extremes of military service. These adaptations influence not only how soldiers perform in combat but also how they respond to injuries, recover from wounds, and cope with various environmental stressors. The soldier's body is a system under persistent challenge—from mountainous terrain and glacial cold to the physiological strain of battlefield trauma and mental stress. Military personnel must maintain optimal performance in conditions that are often far from ideal: irregular meals, limited sleep, high physical loads, and unpredictable psychological strain. These demands shape a unique physiological profile—one that merges strength with resilience, and adaptation with efficiency.

Understanding the physiological distinctions of soldiers can guide more effective medical interventions and help address injuries, physiological strain, and environmental exposure specific to military personnel.

Musculoskeletal System: Strength, Endurance, and Resilience

The musculoskeletal system of soldiers is heavily conditioned through physical training and endurance exercises. This system comprises bones, muscles, ligaments, and tendons, all crucial for load bearing, manoeuvrability, and strength. Due to the physical demands of military tasks, soldiers develop:

- *Increased bone density and strength*: Soldiers typically have a higher bone density than civilians, which aids in handling heavy equipment loads and protecting against fractures. Long-term training induces micro-adaptations in bone structure, increasing resilience and reducing fracture risk.
- *Muscle endurance and fatigue resistance*: Military training emphasizes muscle endurance over short-term power. Soldiers' muscles are trained to resist fatigue through repetitive load-bearing activities, enhancing their ability to maintain performance for extended durations. High levels of muscle endurance are crucial for long marches and prolonged combat engagements.
- *Ligament and tendon strengthening*: Training strengthens ligaments and tendons, which reduces the risk of sprains, strains, and ligament tears. However, repetitive high-impact activities can lead to overuse injuries, a common concern in military settings.

For soldiers in high altitudes and cold environments, muscle endurance and flexibility are vital, as the terrain and temperatures heighten the risk of sprains and strains. However, these adaptations come with risks. Overuse injuries such as shin splints, stress fractures, and chronic tendonitis are common, particularly with repeated high-altitude deployments where uneven terrain and reduced flexibility in cold exacerbate musculoskeletal strain.

Cardiovascular System: Enhanced Circulatory Efficiency

Soldiers require an efficient cardiovascular system to meet the demands of high physical exertion and stressful situations. Key cardiovascular adaptations include:

- *Increased cardiac output and stroke volume*: Regular training enhances cardiac output, allowing soldiers' hearts to pump more blood per beat and deliver oxygen to muscles more efficiently. This improvement is crucial during high-stress situations requiring quick reflexes and sustained physical activity.
- *Lower resting heart rate*: Soldiers often develop a lower resting heart rate, a result of cardiovascular conditioning. This lowers baseline energy expenditure and enhances the ability to tolerate stress during combat. However, this adaptation can complicate trauma assessments, as shock symptoms might be less obvious due to the lower baseline heart rate.
- *Vascular adaptations for blood flow control*: Soldiers exposed to varied climates have better-developed vascular control mechanisms, which help redirect blood flow to critical areas during intense activity. This is particularly useful in combat scenarios requiring quick physical action and situational awareness.
- *Increased risk of thrombosis*: For soldiers deployed in high altitudes, the cardiovascular system undergoes adaptations to cope with low oxygen levels, including increased red blood cell count. However, this also raises blood viscosity, increasing the risk of clot formation, especially during injury or immobilization.

Pulmonary System: Adaptations for Oxygen Demand

The pulmonary system is central to providing oxygen during physical exertion. Soldiers' lungs are conditioned to maximize oxygen uptake and efficiency in various settings:

- *Enhanced respiratory efficiency*: Through training, soldiers develop the ability to take in and utilize more oxygen with each breath, a crucial adaptation for managing stress and physical exertion. This efficiency allows soldiers to delay the onset of fatigue and maintain performance levels.
- *Ventilation control*: Soldiers often develop greater control over their respiratory rate, adjusting breathing to meet the demands of different activities. This adaptation is essential for handling moments of intense exertion, where controlling oxygen intake can prevent early exhaustion.
- *Higher tolerance to hypoxia*: Training in hypoxic or low-oxygen environments enables soldiers to perform effectively with lower oxygen availability. This adaptation helps soldiers maintain alertness and functionality even when oxygen levels are reduced, such as in combat situations involving smoke or restricted breathing conditions.
- *Risk of high-altitude pulmonary oedema (HAPE)*: Soldiers in high-altitude regions face extreme hypoxia, which increases their risk for conditions like high-

altitude pulmonary oedema (HAPE). HAPE is characterized by fluid accumulation in the lungs. Prevention includes gradual ascent and pharmacological prophylaxis (e.g., nifedipine), while treatment requires immediate descent and oxygen.

Neurological and Psychological Resilience

Soldiers face constant high-stress environments, requiring both neurological and psychological resilience:

- *Enhanced stress response*: Soldiers often experience heightened reflexes and quicker response times due to training that conditions the nervous system for rapid decision-making. This adaptation is supported by improved synaptic connections in the brain, which helps soldiers remain calm and effective under stress.
- *Reduced sensitivity to pain*: The military environment conditions soldiers to withstand physical pain, a critical adaptation for enduring injuries and remaining functional in combat. However, this can lead to challenges in assessing injuries, as soldiers may underreport pain levels.
- *Cognitive adaptation and emotional regulation*: Soldiers are trained to regulate their emotions, making quick, clear-headed decisions under pressure. This adaptation is achieved through repeated exposure to simulated combat stressors, enhancing resilience to combat fatigue and shock.
- *Risk of high-altitude cerebral oedema (HACE)*: Soldiers are at risk for HACE, characterized by headache, confusion, and decreased consciousness. Immediate descent, corticosteroids and oxygen administration are essential in managing HACE in injured soldiers.

Endocrine System: Hormonal Adaptations to Stress

The endocrine system regulates hormonal responses to stress and exertion, which are crucial for soldiers in combat:

- *Increased stress hormones*: During combat, soldiers experience elevated cortisol and adrenaline levels, which enhance focus, alertness, and reaction times. While these hormones prepare soldiers for combat, long-term exposure can increase fatigue and reduce immunity.
- *Regulation of blood sugar levels*: Stress hormones maintain glucose availability for the brain and muscles. In prolonged engagements or survival situations, this hormonal regulation is vital for maintaining energy levels and preventing hypoglycaemia.
- *Electrolyte and fluid balance*: Soldiers' endocrine systems are conditioned to preserve electrolytes and fluid balance, critical in environments with limited water supplies. Hormonal control over sodium, potassium, and water levels helps

soldiers avoid dehydration and maintain endurance. However, at high altitudes, the increased metabolic rate and cold conditions can lead to dehydration and electrolyte loss.

Chronic cortisol elevation from repeated deployments or training cycles can lead to adrenal fatigue, weight loss, irritability, and sleep disturbances, all requiring early detection and recovery protocols.

Metabolic System: Energy Utilization and Thermal Regulation

Military tasks require efficient metabolic function to sustain prolonged physical effort and endure harsh climates:

- *Enhanced metabolic flexibility*: Soldiers' metabolism adapts to use both glycogen and fat stores effectively, allowing for sustained performance over extended durations. This adaptation minimizes energy crashes and supports endurance, even in food-scarce environments.
- *Increased caloric needs*: Soldiers at high physical demand have higher caloric needs, which is supported by an increased basal metabolic rate. This adaptation ensures that soldiers' energy demands are met, even during high-stress conditions.
- *Cold adaptation*: The metabolic rate increases in cold environments to generate heat through thermogenesis. This adaptation is particularly critical for soldiers in extreme cold, where prolonged exposure can lead to hypothermia if energy reserves are depleted.

Poor thermal regulation or energy depletion can lead to hypothermia, particularly dangerous during evacuation delays. Prevention includes insulated gear, calorie-dense emergency rations, and active warming techniques.

Immune System: Enhanced Defence Mechanisms

Military personnel face increased exposure to environmental pathogens, and good immunity is vital:

- *Wound healing and inflammation control*: At high altitudes, hypoxia delays collagen synthesis and reduces immune cell efficiency, slowing down the healing process. Field wound care should prioritize clean, sterile management and, if feasible, oxygen therapy to expedite recovery.
- *Heightened susceptibility to infections*: Cold, crowded living conditions increase infection risks. Soldiers face a heightened risk of respiratory infections in high-altitude camps, necessitating vigilant monitoring for early infection signs in open wounds.

- *Environmental contaminants*: Battlefield injuries may involve foreign particles, increasing infection risks. Rigorous debridement and early antibiotic administration are crucial in field care.

Combat trauma care protocols must be adapted for immunocompromised states. Evacuation timelines, antibiotic stewardship, and sterile field improvisation are essential to reduce morbidity.

Thermoregulation: Cold Adaptations and Hypothermia Resistance

Thermal regulation is critical for soldiers operating in extreme climates:

- *Thermoregulatory efficiency*: Soldiers at high altitudes undergo physiological acclimatization, including increased shivering thermogenesis to generate heat. However, rapid cooling from snow exposure or prolonged immobility can quickly lead to hypothermia in injured soldiers.
- *Risk of frostbite and cold injuries*: Frostbite can be seen in soldiers working in high altitudes. Immediate rewarming with non-direct heat sources is essential, alongside careful monitoring to prevent further tissue damage.
- *Hypothermia management*: Cold conditions exacerbate hypothermic responses in trauma patients, complicating resuscitation. The "hypothermia triad"—hypothermia, acidosis, and coagulopathy—requires rapid and continuous warming strategies, insulated transport, and heated IV fluids if available.

FORCE Tactical Pearls

1. *Holistic approach*: Recognize that a soldier's physical condition is influenced by intensive training and adaptability. Recognize adaptations specific to high-altitude and low-temperature settings, including hypoxia, thermoregulation, and acclimatization.
2. *Assessment techniques*: Adapt trauma assessments for field conditions, accounting for elevated physical resilience and stress responses.
3. *Consider environmental and psychological stress*: Factor in the cumulative impact of sleep deprivation, cold exposure, and combat stress on soldiers' physiology.
4. *Immediate management*: Prioritize rewarming, and monitoring for altitude sickness, specific to high-altitude operations

Case Resolution

Upon initial stabilization, the soldier was moved to a wind-sheltered area. A hypothermia prevention kit was immediately employed—he was changed into dry clothing, wrapped in thermal layers, and warmed passively using body-to-body heat and hot water bottles wrapped in cloth. A heated IV fluid line was connected, and warmed Ringer's Lactate was administered slowly through an 18-G cannula to avoid complications from cold-induced vasoconstriction.

Airway was patent and supplemental oxygen was provided via a portable concentrator at 4 L/min, which improved SpO_2 to 90% 94. Given the high-altitude setting and clinical signs—fatigue, headache, dyspnea—there was strong suspicion of early high-altitude pulmonary oedema (HAPE), especially in the context of recent ascent and concurrent chest trauma. The absence of fever and presence of hypoxia further supported this. High-altitude conditions introduced several physiological and logistical challenges to trauma care. Hypobaric hypoxia can significantly worsen even moderate thoracic injuries, while cold exposure alters circulatory dynamics and reduces the reliability of clinical signs like peripheral perfusion. Recognizing shock becomes difficult, as cold-induced vasoconstriction mimics hypovolemia, and pulse oximetry may be unreliable. These environmental factors complicate both diagnosis and triage, demanding clinical judgment that accounts for both trauma and altitude pathophysiology.

Persistent hypoxia and worsening breath sounds on the left side, despite oxygen supplementation, prompted a focused re-evaluation. Needle decompression was cautiously performed at the 5th intercostal space in the anterior axillary line, which led to slight but noticeable clinical improvement, indicating a likely pneumothorax coexisting with HAPE. The soldier remained hemodynamically stable but mentally foggy, raising concern for high-altitude cerebral oedema (HACE). Dexamethasone 8 mg IM was administered to mitigate neurological deterioration. Given the uncertain fluid status and the risks of worsening pulmonary oedema, no mannitol or diuretics were administered.

At this altitude, fluid resuscitation strategies had to be carefully tailored. While the cold and injury profile might suggest hypovolaemia, aggressive fluid loading could exacerbate pulmonary or cerebral oedema. The decision to administer warmed fluids slowly was based on cautious reassessment of perfusion markers, mental status, and pulse quality—recognizing that cold stress, hypoxia, and trauma each independently influence these indicators. These adaptations signify how high-altitude physiology demands that resuscitation be both conservative and responsive to subtle clinical cues.

Once weather permitted, evacuation was coordinated via aerial CASEVAC. Descent to below 9000 ft was prioritized to reduce the burden of hypobaric hypoxia and improve systemic oxygenation. Oxygen support was continued throughout transport, and warming measures were maintained to prevent rebound hypothermia.

This case reflects the need for an integrated approach that combines environmental awareness, trauma management, and physiological insight. Despite the absence of overt external haemorrhage, the soldier's hypoxia, cold exposure, and altered mentation necessitated prompt multi-system interventions. Careful prioritization of oxygen delivery, cautious fluid use, needle decompression, and pharmacologic support ensured that the casualty was stabilized and safely evacuated from one of the most austere operational environments.

Key Messages

- Military service demands unique physiological adaptations that optimize endurance, strength, and cognitive performance under extreme environmental and psychological stressors, especially in high-altitude and cold-weather deployments.
- Musculoskeletal and cardiovascular systems in soldiers are highly conditioned, with increased bone density, muscle fatigue resistance, stroke volume, and oxygen-carrying capacity—essential for prolonged operational performance and survival.
- Pulmonary adaptations enable efficient oxygen utilization and hypoxia tolerance, critical for sustaining physical exertion at altitude and in austere conditions where oxygen supply may be compromised.
- Neurological and psychological resilience is as vital as physical fitness, with enhanced reflexes, memory retention, and emotional regulation being developed through tactical training and cognitive stress conditioning.
- These adaptations can also predispose soldiers to specific injuries and illnesses, such as high-altitude pulmonary/cerebral oedema, overuse syndromes, and stress-induced mental health disorders, requiring anticipatory and context-specific medical strategies.
- A comprehensive understanding of soldier physiology enhances battlefield medical care, allowing clinicians to anticipate complications, tailor treatment, and support recovery with strategies grounded in operational realities.

Conclusion

Soldiers operate under extreme physical, environmental, and psychological conditions that demand unique anatomical and physiological adaptations. Their bodies develop enhanced endurance, cardiovascular efficiency, respiratory resilience, and metabolic flexibility to withstand high-altitude hypoxia, cold exposure, and combat stress. However, these adaptations also pose specific medical challenges. Understanding these physiological distinctions is crucial for military doctors, as it enables more effective trauma management, rapid intervention, and improved recovery strategies.

Bibliography

1. Anderson MK, Hall SJ, Parr GP. Foundations of Athletic Training: Prevention, Assessment, and Management. 4th ed. Philadelphia: Lippincott Williams & Wilkins; 2008. ISBN: 978-0781784450
2. Auerbach PS, Cushing TA, Harris NS. Auerbach's Wilderness Medicine. 7th ed. 2 vols. Philadelphia: Elsevier; 2016. ISBN: 9780323359429
3. Bärtsch, Peter, and Erik R Swenson. "Clinical practice: Acute high-altitude illnesses." The New England journal of medicine vol. 368,24 (2013): 2294–302. doi:https://doi.org/10.1056/NEJMcp1214870
4. Benedek, David M et al. "First responders: mental health consequences of natural and human-made disasters for public health and public safety workers." Annual review of public health vol. 28 (2007): 55–68. doi:https://doi.org/10.1146/annurev.publhealth.28.021406.144037
5. Hackett, P H, and R C Roach. "High-altitude illness." The New England journal of medicine vol. 345,2 (2001): 107–14. doi:https://doi.org/10.1056/NEJM200107123450206
6. Joyner, Michael J, and Carsten Lundby. "Concepts About V˙O2max and Trainability Are Context Dependent." Exercise and sport sciences reviews vol. 46,3 (2018): 138–143. doi:https://doi.org/10.1249/JES.0000000000000150
7. Morgan, Charles A 3rd et al. "Stress-induced deficits in working memory and visuo-constructive abilities in Special Operations soldiers." Biological psychiatry vol. 60,7 (2006): 722–9. doi:https://doi.org/10.1016/j.biopsych.2006.04.021
8. West, John B. "High-altitude medicine." American journal of respiratory and critical care medicine vol. 186,12 (2012): 1229–37. doi:https://doi.org/10.1164/rccm.201207-1323CI

Tactical Combat Casualty Care: Core Principles

3

Aaditya Katyal

Learning Objectives

By the end of this chapter on Tactical Combat Casualty Care: Core Principles, readers should be able to:

- Understand the historical context and evolution of TCCC and its significance in modern military medicine, particularly in reducing preventable deaths on the battlefield
- Identify and explain the core principles of TCCC, specifically the primary causes of preventable combat deaths: hemorrhage, airway obstruction, and tension pneumothorax
- Describe the three phases of TCCC—Care Under Fire, Tactical Field Care, and Tactical Evacuation Care—and understand the key interventions appropriate to each phase
- Demonstrate knowledge of lifesaving interventions, including hemorrhage control techniques (tourniquets, hemostatic agents), airway management, and needle decompression for tension pneumothorax
- Understand adaptations and applications of TCCC in diverse environments, with an emphasis on the Indian context, including unique challenges faced by Indian forces in high-altitude and remote combat zones
- Recognize the influence of TCCC principles in civilian trauma care and their adaptation for high-risk civilian settings, such as disaster response, law enforcement, and emergency medical services

A. Katyal (✉)
Department of Emergency Medicine, Kasturba Medical College, Manipal, Karnataka, India

N. T. Rai, S. Misra (eds.), *Frontline Operational Resuscitation and Combat Emergencies (FORCE) Manual*, https://doi.org/10.1007/978-981-92-1622-2_3

Introduction

You don't have to be a medic to save a life; you just have to know what to do.

Historical Context and Evolution

Tactical Combat Casualty Care (TCCC) was conceived in the early 1990s by the US military, primarily as a response to the inadequacy of civilian trauma care practices on the battlefield. Military conflicts prior to this period highlighted a pressing need for a trauma care protocol that could address the unique conditions faced by soldiers in combat. This led the US Special Operations Command (USSOCOM) to begin developing a model of care that prioritized interventions specific to battlefield scenarios. TCCC emerged with a strong emphasis on reducing preventable deaths by focusing on immediate, field-adapted techniques for managing severe hemorrhage, tension pneumothorax, and airway obstruction—conditions frequently encountered in combat but less common in civilian emergency care settings.

The development of TCCC marked a major shift in military medicine, emphasizing rapid, practical interventions that could be applied by soldiers and medics with limited resources and under hostile conditions. The core framework for TCCC was established with the aim of allowing lifesaving procedures to be implemented immediately on the battlefield, often with minimal equipment. These interventions were organized around three main phases: *Care Under Fire, Tactical Field Care, and Tactical Evacuation Care*. Each phase was specifically designed to address the different stages of casualty care in combat, balancing the need for medical intervention with tactical considerations to ensure the safety of both the provider and the casualty. The practical results seen in these lines contributed significantly to the evolution of TCCC, affirming its critical role in saving lives on the battlefield. Furthermore, the success of TCCC in reducing preventable deaths led to its adoption by other military organizations worldwide, establishing it as a gold standard in battlefield trauma care.

The Committee on Tactical Combat Casualty Care (CoTCCC) was established to ensure that TCCC guidelines remain effective, evidence-based, and aligned with the realities of modern combat. Comprising experts from military medicine, the CoTCCC continuously updates TCCC protocols, integrating new research, technology, and feedback from the field. This process ensures that TCCC guidelines continuously evolve through battlefield feedback and research, ensuring that protocols remain effective and relevant. Each TCCC component is regularly reassessed based on data from combat engagements, allowing for adaptations like the inclusion of newer hemostatic agents and refined needle decompression techniques. CoTCCC's commitment to evidence-based revisions has made TCCC a dynamic and adaptable model that reflects the latest advancements in trauma care while meeting the practical needs of the battlefield.

TCCC, while primarily developed by the US military, is also highly relevant to the Indian forces, especially given India's complex border conflicts, counter-insurgency operations, and engagements in diverse environments. Indian forces face unique challenges in providing immediate medical care in high-altitude areas like the Himalayas and remote, under-resourced regions that demand robust, adaptive casualty care protocols similar to TCCC. Although not fully implemented on the same scale as in US forces, TCCC principles are being adapted to meet the logistical and operational realities of Indian combat zones. Field experiences and post-combat reports indicate that hemorrhage control, airway management, and timely evacuation are critical areas where TCCC principles can substantially reduce preventable combat fatalities.

The development of protocols similar to TCCC within Indian forces has been influenced by practical needs for rapid and effective casualty care in high-stakes environments. This involves equipping and training all personnel, not just medical staff, in essential lifesaving techniques such as the use of tourniquets, hemostatic dressings, and basic airway management tools, which are adaptable across different terrains and climates. To facilitate this, Indian forces have also started to incorporate capsule training programs and specialized trauma care equipment designed for high-altitude operations and austere environments.

Philosophy and Purpose of TCCC

The philosophy of TCCC is based on the idea "*to combine good medicine with good tactics*," aiming to provide effective care without compromising the safety of providers or operational goals. Unlike conventional trauma protocols, TCCC is uniquely designed for combat environments, where ongoing threats and limited resources constrain medical responses. TCCC's phased approach—moving from Care Under Fire to Tactical Field Care and finally Tactical Evacuation Care—ensures that interventions are contextually appropriate, enabling personnel to perform critical actions even in high-stress, high-risk situations.

One of the most important aspects of TCCC is its focus on immediate, lifesaving interventions that are simple to execute and require minimal equipment. The priority given to hemorrhage control exemplifies this approach. Tourniquets, which can be rapidly applied even by nonmedical personnel, are a cornerstone of TCCC's hemorrhage control protocol, especially during the Care Under Fire phase. By emphasizing high-impact, straightforward techniques, TCCC empowers combat soldiers and medics to make rapid decisions, delivering essential care in seconds or minutes—timeframes critical for survival in combat. This philosophy has distinguished TCCC from traditional trauma care by tailoring its interventions to the challenges of battlefield medicine.

Moreover, TCCC fills a gap left by traditional civilian emergency protocols, which are often impractical in combat environments. Civilian trauma protocols assume access to extensive medical resources and stable environments, which are rarely available in combat. TCCC's model, therefore, represents a departure from conventional approaches by addressing only the most common preventable causes of death, ensuring that these are immediately targeted and managed, often before a casualty can be transported to a medical facility.

Global and Civilian Applications

Beyond the military, TCCC concepts are gaining traction within India's paramilitary and civilian emergency response sectors. India's paramilitary forces, such as the Border Security Force (BSF) and the Central Reserve Police Force (CRPF), operate in high-risk areas and are frequently the first responders to traumatic injuries in these regions. Recognizing this, TCCC training has been adapted to provide these forces with essential skills in hemorrhage control, airway management, and self-aid techniques, enabling them to act swiftly and effectively in the face of traumatic injuries.

There has also been a growing movement to incorporate TCCC principles within civilian emergency response in high-risk areas prone to natural disasters or terrorist attacks. Efforts are underway to integrate TCCC-informed training into disaster management and emergency medical services to better equip providers with practical, lifesaving skills during large-scale emergencies. In major urban centers, including Delhi and Mumbai, where civilian emergency personnel may face mass casualty incidents, TCCC's rapid-response framework is being adapted to ensure that providers can manage trauma effectively even before casualties reach hospitals.

Core Principles

Good medicine with bad tactics is still bad medicine.

Principles of TCCC

The Tactical Combat Casualty Care (TCCC) framework is fundamentally aligned with the MARCH algorithm (Fig. 3.1), which systematically addresses the leading causes of preventable death on the battlefield. By prioritizing interventions for massive hemorrhage, airway obstruction, respiratory compromise, circulatory support, and head injury/hypothermia prevention, MARCH ensures a focused and lifesaving approach to trauma care in austere, combat environments.

M—Massive Hemorrhage

Uncontrolled bleeding, particularly from extremity injuries, remains the leading preventable cause of death in combat. MARCH prioritizes rapid hemorrhage control through the use of Combat Application Tourniquets (CATs) and hemostatic dressings. Gunshot wounds and blast injuries to limbs can result in fatal exsanguination within minutes. Evidence from modern conflicts has demonstrated a significant reduction in mortality with early, effective use of tourniquets, reinforcing their essential role in frontline trauma care.

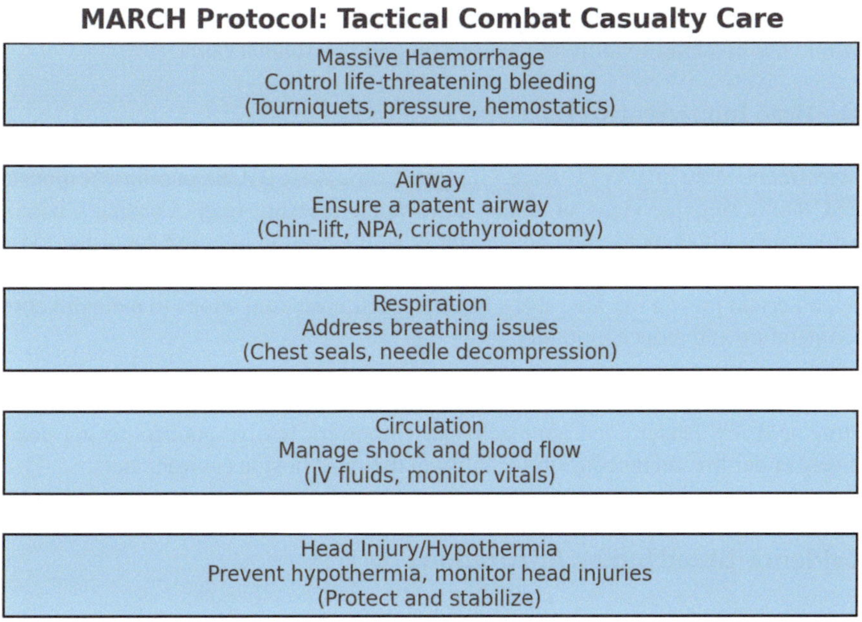

Fig. 3.1 MARCH protocol

A—Airway

Airway obstruction, often caused by maxillofacial trauma, unconsciousness, or severe head injuries, is the second critical threat. MARCH protocol recommends simple airway adjuncts such as the nasopharyngeal airway (NPA) for maintaining patency in semiconscious patients. In most severe cases, emergency cricothyroidotomy is employed to establish a definitive airway. These techniques are designed to be rapidly deployable by trained providers and are vital to preventing hypoxic death.

R—Respiration

Combat chest trauma can result in tension pneumothorax, a condition where accumulating air in the pleural space compresses the lung and mediastinum, impairing ventilation and circulation. MARCH protocols include needle thoracostomy (decompression) as a lifesaving intervention. Prompt recognition and decompression of tension pneumothorax can prevent cardiopulmonary collapse and significantly improve survival in cases of penetrating thoracic injuries.

C—Circulation

Beyond controlling visible hemorrhage, the MARCH algorithm supports restoring and maintaining adequate circulation. While definitive fluid resuscitation strategies depend on evacuation timelines and resources, the emphasis remains on permissive hypotension and intravenous/intraosseous access for administration of blood products or fluids when needed. Tranexamic acid (TXA) may also be considered within the first hour to limit internal bleeding in polytrauma cases.

H—Head Injury/Hypothermia
Combat casualties with traumatic brain injury (TBI) require vigilant neurological assessment, including AVPU scale, Glasgow Coma Scale (GCS), pupillary response, and monitoring for signs of rising intracranial pressure (e.g., Cushing's triad). Simultaneously, hypothermia prevention is vital—even in hot climates—due to its profound impact on coagulation and survival. Casualties must be insulated using hypothermia prevention kits, space blankets, or improvised wraps to maintain core temperature and reduce mortality.

By integrating the MARCH sequence into combat casualty care, TCCC offers a structured, evidence-based approach that empowers first responders to act decisively under fire, enhancing survivability in the most hostile environments.

Evidence-Based Indian Adaptations

Hemorrhage control is a key focus within the Indian military's approach to casualty care. Given that severe extremity wounds are common in border conflicts and counterinsurgency operations, the need for effective hemorrhage control has been highlighted by both medical data and field reports. Tourniquets, hemostatic agents, and pressure dressings are increasingly recognized as indispensable tools for Indian soldiers in combat. Adaptations to these tools—such as lighter, more compact designs suitable for high-mobility operations—are becoming a standard component of the Indian forces' medical kits, especially for units stationed in remote regions.

Airway management is equally challenging, particularly in the high-altitude areas where respiratory issues are compounded by hypoxia. The Indian military has begun incorporating airway adjuncts, such as nasopharyngeal and oropharyngeal airways, in standard issue kits for units operating in these areas. Further, a focus on training in cricothyroidotomy procedures provides a last-resort measure for maintaining an airway in extreme cases. These adaptations are crucial for addressing the particular demands of high-altitude combat zones and are drawn from TCCC's focus on rapid, lifesaving interventions suitable for remote, austere environments.

Combat casualties in India, especially those in the northern and eastern frontiers, face a heightened risk of hypothermia due to extreme cold conditions. The prevention of hypothermia is thus a critical component of casualty care, particularly in operations conducted in regions with sub-zero temperatures. Hypothermia exacerbates blood loss, impairs clotting, and increases the risk of mortality, emphasizing the need for Indian forces to integrate hypothermia management into their field care protocols. To address this, TCCC-inspired adaptations include the issuance of insulated blankets, advanced warming devices, and modified intravenous fluid warmers designed for use in extreme climates. Standardizing these measures is challenging due to the logistical limitations of supplying these resources in remote areas. The

Indian military has made strides in securing portable and durable equipment that can withstand the harsh conditions, such as battery-operated warming blankets and compact IV warmers, to help stabilize casualties in extreme cold environments before evacuation.

Approach to Casualty Care in the Combat Field

In combat, courage is just as much about stepping back as it is stepping in.

Overview of TCCC Phases of Care

TCCC framework is structured around *three distinct phases: Care Under Fire, Tactical Field Care, and Tactical Evacuation Care.* Each phase is designed to address specific needs, challenges, and risks encountered at different stages of combat casualty care (Fig. 3.2). These phases enable military providers to provide context-appropriate interventions, prioritizing immediate survival in high-threat environments and allowing for more comprehensive care as the tactical situation stabilizes.

1. *Care Under Fire*: This initial phase occurs at the point of injury, where active combat and immediate threats restrict the scope of medical intervention. The primary objective in Care Under Fire is rapid hemorrhage control, typically through the application of a tourniquet. This intervention is prioritized as it addresses the leading cause of preventable death—exsanguination—while minimizing exposure to enemy fire. Self-aid and buddy-aid play a crucial role here, as casualties may be required to apply their own tourniquets if capable.
2. *Tactical Field Care*: Once the immediate threat has subsided, providers move to the Tactical Field Care phase, which allows for a broader range of medical interventions. This phase focuses on airway management, hemorrhage control beyond extremity injuries, fluid resuscitation, hypothermia prevention and pain management. Providers are able to use additional medical resources and take more time to assess the casualty's condition, which enhances the quality of care.
3. *Tactical Evacuation Care*: The final phase involves transferring the casualty to a higher level of care, typically via medical evacuation (MEDEVAC). During Tactical Evacuation Care, stabilization techniques and advanced interventions, such as IV fluid and blood administration, are employed to keep the casualty stable until they reach a medical facility. This phase highlights the need for effective communication between field medics and evacuation personnel, ensuring continuity of care and reducing the risk of complications during transport.

The three-phase approach of TCCC is essential for adapting medical interventions to the realities of combat, *prioritizing immediate survival actions, and progressively increasing the complexity of care as conditions allow.*

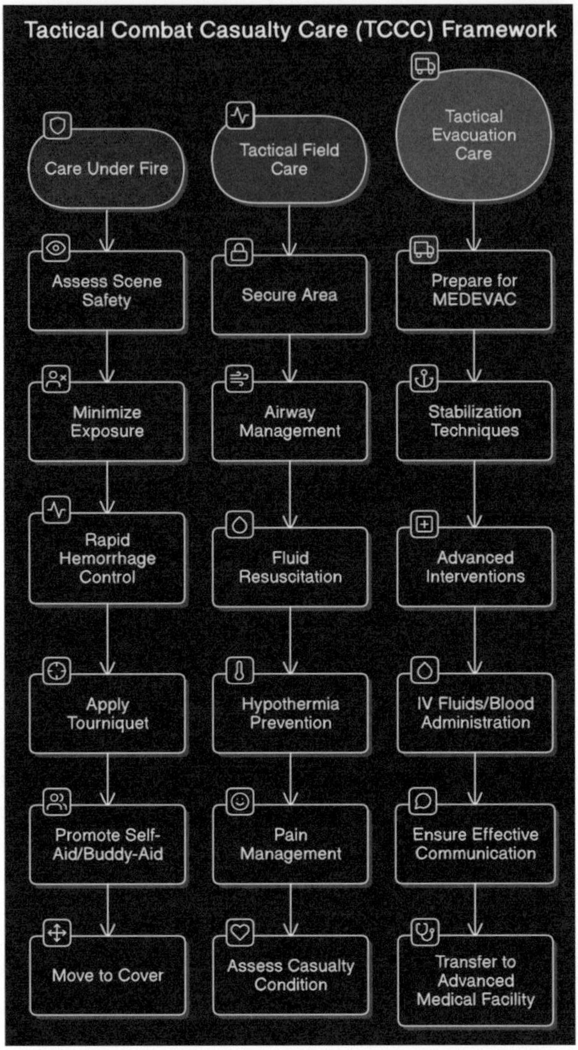

Fig. 3.2 TCCC phases of care. (Figure illustrated using AI tools with OpenAI, ChatGPT-4, 2025)

1. *Care Under Fire*

Immediate Threats and Tactical Priorities: In the Care Under Fire phase, the provider's ability to provide medical care is heavily constrained by active combat. Ensuring the safety of both the injured and the provider is paramount, limiting interventions to those that can be executed swiftly without exposing personnel to additional danger. This phase emphasizes situational awareness and quick decision-making, balancing the need for hemorrhage control with the immediate threat posed by enemy forces.

Hemorrhage Control with Tourniquets: Tourniquet application is central to the Care Under Fire phase, as hemorrhage from extremity wounds is the leading cause of preventable death on the battlefield. The use of tourniquets, such as the Combat Application Tourniquet (CAT), allows soldiers to quickly stop bleeding in major extremity injuries. The efficacy of tourniquets in this context has been well-documented, with studies showing that rapid application can reduce mortality by preventing exsanguination within minutes of injury. Proper placement and application techniques are critical, as improper use can lead to ineffective hemorrhage control or additional injury.

Self-Aid and Buddy-Aid: Given the constraints of active combat, TCCC emphasizes the importance of self-aid and buddy-aid in the Care Under Fire phase. Self-aid enables casualties who are still physically capable to apply their own tourniquets, conserving the medic's attention for casualties unable to assist themselves. Buddy-aid allows soldiers to help each other in situations where self-aid is not feasible. This approach not only expedites hemorrhage control but also supports unit cohesion and resilience under fire.

Case Scenario

A soldier suffers a gunshot wound to the thigh during active combat, resulting in heavy bleeding from the thigh.

- *Response*: The soldier applies a CAT proximal to the injury while remaining in cover. Another nearby soldier provides buddy-aid, securing the tourniquet and ensuring bleeding control before moving the injured to a safer location.
- *Key message*: Rapid tourniquet application prevents further blood loss, increasing the soldier's chance of survival until Tactical Field Care is available.

2. *Tactical Field Care*

Airway Management

In the Tactical Field Care (TFC) phase, soldiers and medics are tasked with securing a casualty's airway as a top priority to prevent asphyxiation, which is crucial for sustaining life in combat situations. This phase allows soldiers and medics the opportunity to perform a more thorough assessment of the casualty's airway and take necessary measures to ensure it remains open and functional. In cases where a casualty has only a mild airway obstruction, such as due to swelling or minor trauma, soldiers and medics often use a nasopharyngeal airway (NPA). The NPA, a soft rubber tube inserted through the nose into the throat, helps to keep the airway open without requiring extensive manipulation, making it suitable for cases where the casualty is semiconscious or mildly injured.

For casualties suffering from severe facial or neck trauma, where traditional airway management techniques may be inadequate, a cricothyroidotomy may be performed. This surgical procedure involves creating an opening in the cricothyroid membrane to establish an alternate route for air to reach the lungs. Given the technical complexity and risks associated with cricothyroidotomy, a protocolized approach is needed for soldiers and medics in evaluating when this intervention is appropriate based on the casualty's injuries and overall condition.

Breathing and Ventilation Management

In the Tactical Field Care (TFC) phase, breathing management is critical for stabilizing casualties with chest injuries to maintain oxygen delivery to vital organs. Soldiers and medics first assess breathing by observing chest movement, listening for breath sounds, and noting any abnormalities such as shallow or irregular breathing. Signs like decreased breath sounds on one side of the chest or difficulty breathing can indicate life-threatening conditions, including pneumothorax, which requires immediate intervention.

A major threat in combat chest trauma is tension pneumothorax, where air trapped in the pleural space compresses the lung and heart, impeding both respiration and circulation. To manage this, a needle decompression is performed, inserting a large-bore needle into the chest at specific points (usually the second intercostal space at the midclavicular line or fifth intercostal space at the anterior axillary line) to release trapped air. This procedure often provides rapid relief and prevents further complications from lung compression.

For open chest wounds, which allow air to enter the chest cavity abnormally, vented chest seals are used to cover the wound. These seals feature a one-way valve that prevents additional air from entering but allows trapped air to escape, reducing the risk of a secondary tension pneumothorax.

If supplemental oxygen is available, it is administered to enhance oxygen saturation and support tissue oxygenation. For casualties unable to breathe effectively on their own, a bag valve mask (BVM) may be needed to assist with manual ventilation, although this can be challenging in a tactical setting.

Shock Prevention

Preventing shock is another essential component of Tactical Field Care, as shock can rapidly decrease a casualty's chances of survival due to the resulting inadequate blood flow and oxygen supply to vital organs. In the TFC phase, fluid resuscitation plays a significant role, as it helps to maintain blood pressure and perfusion. When available, blood products are prioritized due to their effectiveness in supporting circulation and carrying oxygen. If blood products are not accessible, limited amounts of crystalloid solutions may be used temporarily to stabilize the casualty, although these are less effective than blood products for managing shock.

TCCC protocols also advocate the use of tranexamic acid (TXA), a medication that helps to stabilize blood clots, in cases where a casualty is at high risk of severe hemorrhage. Research has demonstrated that TXA can significantly improve survival rates, especially in situations where prolonged field care is necessary due to delayed evacuation. Administering TXA within three hours of injury is particularly beneficial, as it assists in controlling internal bleeding and reduces the likelihood of hemorrhagic shock, providing a critical bridge until more advanced care is available.

Hypothermia Management
Hypothermia is a significant risk for combat casualties, even in warm climates, as the body can lose heat rapidly due to factors such as exposure, blood loss, and immobilization. TCCC emphasizes hypothermia prevention during Tactical Field Care to counteract this risk, as cold exposure can exacerbate blood loss and interfere with clotting mechanisms, both of which increase mortality risk. Combat medics are instructed to use specialized insulating blankets and other warming equipment to maintain a casualty's body temperature.

In addition, warm intravenous (IV) fluids are recommended to further support body temperature and prevent the complications associated with hypothermia. This approach ensures that casualties maintain sufficient warmth to support clotting and immune function, reducing the likelihood of secondary complications. TCCC guidelines highlight that even slight drops in body temperature can have significant impacts on casualty outcomes, making hypothermia prevention a critical component of Tactical Field Care.

Pain Management and Medication Protocols
In the Tactical Field Care (TFC) phase, pain management is critical not only for alleviating physical discomfort but also for maintaining a casualty's psychological stability and ensuring cooperation in potentially high-stress, life-threatening conditions. Effective pain management can improve overall outcomes by reducing shock risk and calming the casualty, which is essential for their survival and ease of transport. TCCC guidelines prioritize safe, effective pain relief that does not compromise respiratory function, a crucial consideration in battlefield settings.

TCCC-approved analgesics in the TFC phase include ketamine and fentanyl, each carefully selected for its balance of effectiveness and safety, particularly in environments where advanced monitoring is limited. These medications are chosen specifically because they do not induce significant respiratory depression—a key risk factor in pain management on the battlefield, where maintaining airway and breathing stability is often challenging.

Case Scenario
A soldier with a gunshot wound to the chest is experiencing difficulty breathing and shows signs of shock.

- *Response*: The provider performs needle decompression to relieve tension pneumothorax and administers TXA to help prevent further blood loss.
- *Key message*: Early intervention stabilizes the casualty, enabling safe transport during the Tactical Evacuation Care phase.

3. *Tactical Evacuation Care*

The Tactical Evacuation Care (TACEVAC) phase is the final stage in the TCCC process, focused on safely moving casualties from the battlefield to a higher level of medical care. During this phase, soldiers and medics prioritize stabilizing casualties for transport, managing life-threatening injuries, and providing continuous monitoring, all while navigating the unique logistical and tactical challenges of evacuation. TACEVAC typically occurs in *two forms*: *CASEVAC (Casualty Evacuation)*, where transport is provided by nonmedical vehicles, and *MEDEVAC (Medical Evacuation)*, which involves medical units and more comprehensive equipment.

Key Components of TACEVAC

1. *Patient stabilization and monitoring*: Soldiers and medics continuously assess and stabilize the casualty's airway, breathing, and circulation to maintain vital functions during transport. Hemorrhage control and reassessment of wounds are also prioritized to prevent worsening of injuries en route.
2. Advanced airway and breathing management: Soldiers and medics ensure that airways remain open, performing advanced interventions like cricothyroidotomy if necessary. In air evacuations, they monitor for respiratory issues like tension pneumothorax and use needle decompression or portable ventilators if needed.
3. *Hemorrhage control*: Managing bleeding remains critical. Soldiers and medics may adjust tourniquets, use hemostatic agents, and, if available, administer blood products or tranexamic acid (TXA) to control hemorrhage during evacuation.
4. *Hypothermia prevention*: Combat casualties are vulnerable to hypothermia due to blood loss and exposure, even in warm climates. Soldiers and medics use insulating blankets, heat packs, and warmed IV fluids to maintain body temperature, reducing risks associated with hypothermia.
5. *Pain and sedation management*: Effective pain relief is crucial for casualty comfort and stability during evacuation.
6. *Documentation and handover*: Accurate records of treatments and complications are essential for a smooth transition to advanced medical care. Soldiers and medics prepare detailed reports to ensure continuity of care upon arrival at the receiving facility.

Tactical Combat Casualty Care in the Indian Scenario

In combat medicine, you aren't just fighting for one life—you're fighting for every life on the line.

Adapting TCCC to India's Operational Environment

India's armed forces operate in some of the most challenging environments globally, from high-altitude zones like the Himalayas to arid deserts and dense jungles.

This variety of terrain, combined with the nature of regional conflicts, necessitates unique adaptations of TCCC principles. The operational environment in high-altitude regions, such as the Line of Actual Control (LAC) bordering China, presents specific medical challenges including altitude sickness, hypothermia, and delayed evacuation times due to rugged terrain and extreme weather conditions. These conditions demand that TCCC protocols be adapted to include prolonged field care and high-altitude medical interventions.

The Indian military medical corps has thus tailored TCCC protocols to incorporate strategies for managing high-altitude sickness, frostbite, and hypothermia as part of routine trauma care. This adaptation ensures that soldiers can receive comprehensive first aid and stabilization, even in the absence of immediate evacuation options. India's military medical community is also investing in specialized cold-weather and altitude-related trauma training for personnel stationed in these regions, reinforcing the importance of TCCC principles with a local adaptation suited to the environment.

Current TCCC Training and Implementation in India

Recognizing the value of TCCC in combat casualty care, the Indian forces have adapted and integrated core principles of TCCC in officers training. This training includes essential skills such as hemorrhage control, airway management, and hypothermia prevention, with a focus on field improvisation due to resource constraints in certain regions. For instance, soldiers in remote areas are trained to use improvised methods for hemorrhage control and stabilization when specialized equipment like advanced tourniquets and hemostatic dressings may not be available.

The Indian military has increasingly collaborated with allied countries, such as the United States, Israel and Kazakhstan, to enhance its TCCC training protocols. Joint exercises have allowed Indian forces to learn from the TCCC practices of other nations, especially in areas like hemorrhage control, the use of tourniquets, and field medical evacuations. These exchanges have been beneficial for transferring knowledge on self-aid and buddy-aid techniques, critical in situations where immediate medical assistance may be unavailable.

India's operational dynamics, which often involve joint operations with paramilitary forces like the Border Security Force (BSF) and the Central Reserve Police Force (CRPF), necessitate a unified approach to casualty care that can be implemented across agencies. Tactical evacuation in India is further complicated by limited infrastructure in many of the combat zones, where helicopter-based MEDEVAC is not always available due to terrain and weather conditions. Basic lifesaving training in TCCC has been extended to these forces to ensure they can handle traumatic injuries in areas with ongoing insurgencies or difficult-to-access locations. As a result, soldiers and officers in these units are becoming more adept at managing life-threatening injuries until further medical assistance arrives, enhancing their resilience and operational effectiveness.

Coordination between military and paramilitary units is also essential to ensure that the standards of care are consistent. Recent initiatives aim to establish standardized protocols and shared training for both military and paramilitary personnel, ensuring that all providers have a common understanding of basic TCCC principles. These efforts are crucial for enhancing casualty care during joint operations and have led to improved survival rates in combat zones where swift and coordinated evacuation can be challenging.

Challenges and Future Directions in Implementing TCCC

Implementing TCCC protocols in India involves significant logistical and geographical challenges. High-altitude areas, such as those in the northern borders, not only complicate medical evacuation but also pose risks of altitude-related illnesses. To address these challenges, Indian military soldiers and medics are trained in prolonged field care techniques, with an emphasis on stabilizing patients for extended periods. Protocols are being adjusted to account for limited evacuation capabilities, especially in regions where helicopters cannot access due to high altitude or inclement weather.

Moreover, resource limitations in some remote outposts mean that advanced TCCC equipment may not be readily available. Indian forces have therefore incorporated training on improvisational techniques, teaching soldiers how to make use of available materials for hemorrhage control and basic airway management. This approach ensures that soldiers have the skills needed to manage injuries effectively, even with minimal equipment. Additionally, the Indian military is exploring the potential of telemedicine to support TCCC, allowing field medics to communicate with specialists remotely, receiving guidance on complex trauma cases when traditional evacuation is not feasible.

The impact of TCCC principles is not limited to military applications; its core concepts are increasingly being integrated into India's civilian emergency response framework. Given the high incidence of traumatic injuries in India due to industrial accidents, road accidents, and natural disasters, there is significant potential for TCCC's hemorrhage control, airway management, and shock prevention techniques to improve civilian prehospital care. Initiatives are underway to adapt TCCC principles for civilian use, with training programs targeted at first responders, paramedics, and disaster response teams.

In India, collaborative efforts between the military, government agencies, and medical institutions are leading to the development of training modules for nonmilitary emergency providers that mirror TCCC's approach to trauma care in high-risk environments. This civilian-military collaboration has the potential to strengthen India's overall trauma response capabilities, benefiting both combat and civilian populations alike.

Key Messages

- Tactical Combat Casualty Care was created to address gaps in civilian trauma care on the battlefield, emphasizing immediate, lifesaving interventions tailored to combat conditions.
- TCCC targets the leading preventable causes of death in combat, including severe hemorrhage, airway obstruction, and tension pneumothorax, through high-impact, simple techniques.
- The TCCC model is organized into *three phases—Care Under Fire, Tactical Field Care, and Tactical Evacuation Care*—allowing providers to provide appropriate care while prioritizing safety and tactical awareness.
- Care Under Fire prioritizes immediate hemorrhage control using tourniquets, often with self-aid or buddy-aid to minimize exposure to threats while stabilizing the casualty until more advanced care is possible.
- Tactical Field Care allows for more thorough assessment and interventions, including airway management, fluid resuscitation, and hypothermia prevention, tailored to the casualty's condition and the tactical environment.
- Tactical Evacuation Care focuses on safe transport to a medical facility, requiring coordination, stabilization techniques, and continued support, with adaptations for environments where traditional evacuation may be challenging.
- In the Indian context, TCCC principles are adapted to diverse operational environments, from high-altitude border regions to dense forests, integrating specific solutions like hypothermia prevention and improvised evacuation methods to address local challenges.
- Beyond the military, TCCC principles are being incorporated into training for Indian paramilitary and civilian providers, enhancing trauma response in high-risk environments like disaster zones and areas with conflict.

Conclusion

Tactical Combat Casualty Care (TCCC) has revolutionized battlefield medicine by addressing the most preventable causes of death—massive hemorrhage, airway obstruction, and tension pneumothorax—through simple, evidence-based, and scalable interventions. Structured across three dynamic phases—Care Under Fire, Tactical Field Care, and Tactical Evacuation—TCCC ensures that lifesaving actions are prioritized without compromising tactical safety. Its growing adoption within the Indian forces, especially in high-altitude and resource-limited settings, reflects its adaptability to diverse combat environments. By empowering all personnel with core trauma skills and incorporating innovations like prolonged field care and hypothermia prevention, TCCC enhances survivability in the golden minutes after injury.

Moreover, its integration into civilian disaster response and emergency services signifies its broader relevance. As operational challenges evolve, continued refinement and widespread training in TCCC principles will be essential to ensure that every provider—military or civilian—is equipped to save lives when seconds matter most.

Bibliography

1. Auerbach PS, Cushing TA, Harris NS. Auerbach's Wilderness Medicine. 7th ed. 2 vols. Philadelphia: Elsevier; 2016. ISBN: 9780323359429
2. Butler, Frank K et al. "Tactical Combat Casualty Care and Wilderness Medicine: Advancing Trauma Care in Austere Environments." *Emergency medicine clinics of North America* vol. 35,2 (2017): 391–407. doi:https://doi.org/10.1016/j.emc.2016.12.005
3. Butler, Frank K Jr et al. "Tactical combat casualty care 2007: evolving concepts and battlefield experience." *Military medicine* vol. 172,11 Suppl (2007): 1–19. doi:https://doi.org/10.7205/milmed.172.supplement_1.1
4. Butler, Frank K Jr. "Fluid Resuscitation in Tactical Combat Casualty Care: Yesterday and Today." *Wilderness & environmental medicine* vol. 28,2S (2017): S74–S81. doi:https://doi.org/10.1016/j.wem.2016.12.007
5. Giebner, Stephen D. "The Transition to the Committee on Tactical Combat Casualty Care." *Wilderness & environmental medicine* vol. 28,2S (2017): S18–S24. doi:https://doi.org/10.1016/j.wem.2016.11.005
6. Giebner, Stephen. "TCCC Updates: Tactical Combat Casualty Care Curriculum Annual Update 2014." *Journal of special operations medicine: a peer reviewed journal for SOF medical professionals* vol. 14,4 (2014): 144–145. doi:https://doi.org/10.55460/W2P1-7IUE
7. Gurney, Jennifer M et al. "Tactical Combat Casualty Care Training, Knowledge, and Utilization in the US Army." *Military medicine* vol. 185,Suppl 1 (2020): 500–507. doi:https://doi.org/10.1093/milmed/usz303
8. Remley, Michael A et al. "Prolonged Casualty Care Guidelines 21 December 2021." *Journal of special operations medicine: a peer reviewed journal for SOF medical professionals* vol. 22,1 (2022): 18–47. doi:https://doi.org/10.55460/8IUQ-907J
9. Savage, Erin et al. "Tactical combat casualty care in the Canadian Forces: lessons learned from the Afghan war." *Canadian journal of surgery. Journal canadien de chirurgie* vol. 54,6 (2011): S118–23. doi:https://doi.org/10.1503/cjs.025011
10. Tien, Homer C et al. "An evaluation of tactical combat casualty care interventions in a combat environment." *Journal of the American College of Surgeons* vol. 207,2 (2008): 174–8. doi:https://doi.org/10.1016/j.jamcollsurg.2008.01.065

Understanding Battlefield Injury Mechanisms

4

Milandeep

Learning Objectives

By the end of this chapter, readers will be able to:

- *Identify common mechanisms of injury*: Recognize and differentiate various battlefield injuries—including ballistic trauma, blast injuries, penetrating trauma, and blunt force trauma—while understanding their anatomical and physiological consequences.
- *Analyze physiological effects*: Comprehend how these injuries disrupt core systems (respiratory, circulatory, neurological) and influence treatment priorities in the context of combat medicine.
- *Develop systematic assessment approaches*: Apply battlefield-appropriate triage protocols such as the ABC and MARCH frameworks to rapidly assess, prioritize, and intervene in complex trauma cases under fire.
- *Apply theoretical knowledge in tactical contexts*: Utilize case-based simulations to practice decision-making, resource prioritization, and casualty stabilization in operationally realistic scenarios, preparing for prolonged field care and delayed evacuation settings.

Introduction

Combat zones represent some of the most demanding environments for medical response. Unlike civilian trauma, battlefield injuries are often caused by high-velocity projectiles, fragmentation, pressure waves from explosions, and prolonged

Milandeep (✉)
Department of Trauma Surgery and Critical Care, JPN Apex Trauma Centre, AIIMS, New Delhi, India

N. T. Rai, S. Misra (eds.), *Frontline Operational Resuscitation and Combat Emergencies (FORCE) Manual*, https://doi.org/10.1007/978-981-92-1622-2_4

environmental exposure. These injuries are frequently complex, polytraumatic, and complicated by delayed evacuation timelines, limited resources, and ongoing tactical threats.

The mechanisms of injury in combat medicine are diverse and situationally dependent. Ballistic trauma from rifles or handguns leads to extensive soft tissue and bony damage due to high kinetic energy transfer and cavitation effects. Blast injuries from improvised explosive devices (IEDs) and grenades compound trauma through a combination of pressure waves, thermal injuries, and secondary projectiles. Penetrating trauma introduces the risk of internal organ damage and infection, while blunt trauma and environmental injuries (e.g., hypothermia, burns) may exacerbate physiological instability.

Medical personnel deployed in such environments must be adept not only at recognizing injury types but also at executing rapid, context-sensitive triage and interventions. Tactical Combat Casualty Care (TCCC), supported by tools such as the MARCH protocol and the ABCDE approach from ATLS, equips first responders and medics to deliver lifesaving care while maintaining operational safety.

This chapter leverages combat case scenarios to explore injury mechanisms in-depth, emphasizing the principles of structured assessment, priority-based interventions, and trauma-informed evacuation planning. The aim is to build competence and confidence in combat trauma care—enabling faster recognition, better outcomes, and greater survivability for those injured on the battlefield.

Case Scenarios

Case 1: Shrapnel Injuries from an Ambush Blast

During a night convoy halt, a mechanized infantry unit is ambushed by an IED blast (Fig. 4.1). In the immediate aftermath of the blast, enemy fire remains active, and visibility is severely compromised. The casualty takes shelter behind available cover, and with no access to advanced medical support, the only aid available in those critical initial moments is from a fellow soldier providing buddy care.

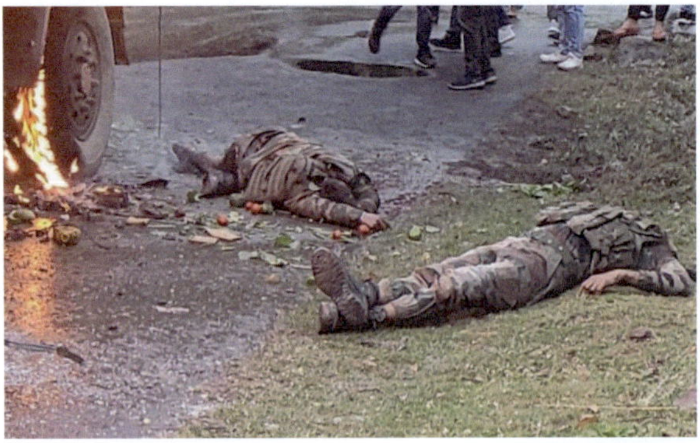

Fig. 4.1 IED ambush on mechanized infantry unit

- *Care Under Fire (CUF)*
  Immediate tourniquet application to control limb hemorrhage while under active fire. No further care provided until suppression is achieved.
- *Tactical Field Care (TFC)*
  After suppression, detailed assessment and airway/breathing management begin.

MARCH Assessment

M—massive hemorrhage: Tourniquet applied to left thigh in CUF phase. Abdominal wound managed with hemostatic gauze and compression dressing.

A—airway: Assessed and confirmed patent; monitored continuously.

R—respiration: Clear bilateral breath sounds; supplemental oxygen provided.

C—circulation: Two IV lines inserted in TFC phase. Fluids initiated; TXA administered.

H—head injury/hypothermia: Patient insulated immediately. Consciousness preserved.

- *Tactical Evacuation Care (TACEVAC)*
  Evacuation initiated under low light to Casualty Collection Point (CCP). TACEVAC via armored vehicle with ongoing IV therapy and vital signs monitoring every 5 min during transit. Enemy fire delayed care. Suppressive fire allowed casualty movement. Interventions prioritized for speed and effectiveness under fire.

Case 2: Gunshot Wound to the Chest

In an urban combat environment, a male squad leader is struck while maneuvering across a rooftop (Fig. 4.2). With limited cover available at the point of injury and the risk of sniper fire still present, a casualty drag is immediately performed by a team member to bring him to below-deck cover. Although the air threat is minimal, the persistent danger from enemy snipers dictates cautious movement and limited exposure during the rescue.

- *Care Under Fire (CUF)*
  No intervention possible during CUF. He is dragged immediately by a team member to bring him to below-deck cover.
- *Tactical Field Care (TFC)*
  - Patient is reached after 3 minutes. Field medic provides full trauma workup and intervention.

MARCH Assessment

M—massive hemorrhage: No major bleeding; body check confirms.

A—airway: Maintained and monitored. Alert and speaking.

R—respiration: Clinical suspicion of tension pneumothorax. Immediate needle decompression performed, followed by vented chest seal.

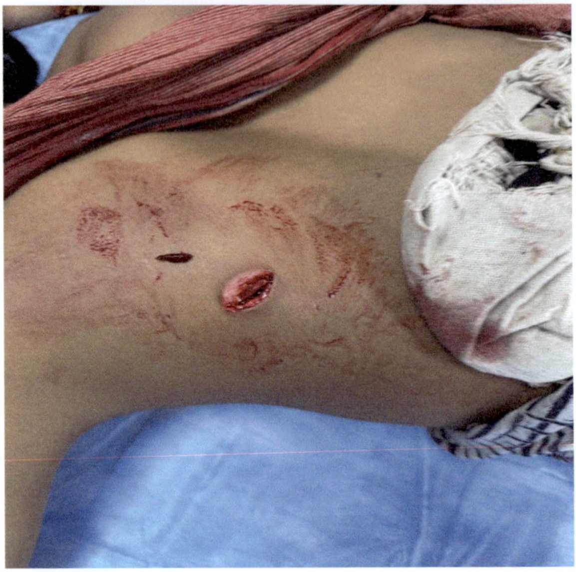

Fig. 4.2 Soldier with entry wound over left side of chest posteriorly

C—circulation: IV access achieved; hypotension treated with warmed crystalloids. TXA considered but deferred due to controlled bleeding.

H—head injury/hypothermia: Conscious; cognitive baseline established. Body wrapped to prevent heat loss.

- *Tactical Evacuation Care (TACEVAC)*
  Helicopter-based TACEVAC not viable. Rooftop casualty extraction required rope-lowering. Scene had limited light and need to do a rapid exfil. Casualty carried down to armored vehicle with reassessment every 5 min. Risk of further exposure minimized by suppressive cover during TFC and TACEVAC.

Case 3: Polytrauma from IED Blast

During a jungle patrol through insurgency-prone terrain, an improvised explosive device (IED) detonates as a soldier advances along a narrow trail (Fig. 4.3). The scene remains unstable, with a high risk of secondary IEDs potentially targeting rescue attempts. The casualty lies approximately 10 m away in exposed terrain, complicating immediate access and necessitating a cautious approach for extraction while maintaining situational awareness and force protection.

- *Care Under Fire (CUF)*: Buddy applies tourniquet to leg and drags casualty behind rock formation.
- *Tactical Field Care (TFC)*
  Once area is cleared by EOD team, medic begins a full MARCH assessment.

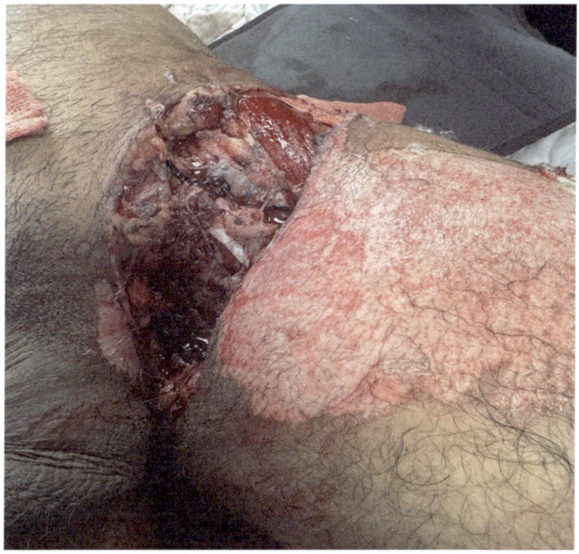

Fig. 4.3 Soldier with groin injury due to IED blast

MARCH Assessment

M—massive hemorrhage: Femoral bleed controlled by tourniquet; abdominal shrapnel packed with hemostatic dressing.

A—airway: Singed facial hair suggests blast inhalation. O_2 applied. Intubation kit ready.

R—respiration: Breath sounds intact; oxygen continued.

C—circulation: Hypotensive; 2 IVs established. TXA administered early. No radial pulse.

H—head injury/hypothermia: Burns covered with dry dressings. Patient wrapped with hypothermia kit. Confusion managed as mild TBI.

- *Tactical Evacuation Care (TACEVAC)*
  Jungle terrain complicates movement. Helicopter LZ 300 m away. Medic manages for Prolonged Field Care (~90 min) before TACEVAC. Patient manually carried through dense trail. One medic, one litter bearer, and one armed escort assigned.

Case 4: Environmental Injury—Hypothermia During High-Altitude Patrol

While on a high-altitude patrol along the Siachen Glacier, a soldier remains stationary for over three hours in sub-zero wind chill conditions as part of a concealment posture. There is no active combat engagement, but movement is deliberately restricted to avoid detection by opposing forces.

Table 4.1 Summary of case scenarios

Case	Primary threat	Tactical challenge	Evacuation plan
1. Shrapnel (ambush)	Extremity + torso bleeding	Under fire; partial cover	Armored vehicle with medic
2. Gunshot wound to chest	Tension pneumothorax	Rooftop exposure	Vehicle evac with reassessments
3. IED polytrauma	Burns, fracture, shrapnel	Jungle terrain, delayed evac	Carried to LZ, then air evac
4. Hypothermia	Cold exposure	No active fire, but immobilized long and sub-zero temperature	Snowmobile to forward aid post

- *Care Under Fire (CUF)*: No active combat engagement.
- *Tactical Field Care (TFC)*
  Medical attention initiated 20 minutes post-immobilization, during pause in mission.

MARCH Assessment

M—massive hemorrhage: No visible injuries; trauma excluded.

A—airway: Patent but monitored. Risk of airway collapse in deeper hypothermia.

R—respiration: Bradypnea; supplemental oxygen provided.

C—circulation: Weak pulse, early bradycardia; IV access obtained and warmed fluids started.

H—head injury/hypothermia: Core body temperature ~34 °C. Rewarming initiated using hot packs, insulated layers, and passive warming.

- *Tactical Evacuation Care (TACEVAC)*
  Mission constraints delayed care. Patient hidden under thermal tarp to avoid IR detection. Gear soaked; gloves frozen—necessitating buddy assistance. Immediate return planned to forward base via snowmobile. Continued rewarming en route. Passive + active warming techniques maintained (Table 4.1).

Approach to an Injured Soldier

The approach to a battlefield casualty must be *rapid, repeatable, and tactically sound.* Unlike civilian trauma environments, combat zones introduce unique threats that demand *dual focus: safeguarding both the casualty and the provider.*

Tactical Considerations: Safety First

The first and most critical step in combat casualty care is ensuring the safety of the rescuer and the casualty. This principle—integral to the *Care Under Fire (CUF)* phase of TCCC—prioritizes immediate threat suppression over medical intervention.

Table 4.2 ABC → MARCH assessment

ABC	MARCH equivalent	Purpose
Airway	A—airway	Maintain patency under duress
Breathing	R—respiration	Identify and manage chest trauma
Circulation	M and C	Control bleeding, maintain perfusion

- *Is the firefight ongoing?* Immediate care is limited to lifesaving actions (e.g., applying a tourniquet).
- *Can the casualty move?* If responsive, instruct the casualty to self-apply tourniquet or crawl to cover.
- *Is buddy drag feasible?* If the casualty is unresponsive, consider tactical drags using a belt, rifle sling, or casualty harness.

Only once a safe perimeter is established does the TCCC phase transition from CUF to Tactical Field Care (TFC).

Primary Survey: ABC → MARCH Assessment

Traditionally, trauma surveys follow the ABC approach—airway, breathing, and circulation. In battlefield settings, however, MARCH is the preferred structure, encompassing and expanding ABC (Table 4.2) in an order of battlefield priority:

The MARCH algorithm is the cornerstone of Tactical Combat Casualty Care. Designed for hostile, resource-scarce environments, it enables structured triage of multiple simultaneous threats to life.

M—Massive Hemorrhage

- Apply tourniquets within 60 s for extremity bleeds.
- Use hemostatic agents (e.g., Celox, QuikClot) for junctional bleeding.
- Prioritize blood loss control before airway or breathing in trauma care under fire.

A—Airway

- Confirm patency via verbal check or visible chest rise.
- Use:
  - NPA in semiconscious casualties
  - OPA if unconscious without gag reflex
  - Surgical airway if obstruction is unrelievable

R—Respiration

- Expose the chest. Assess breath sounds, rise, and symmetry.
- Interventions:
  - Needle decompression for tension pneumothorax
  - Vented chest seals for open wounds
  - Oxygen if available

C—Circulation

- Evaluate for signs of shock: delayed capillary refill, weak radial pulse, confusion.
- Establish IV/IO access.
- Start fluid resuscitation (Hextend, crystalloids, or blood).
- Administer TXA if within 3 h of injury.

H—Head Injury/Hypothermia

- Monitor for TBI (GCS ≤13, unequal pupils, vomiting).
- Prevent heat loss in all trauma patients—even in warm climates.
- Insulate casualty with space blankets, jackets, or body-to-body warming.

MARCH is reassessed after every intervention and at every stage shift (CUF → TFC → TACEVAC).

Secondary Survey

Once life-threatening conditions have been addressed during the MARCH-based primary survey, a systematic secondary survey is initiated during the Tactical Field Care (TFC) phase. This ensures no injuries are missed, and the casualty is prepared for evacuation.

Head-to-Toe Physical Examination

Conduct a tactile and visual examination with gloves on, feeling for:

- Deformities
- Tenderness
- Lacerations
- Swelling
- Crepitus (in fractures)

Begin at the head and progress downward:

- *Head*: Palpate scalp for bleeding or skull depression.
- *Neck*: Look for tracheal deviation, JVD, subcutaneous air.
- *Chest*: Confirm bilateral rise, reassess seal placements.
- *Abdomen*: Check for distension, rigidity, or rebound tenderness.
- *Pelvis*: Gently compress only once—avoid repeated palpation.
- *Limbs*: Check pulses, movement, sensation.
- *Back*: Logroll if spinal precautions apply; inspect for entry wounds or abrasions.

Field Diagnostics

In advanced combat setups or specialized units, basic diagnostics may be available:

- *Pulse oximetry*: Helps monitor response to interventions.
- *Glucose check*: Important in altered consciousness without trauma.
- *Portable ultrasound (FAST exam)*: Assess for internal bleeding.

Once life-threatening conditions have been addressed using the MARCH-based primary survey and systematic secondary survey in Tactical Field Care (TFC) phase, focus shifts to bleeding control, stabilization, and packaging the casualty for safe evacuation.

Key Field Interventions

1. *Hemorrhage Control*
   Uncontrolled hemorrhage remains the leading cause of preventable battlefield deaths. First-line measures must be decisive and efficient:
   - *Direct pressure*: Always attempt with gloved hands, gauze, or trauma pads.
   - *Tourniquet (CAT/SOF-T)*: Apply high and tight for limb injuries; document time of application.
   - *Junctional bleeding (groin, axilla, neck)*: Requires wound packing with hemostatic gauze and firm pressure dressings.
   - *TXA (tranexamic acid)*: 1 g IV/IO within 3 h of injury improves survival by promoting clot stability.

FORCE Tactical Pearl

Reassess tourniquets every 15 min. *If bleeding is controlled and time to evac is short, do not remove in the field.*

2. *Fracture Stabilization*
   Fractures—especially open ones—risk worsening bleeding, infection, and neurovascular injury if left unsupported.
   - *Limb fractures*: Splint in position of comfort. Use SAM splints or improvised rigid materials.
   - *Open fractures*: Cover with sterile dressing; control bleeding first.
   - *Pelvic fractures*: Suspect in blast/blunt trauma with groin bruising or leg malrotation. Apply pelvic binder (if available) or improvise with cravat + windlass method.

FORCE Tactical Pearl

Immobilized limbs make transport safer and reduce pain-related movement that may disrupt clots.

3. *Packaging and Prep for Evacuation*
   Evacuation preparation starts *before the transport team arrives*:
   - Protect IV sites, airway adjuncts, chest seals.
   - Rewarm casualty using hypothermia prevention kits.
   - Create improvised stretchers if needed (e.g., poncho + poles).
   - Document all findings and interventions (MIST).

FORCE Tactical Pearl
Avoid white light or loud comms during night extractions. Flashlights should be red-filtered; hand signals or pre-briefed gestures are preferred.

Once stabilized, transition the casualty toward Tactical Evacuation Care (TACEVAC):

- Document all interventions (MIST format):
  M—mechanism of injury
  I—injuries found
  S—signs/vitals
  T—treatment rendered
- Recheck all interventions:
  - Are tourniquets still effective?
  - Are seals still intact?
  - Is the IV line secured?
- Bundle casualty using hypothermia wrap.
- Assign roles during extraction:
  - One maintains vitals.
  - One handles documentation.
  - One provides cover/fire support if in active zones.

Injury Mechanisms

Understanding how battlefield injuries occur helps predict associated complications and guides management even in the absence of diagnostics. The *three major types—ballistic, blast, and penetrating trauma*—often overlap in combat scenarios with added environmental factors (Table 4.3).

Table 4.3 Injury mechanisms with key features, common injuries, and field care priorities

Injury mechanism	Key features	Common injuries	Field care priorities
Ballistic trauma	Caused by projectiles transferring kinetic energy (bullets, fragments) Severity depends on: Projectile velocity (high > low) Tissue density (muscle ≠ liver) Yaw, tumble, fragmentation increase damage	Thoracic gunshot → pneumothorax, hemothorax Abdominal penetration → bowel perforation, peritonitis Long bone injuries → open fractures, neurovascular compromise	Control massive hemorrhage Rapid thoracic decompression Maintain airway and circulation
Blast trauma	Categorized into four types: *Primary*: pressure wave → barotrauma to lungs, GI, ears *Secondary*: flying debris/shrapnel *Tertiary*: body thrown against objects *Quaternary*: burns, inhalation injury, environmental contamination	Hemoptysis, hearing loss, abdominal distension (primary) Shrapnel wounds (secondary) Pelvic instability, blunt trauma (tertiary) Burns, inhalational injury (quaternary)	Recognize multisystem trauma Follow MARCH sequence Monitor for evolving blast lung/TBI overlap
Penetrating trauma	Includes stab wounds, bayonets, traps Depth vs location critical Often seen in close combat/urban warfare High infection risk in field conditions	Neck/chest → airway injury, tension pneumothorax Abdomen → internal bleeding, peritonitis Extremities → neurovascular compromise	Seal open chest wounds Ensure airway patency Early IV antibiotics in prolonged field care

GI gastrointestinal, *TBI* traumatic brain injury

Environmental Factors

In combat, *environmental exposure often compounds traumatic injuries, influencing both physiological responses and field care logistics.* Military personnel must operate in terrains ranging from deserts and jungles to glaciers—each with unique threats (Table 4.4).

Table 4.4 Environmental threats and tactical field care considerations in austere settings

Environment	Potential threats	Physiological/tactical impact	Field care protocols
1. Cold weather and high altitude	Hypothermia Frostbite Altitude sickness (AMS, HAPE, HACE)	Cold impairs clotting → worsens bleeding Shivering raises oxygen use, depletes glucose Hypoxia at altitude → decreased cognition and decision-making Rapid decompensation possible	Rewarm early using active (heating pads) and passive (blankets, insulation) methods Administer oxygen if altitude illness suspected Avoid unnecessary fluid boluses due to cold diuresis risk
2. Hot and arid conditions	Dehydration Heat exhaustion/stroke Electrolyte imbalance	Salt loss and fluid deficit impair thermoregulation Tachycardia and/or hypotension may mimic shock	Oral rehydration if alert IV fluids only if clear hypovolemia Shade casualty, loosen clothing Apply evaporative cooling (wet cloth + breeze)
3. Jungle and tropical environments	Infectious diseases: malaria, leptospirosis Wound maceration due to moisture	Continuous wetness causes trench foot, fungal skin infections Slows wound healing, increases infection risk	Keep feet and wounds dry Use antifungal powders Prioritize wound hygiene Malaria prophylaxis and infection screening as per protocols

AMS acute mountain sickness, *HAPE* high-altitude pulmonary edema, *HACE* high-altitude cerebral edema

FORCE Tactical Pearl

Casualties may require urgent evac not for trauma, but for exposure-related deterioration.

Case Resolution

Case 1: Shrapnel Injuries from an Ambush Blast

Outcome: The soldier's limb bleed was controlled at CUF phase. Abdominal wound required urgent laparotomy upon arrival. Early TXA and warm fluids improved perfusion.

Key Message: Early bleeding control + field insulation can prevent deterioration en route.

Case 2: Gunshot Wound to the Chest

Outcome: Tension pneumothorax resolved with needle decompression. Chest seal maintained function. No hemothorax on arrival. Patient stabilized for transfer to surgical thoracotomy.

Key Message: Chest decompression must be drilled into every soldier and provider—it is often the difference between arrest and survival.

Case 3: Polytrauma from IED Blast

Outcome: Femoral bleeding and abdominal trauma were managed in field. Burns dressed. Confusion partially improved with oxygen and fluids. ORIF of femur + laparotomy done post-evac.

Key Message: Polytrauma requires parallel action on MARCH elements, not sequential.

Case 4: Environmental Injury—Hypothermia During High-Altitude Patrol

Outcome: Responded well to passive rewarming. Vitals normalized within 40 min. No dysrhythmias. Treated conservatively at base.

Key Message: Hypothermia can mimic trauma—never ignore subtle signs (clumsiness, slurred speech).

Long-Term Considerations

Combat injury recovery extends far beyond the battlefield. Survivors must navigate functional recovery, psychological adaptation, and reintegration—requiring both structured rehabilitation and personalized follow-up.

1. *Physical rehabilitation*
   - *Fractures and amputations*:
     - Require staged surgical correction, early mobilization, and prosthetic adaptation.
     - Emphasize balance training and proprioception.
   - *Burns*:
     - Often need grafting, compression therapy, and long-term scar management.
     - Joint contracture prevention is crucial in limb function retention.

> **FORCE Tactical Pearl**
> Include rehab prep in TACEVAC notes—e.g., document splinting method, ROM preserved, dressing status.

2. *Neurocognitive monitoring*
   - *Blast-related TBIs*:
     - May present weeks later with headaches, memory loss, or mood changes.
     - Require serial neurocognitive assessments.
   - *Hypoxia-related decline*:
     - Soldiers with HAPE/HACE may develop mild cognitive lag or coordination deficits.
     - Baseline reestablishment is key in decision about return to duty.

> **FORCE Tactical Pearl**
> Include neurocognitive observations in MIST: e.g., "Anxious but cooperative; verbalizing incident clearly; no memory gaps."

3. *Psychological support*
   - PTSD, survivor's guilt, and depression remain prevalent.
   - Peer debriefs, structured counselling, and family reintegration planning are essential.
   - Combat medics now play a growing role in mental health first aid—identifying early signs and supporting transitions.
4. *Reintegration and duty fitness*
   - Medical boards assess fitness to return to field roles or offer retraining.
   - Focus areas:
     - Mobility/function scores
     - Cardiopulmonary reserve
     - Cognitive/emotional readiness

Forward-thinking units now embed rehab liaisons and case managers to personalize recovery—bridging the gap between surgery and reintegration.

> **Key Messages**
> - Combat trauma is unique in its complexity, mechanism, and environmental influence—requiring structured, battlefield-ready medical response.
> - The MARCH protocol, integrated across TCCC phases (CUF, TFC, TACEVAC), enables rapid, prioritized lifesaving interventions.
> - Tactical awareness is as essential as clinical skill—care must not compromise mission safety.

(continued)

- Environmental factors like hypothermia and heatstroke can be as deadly as physical trauma and must be actively managed.
- Case-based training reinforces protocol memory, improving survival under operational pressure.
- Long-term recovery spans surgical, psychological, and rehabilitative domains—medical planning must account for all.

Conclusion

Understanding battlefield injury mechanisms is not merely academic—it is a matter of survival. Ballistic, blast, penetrating, and environmental injuries present uniquely complex challenges in military operations. By applying a structured, phase-based approach—anchored in Tactical Combat Casualty Care (TCCC) and the MARCH protocol—combat medics and first responders can intervene decisively in resource-limited, high-threat settings. The integration of tactical considerations into medical response ensures that care does not compromise mission integrity. Through scenario-driven training and methodical triage, even non-medical personnel can contribute meaningfully to survival outcomes. Yet, saving a life is only the beginning. Post-trauma recovery demands long-term planning—physical rehabilitation, mental health support, and readiness assessments. This chapter emphasizes that tactical medicine is not just about technique—*it is about mindset, adaptability, and systems thinking under fire.* In every provider lies the power to preserve life when every second, and every action, counts.

Bibliography

1. American College of Surgeons Committee on Trauma. ATLS: Advanced Trauma Life Support. 10th ed. Chicago: American College of Surgeons; 2018. ISBN: 978-0996826235
2. Auerbach PS, Cushing TA, Harris NS. Auerbach's Wilderness Medicine. 7th ed. 2 vols. Philadelphia: Elsevier; 2016. ISBN: 9780323359429
3. Deaton, Travis G et al. "Tactical Combat Casualty Care (TCCC) Guidelines: 25 January 2024." *Journal of special operations medicine: a peer reviewed journal for SOF medical professionals*, QT3B-XK5B. 13 Mar. 2024, doi:10.55460/QT3B-XK5B
4. Feliciano DV, Mattox KL, Moore EE. *Trauma*. 9th ed. New York: McGraw Hill Medical; 2020. ISBN: 978-1260143355
5. Ranger Training Brigade, U.S. Army Infantry School, U.S. Department of the Army. Ranger Handbook: U.S. Army Ranger Handbook SH 21-76. Revised Feb 2011. New York: CreateSpace Independent Publishing Platform; 2013. ISBN: 978-1304107619
6. U.S. Special Operations Command. *Advanced Tactical Paramedic Protocols Handbook*. Revised 11th ed. Tampa, FL: Breakaway Media, LLC; 2024. ISBN: 979-8990225718

Management of Shock and Hemorrhage in the Tactical Settings

5

Debmoy Ghatak and Drishti Batra

Learning Objectives

- Understand that hemorrhagic shock is the leading cause of preventable combat fatalities and the importance of rapid recognition in tactical settings.
- Describe the pathophysiology of hemorrhagic shock, including the body's compensatory mechanisms and the progression to decompensated shock.
- Identify and apply the principles of hemorrhage control across the three phases of Tactical Combat Casualty Care (Care Under Fire, Tactical Field Care, and Tactical Evacuation Care), including the proper application of tourniquets, direct pressure, and hemostatic agents.
- Explain the principles of judicious fluid resuscitation in combat casualties, including the rationale for permissive hypotension and the prioritized use of blood products and tranexamic acid (TXA).
- Recognize the unique challenges of managing shock and hemorrhage in diverse Indian operational environments (high-altitude, desert, jungle/monsoon) and the importance of logistical adaptations.
- Understand the initial management of a casualty in shock upon arrival at a higher echelon of medical care (base/command hospital), including the structured handoff and the principles of Damage Control Resuscitation (DCR) and Damage Control Surgery (DCS).

D. Ghatak (✉)
Department of Trauma and Emergency, AIIMS, Kalyani, West Bengal, India

D. Batra
Department of Trauma Surgery and Critical Care, JPN Apex Trauma Centre, AIIMS, New Delhi, India

N. T. Rai, S. Misra (eds.), *Frontline Operational Resuscitation and Combat Emergencies (FORCE) Manual*, https://doi.org/10.1007/978-981-92-1622-2_5

Introduction

In tactical combat scenarios, shock and hemorrhage present immediate threats to life. *Hemorrhagic shock, defined as shock caused by severe blood loss, is the leading cause of preventable combat fatalities, with nearly 90% of combat fatalities occurring before a casualty reaches a medical treatment facility.* Combat medics and combat casualty care providers must be adept in rapid assessment and intervention to effectively mitigate these risks and stabilize casualties. This is particularly crucial in the Indian forces' context, where wounded personnel need effective management across diverse operational environments, from high-altitude regions to dense jungles and deserts.

Shock is a life-threatening condition wherein the circulatory system fails to supply sufficient oxygenated blood to tissues. In combat, shock most commonly results from blood loss (hypovolemic shock) due to trauma. Understanding the various types of shock, including *hypovolemic* (hemorrhage being the most common cause), *distributive* (e.g., from sepsis), *cardiogenic* (from heart failure), and *obstructive shock* (e.g., tension pneumothorax), is important (Fig. 5.1). However, this chapter will primarily focus on hypovolemic shock and hemorrhage control techniques most relevant in combat settings. Frontline resuscitation needs emphasis on identifying hemorrhage sources, controlling bleeding, and initiating resuscitative measures even under hostile conditions.

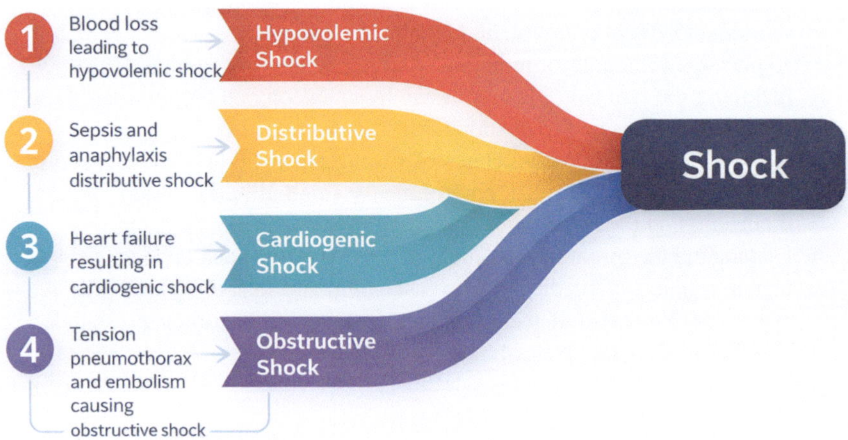

Fig. 5.1 Types of shock

Case Scenarios

Scenario 1: Eastern Manipur—Active Combat Zone

A frontline soldier sustains a gunshot wound to the thigh and suspected torso injury during an ambush in Eastern Manipur. Ongoing firefight and low visibility delay evacuation.

- *Care Under Fire (CUF)*: Immediate hemorrhage control with tourniquet applied under fire. No further interventions until threat suppression.
- *Tactical Field Care (TFC)*: Post-suppression, the casualty is moved to cover for full MARCH assessment and supportive care.

MARCH Assessment

M—Massive hemorrhage:
Tourniquet applied high on thigh under fire. Bleeding controlled before further movement or interventions.
A—Airway:
Casualty is conscious and speaking. No airway compromise; monitored continuously for deterioration.
R—Respiration:
Chest wound suspected. Breathing shallow on reassessment; chest seal prepared for field application.
C—Circulation:
Weak radial pulse. IV access deferred due to ongoing tactical movement; perfusion monitored.
H—Hypothermia prevention:
Reflective sheeting and poncho liner ready. Body insulated after initial bleeding controlled.

- *Tactical Evacuation Care (TACEVAC)*: Fire suppression was necessary before extraction. Casualty evacuated to armored vehicle under low-light conditions. Vital signs monitored en route. No air evacuation possible due to terrain and threat. Movement executed under cover with noise and light discipline. All interventions prioritized for speed

Reflective Questions:

1. What indicators would suggest that the casualty is transitioning into hemorrhagic shock despite initial tourniquet control?
2. How would you determine the need for early blood product transfusion in this field setting?
3. In the absence of IV access, what steps can be taken to maintain perfusion and prevent shock progression?

Scenario 2: Siachen Glacier—Delayed Evacuation in Cold Terrain

A soldier falls off a ridge during a high-altitude patrol. Multiple fractures suspected. Whiteout conditions delay evacuation and access to care.

- *Care Under Fire (CUF)*: No active combat engagement.
- *Tactical Field Care (TFC)*:
  Initial stabilization in snow. Buddy initiates airway management and warming measures.

MARCH Assessment

M—Massive hemorrhage:
No external bleeding. Suspected internal bleeding from pelvic and femur fractures. Improvised pelvic binder considered.
A—Airway:
Jaw thrust maintained in semi-conscious casualty. No adjunct placed. Monitored for gag reflex.
R—Respiration:
Respirations shallow but present. No chest trauma. Hypothermia suspected to depress rate.
C—Circulation:
Radial pulse absent. TXA prepared. IV access delayed due to frozen gear and terrain.
H—Hypothermia prevention:
Reflective blankets, insulation layers, and body heat used. No active warming fluids available.

- *Prolonged Field Care (PFC)*: Sustained management for 90+ min due to delayed evacuation in extreme cold.
- *Tactical Evacuation Care (TACEVAC)*:
  Movement restricted to avoid detection. Snow blindness and icy terrain delayed medical access. Cold gear impaired patient handling and IV access. Casualty was later manually transported to LZ via snowmobile. Continuous passive and active warming during transit. Vital signs checked every 10 min.

Reflective Questions:

1. What signs would confirm internal bleeding as the primary cause of shock in this casualty?
2. How would you prioritize TXA and fluid delivery in a cold environment with difficult vascular access?
3. What are the consequences of delaying hemorrhage control measures like pelvic stabilization in cases of suspected internal bleeding?

Understanding Hemorrhagic Shock in Combat Trauma: Pathophysiology and Classification

Combat injuries from high-velocity projectiles, blasts, and fragmentation typically result in extensive damage to tissues and blood vessels. This leads to rapid and significant blood loss from multiple sites simultaneously. This loss of circulating blood volume is the primary driver of hemorrhagic shock in these scenarios.

Pathophysiology

The development of hemorrhagic shock follows a predictable sequence of physiological events triggered by acute blood loss. Understanding these underlying mechanisms is essential for recognizing early signs of shock, anticipating deterioration, and guiding timely intervention. The cascade begins with the immediate effects of vascular injury and progresses through compensatory responses, cellular dysfunction, and ultimately systemic collapse if bleeding is not controlled. The key components of this pathophysiological progression are outlined below and in Fig. 5.2:

- *Rapid blood volume loss*: The immediate consequence of damaged blood vessels is the escape of blood from the circulatory system. The severity and speed of this loss depend on the size and number of injured vessels.
- *Decreased cardiac output*: Blood volume is crucial for the heart to effectively pump blood. As blood volume decreases, the amount of blood the heart pumps per minute (cardiac output) falls. This means less oxygenated blood is being delivered to the body's tissues.
- *Compensatory vasoconstriction*: The body attempts to counteract this reduced cardiac output through compensatory mechanisms. One of the first responses is the release of catecholamines, leading to vasoconstriction, where blood vessels narrow in the skin, muscles, and visceral organs. This is an attempt to maintain blood pressure and prioritize blood flow to the vital organs like the heart, brain, and kidneys. Clinically, this can manifest as cutaneous vasoconstriction, leading to cool and pale skin. The heart rate also increases (tachycardia) in an attempt to maintain cardiac output despite the reduced stroke volume.
- *Tissue hypoperfusion*: Despite the compensatory vasoconstriction, the overall reduction in blood volume and cardiac output leads to inadequate delivery of oxygen and nutrients to the tissues, a state known as tissue hypoperfusion.
- *Metabolic acidosis*: When tissues do not receive enough oxygen, they switch from aerobic to anaerobic metabolism. This inefficient process produces lactic acid, which accumulates in the blood, leading to metabolic acidosis.
- *Trauma-induced coagulopathy (TIC)*: Severe tissue injury and shock can disrupt the normal blood clotting process, leading to trauma-induced coagulopathy. This makes it harder for the body to form blood clots to stop the ongoing hemorrhage, creating a vicious cycle that exacerbates blood loss. Factors like hypothermia and acidosis can further worsen coagulopathy.

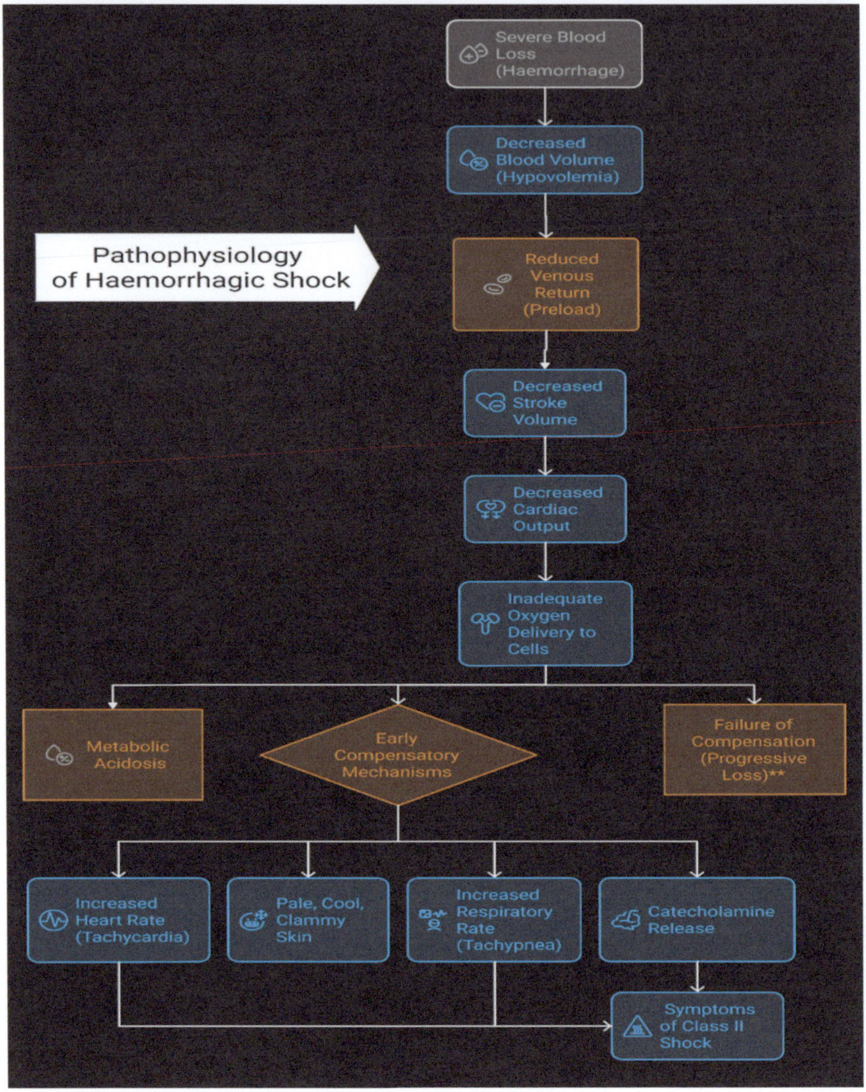

Fig. 5.2 Pathophysiology of compensated hemorrhagic shock. (Figure illustrated using AI tools with OpenAI, ChatGPT-4, 2025)

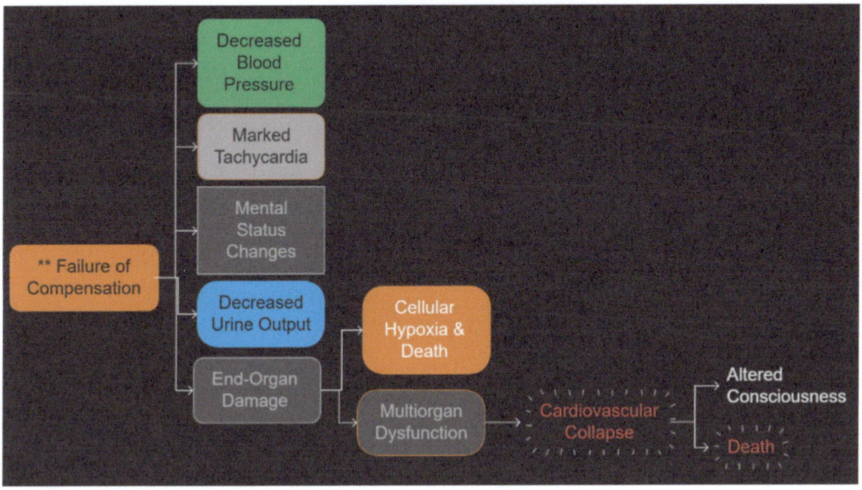

Fig. 5.3 Pathophysiology of decompensated hemorrhagic shock. (Figure illustrated using AI tools with OpenAI, ChatGPT-4, 2025)

As the blood volume continues to decrease, the compensatory mechanisms eventually become overwhelmed and fail, leading to decompensated shock. This is where the signs of shock become more pronounced and life-threatening (Fig. 5.3).

Hemorrhage is traditionally classified into four classes based on blood volume loss (Table 5.1):

- *Class I hemorrhage (<15% blood loss)*: Often minimal signs. Heart rate might be normal or slightly increased. Blood pressure usually remains normal.
- *Class II hemorrhage (15–30% blood loss)*: Tachycardia (increased heart rate) and tachypnoea (increased respiratory rate) are common. Pulse pressure (the difference between systolic and diastolic blood pressure) decreases due to an increase in diastolic pressure from vasoconstriction. The skin might start to become cool and clammy due to vasoconstriction. The patient may exhibit mild anxiety.
- *Class III hemorrhage (31–40% blood loss)*: Increased respiratory rate as the body attempts to compensate for acidosis and hypoxia. *With marked tachycardia and tachypnoea, there is a measurable decrease in systolic blood pressure.* Mental status changes, such as anxiety, confusion, or agitation, become more apparent. Urine output starts to decrease. The skin is typically pale and cold.
- *Class IV hemorrhage (>40% blood loss)*: This represents severe, life-threatening shock. There is profound tachycardia and significant hypotension (low blood pressure). Mental status is severely altered, often with the patient being lethargic or unresponsive. Urine output is minimal or absent. The skin is cold, pale, and clammy. The need for massive transfusion becomes critical at this stage.

Table 5.1 Different classes of shock and clinical manifestations

Class of hemorrhagic shock	Approximate blood loss	Heart rate	Blood pressure	Pulse pressure	Respiratory rate	Mental status	Other clinical symptoms	Need for blood products	Glasgow Coma Scale	Base deficit	Urine output
Class I	<15%/ <750 ml (for a 70 kg male)	↔/<100 bpm	Normal	Normal	↔/14–20	Slightly anxious	Minimal symptoms Minimal tachycardia. No measurable changes in BP or RR	Monitor	↔	0 to –2 mEq/L	↔
Class II	15–30%/750 –1500 ml	↔/↑/100–120 bpm	Normal	Narrowed	↔/20–30	Mildly anxious	Tachycardia, tachypnoea, decreased pulse pressure (due to increased diastolic BP). Subtle CNS changes (anxiety, fear, hostility) Cool extremities with pale skin. Weak peripheral pulse	Possible	↔	–2 to –6 mEq/L	↔
Class III	31–40%/1500 –2000 ml	↑/>120 bpm	↔/↓/ Decrease	Narrowed	↔/↑/30–40	Anxious, confused	Marked tachycardia and tachypnoea, significant changes in mental status, measurable fall in systolic BP. Pale, cool, clammy skin. Rapid, weak pulse. Tachypnoea and air hunger. Decreased urine output	Yes	↓	–6 to –10 mEq/L	↓
Class IV	>40%/>2000 ml	↑↑/>140 bpm	↓/Decreased	Narrowed/ unmeasurable diastolic BP	>35	Confused, lethargic	Marked tachycardia, significant decrease in systolic BP, very narrow or unmeasurable diastolic BP. Bradycardia may develop preterminally. Negligible urine output. Cold and pale skin. Profound hypotension	Massive Transfusion Protocol	↓	–10 mEq/ L or less	↓↓

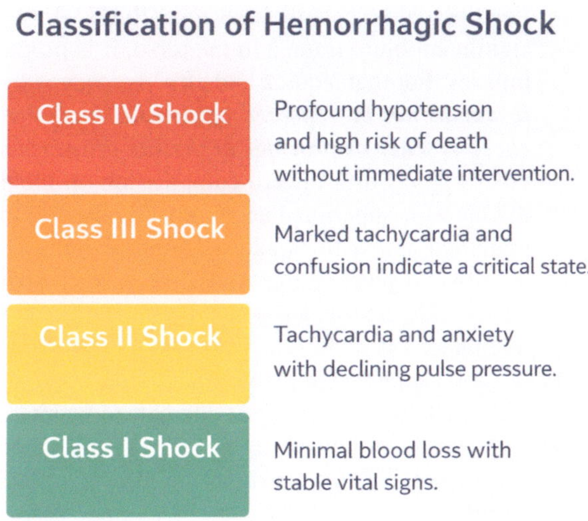

Fig. 5.4 Classification of hemorrhagic shock

Early recognition of these signs and understanding the underlying pathophysiology are crucial for timely and effective interventions, such as rapid hemorrhage control with tourniquets and hemostatic agents, and judicious fluid resuscitation with a priority for blood products in later stages (Fig. 5.4).

FORCE Tactical Pearl
In combat, early identification and intervention in the compensatory or early decompensated phase are critical for casualty survival.

Recognition and Assessment of Shock and Hemorrhage in the Field

Effective shock and hemorrhage management begins with prompt recognition. In combat situations, time is of the essence, and standard diagnostic tools are often unavailable. FORCE providers must rely on *rapid assessment protocols and physical cues* to gauge the severity of blood loss and shock.

Signs and Symptoms of Hemorrhagic Shock

- Telltale signs of obvious hemorrhage like:
  - Obvious bleed from an injured limb or open wound with bleeding, dress soiled with significant bleed, costume laden with clots, open fractures.
  - Obvious long bone fracture with hugely swollen deformed limbs.

Positive pelvic compression test [PCT]—In a case of fall from height or significant blunt trauma to the torso, it is prudent to always rule out pelvic injuries. For that a quick and effective way is to do *pelvic compression test. It should not be repeated afterwards once evaluated by the most experienced rescuer or provider at the site of resuscitation.* During PCT the provider applies firm inward compression on the pelvic girdle with thumb on the anterior superior iliac spine and palm on the outer surface of the iliac bone and assess for tenderness and obvious bony crepitation or unnatural mobility. If positive that raises the suspicion of underlying pelvic fracture and is indicated to put a pelvic binder in place focussing over the greater trochanter.

- Pale, cool, clammy skin [due to peripheral vasoconstriction].
- Rapid, weak pulse [as the heart attempts to maintain perfusion].
- Tachypnea and air hunger [as the casualty tries to compensate for hypoxia].
- Altered mental status, such as confusion or agitation [indicating cerebral hypoxia].

Rapid Assessment Techniques

MARCH Protocol:

This framework prioritizes life-threatening issues in order: *massive hemorrhage, airway, respiration, circulation, and head injury/hypothermia* while doing primary survey of a casualty.

- *Massive hemorrhage*: Immediate control of external bleeding is prioritized, especially for limb and junctional injuries. *Hemorrhage is the most prevalent preventable cause of mortality in combat situations.*
- *Airway and respiration*: Secure airway and assess breathing, as respiratory compromise exacerbates shock. A compromised airway is the second most common cause for preventable combat mortality. A tension pneumothorax must always be ruled out as a contributor to shock. A simple intervention of needle or finger thoracostomy will relieve intrathoracic tension.
- *Circulation*: Monitor pulse and blood pressure if possible. Low blood pressure and high pulse rate suggest hypovolemic shock. Early adoption of damage control resuscitation protocols with permissive hypotension, limited crystalloid infusion, and early initiation of blood and blood products has proven benefits in combat setting.
- *Head injury/hypothermia*: Head injuries may complicate shock management. Hypothermia worsens coagulopathy in hemorrhaging patients. Along with shock and underrunning acidosis, hypothermia culminates into *lethal triad of trauma—hypothermia, acidosis and coagulopathy*. All efforts should be made to prevent hypothermia at all phases of casualty care.

MARCH protocol, which is adopted in military settings, is a modified version of the standard ATLS–ABCDE protocol of primary survey, prioritizing ongoing deficits of circulation with airway and breathing in a C-A-B approach.

In the field environment, especially in austere Indian operational environments where advanced monitoring may be unavailable, recognition of shock must rely on easily detectable clinical signs. *The most reliable field indicators of shock are altered mental status, provided there is no associated head injury, and the presence of weak or absent peripheral (radial) pulses.*

Combat Casualty Care (CCC) Phases and Specific Considerations for Hemorrhage Control

Combat Casualty Care (CCC) is structured around *three phases of care*, each with specific considerations for hemorrhage control and shock management.

Care Under Fire (CUF)

This phase occurs while both the casualty and care provider remain *under effective hostile fire*. The primary considerations include suppression of hostile fire, moving the casualty to a safe position, and treatment of immediate life-threatening hemorrhage.

- *Key interventions*: *tourniquet application*
  A tourniquet is a device designed to constrict a limb with the purpose of controlling severe bleeding from extremities. It can either be an improvised tool or a commercially manufactured product. *Tourniquets are an indispensable tool in a life-threatening extremity hemorrhage.* The widespread introduction of the Combat Application Tourniquet (CAT) (Fig. 5.5) has significantly increased tourniquet use. Studies have shown that tourniquet use in military settings is associated with high survival. Guidelines now endorse tourniquet application when direct pressure is ineffective or impractical.

It is an essential item in medi-kit in frontline deployment. In cases of CUF the tourniquet can be applied by self or by buddy on site. *Often in CUF scenario, packing of any wound is time consuming and impractical.*

Few pertinent things to keep in mind regarding tourniquets in CUF scenario:

- Very much effective in injury of a limb.
- Apply over the garment; apply as "*high and tight*" irrespective of how distal the wound is. Remember to reassess and modify position when tactically feasible.
- Tighten until bleeding stops and the distal pulse is eliminated.
- If one tourniquet fails to stop side-by-side application, another tourniquet proximal to the wound is advised.

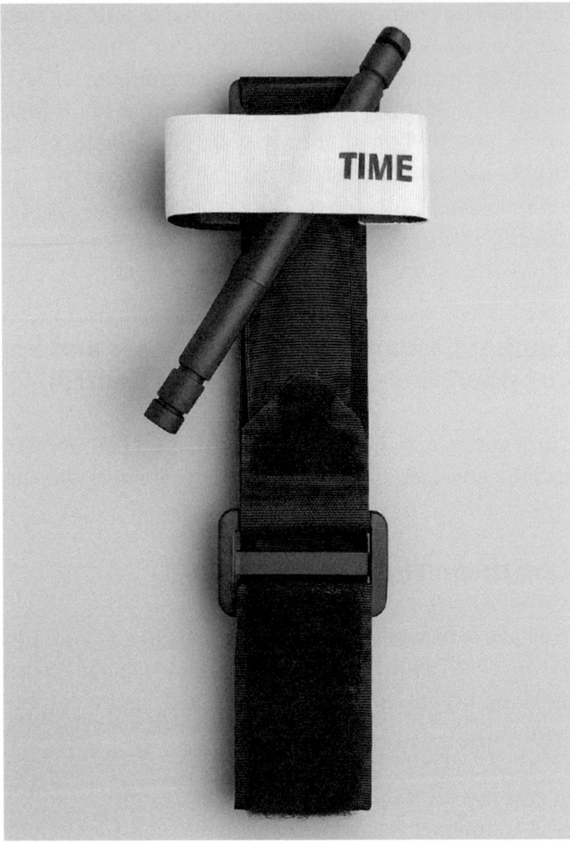

Fig. 5.5 CAT tourniquet

- *Document the time of application.* Do not leave tourniquets continuously for *more than 1 h* at a stretch for the risk of rhabdomyolysis and distal limb ischemia.
- A*void placing and carrying tourniquets too distally in the lower limbs.* Often a number of tourniquets are limited and an IED impact may involve the distal most limb itself.

The Indian forces may consider tourniquet alternatives like Israeli Bandage (Fig. 5.6) and improvisation techniques like a carabiner as windlass when standard equipment is unavailable, particularly in remote border posts. Common errors like positioning the tourniquet too low or not applying enough pressure should be avoided.

Indian-specific considerations include the use of indigenously manufactured tourniquets (Fig. 5.7) and tactical challenges specific to counterinsurgency operations in urban, jungle, or mountain environments. Shock management is typically postponed until a safer environment is reached.

The essential parts of a tourniquet are:

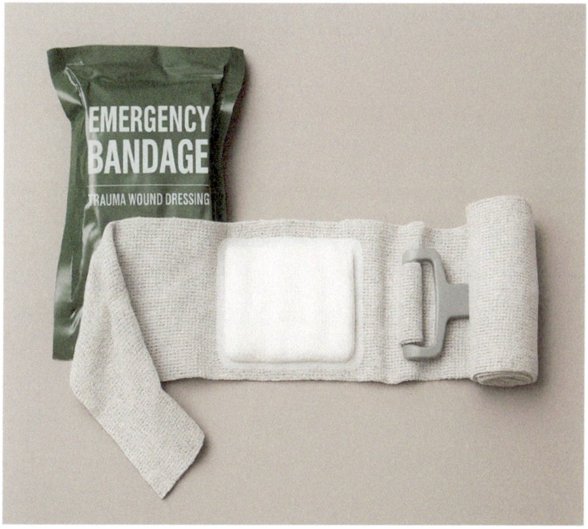

Fig. 5.6 Israeli bandage

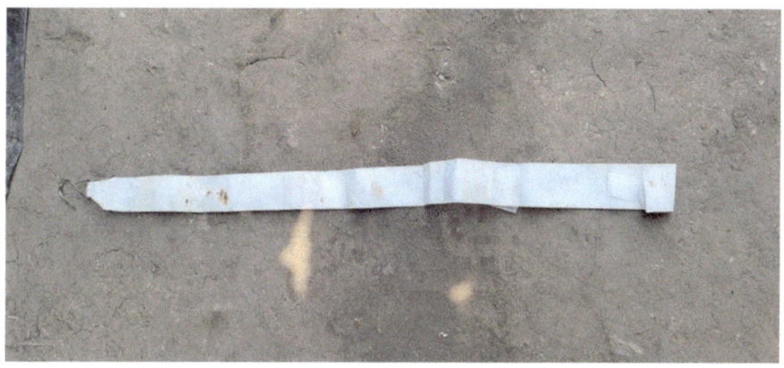

Fig. 5.7 Indian field tourniquet

1. *A constricting band* to wrap around the extremity. This band should ideally be *at least one and a half inches in width* to effectively compress blood vessels and reduce the risk of nerve damage.
2. *A windlass (or twist stick)* which is a rigid object used to twist the material and generate the mechanical advantage necessary to tighten the constricting band enough to eliminate arterial blood flow past the device. *Simply tying a constricting band tightly is usually insufficient to stop arterial flow.*
3. *A securing mechanism* to keep the windlass from unwinding and maintaining the pressure.

Commercial tourniquets are always better than improvised tourniquets because they are specifically designed and tested to occlude arterial flow effectively and reliably. Improvised tourniquets are poor substitutions and should be converted to a commercial tourniquet as soon as possible. Commercial windlass, pneumatic, or ratcheting devices have demonstrated effectiveness in occluding arterial flow.

To improvise a tourniquet when a commercial one is unavailable, you will need material for the band, a windlass, and a way to secure the windlass.

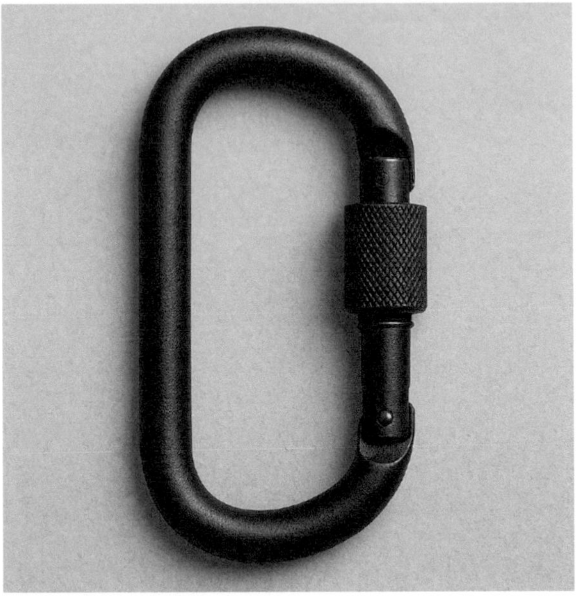

Fig. 5.8 Carabiner

- Good options for the *band material* include:
  - Neckties
  - Neckerchiefs, scarves, bandanas
  - Fabric long enough to wrap around the limb
  - Nylon webbing
  Triangular bandages folded into a strip

Poor options for material include *belts* (which are difficult to tighten adequately) and *zip ties* (which can cause significant tissue and nerve damage) and inelastic thin nylon ropes.

- Good options for the windlass include:
  - Carabiners—if sturdy (Fig. 5.8)
  - Sticks (sturdy enough not to break)
  - Jack handles (from vehicles)
  Broom handles (may need to be shortened)
- *Poor windlass options include pens/pencils (likely to break) and relying on hands alone (ineffective).*

It is critical to understand that inadequate pressure applied by a tourniquet will only impede venous return while arterial flow continues, potentially increasing blood loss and turning a non-life-threatening injury into a fatal one. *Material wrapped tightly without a windlass is a venous constricting band, not an effective tourniquet.* Studies show significantly higher failure rates for improvised tourniquets without a windlass.

- *Steps to improvise a tourniquet:*

1. Wrap the chosen material around the injured limb above the bleeding site (Figs. 5.9 and 5.10).
2. Tie the material in a knot.
3. Insert the windlass into the knot.

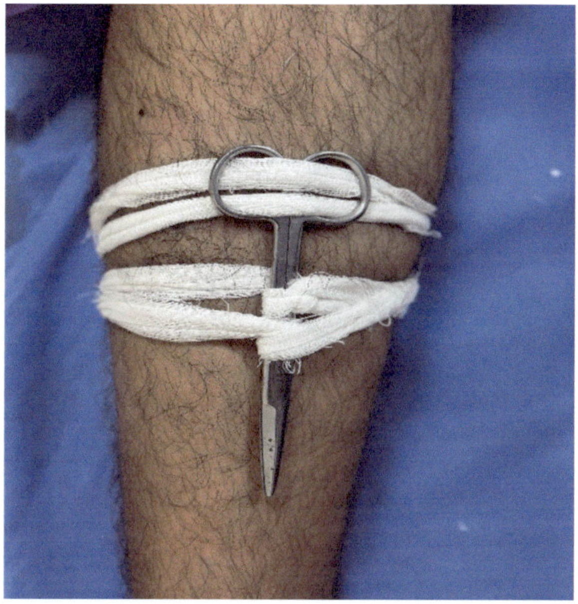

Fig. 5.9 A pair of scissors is used as a windlass and fixed so that it does not unwind

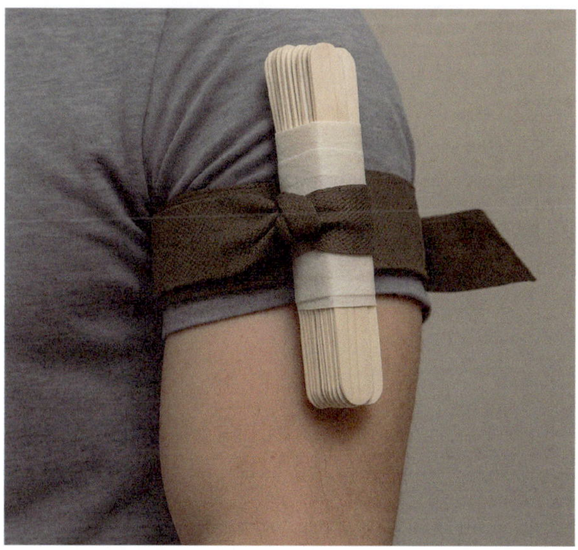

Fig. 5.10 A pack of tongue spatulas are taped together and act as a windlass

4. Twist the windlass to tighten the band until the bleeding stops or slows to an inconsequential amount. *A helpful tip is that the pulse should not be present below the tourniquet.*
5. Secure the windlass in place to prevent it from unwinding.
6. Note the time of tourniquet application, ideally by writing a "T" and the time on the casualty's forehead.

Junctional Bleed

For bleeding from a junctional region (like neck, groin and axillae), CAT is ineffective and bleeding from these sites needs direct sustained pressure for immediate bleeding control in the CUF phase. There are specialized tourniquets like SAM Junctional Tourniquets that can be applied to these areas once an underlying blunt pelvic fracture is ruled out in a later phase.

Tactical Field Care (TFC)

This phase begins when both the casualty and care provider are no longer exposed to significant hostile fire; however, medical care is still constrained by the tactical situation, the resources at hand, and the surrounding conditions.

Key interventions include reassessment of tourniquets applied during CUF; control of other sources of bleeding through direct pressure, wound packing with hemostatic gauze, and pressure dressings; assessment for hemorrhagic shock (using altered mental status and weak/absent radial pulse); and initiation of fluid resuscitation based on shock status.

1. *Reassessment of the Tourniquet placed in the CUF Phase*

   If there is a bleeding wound in the extremity, then the tourniquet that was paced over the garment in the CUF phase needs to be repositioned just on to the skin *2–3 in proximal to the bleeding site unlike the "high and tight" approach in CUF*. This repositioning helps in better hemorrhage control and prevents unintentional ischemia of an uninjured proximal segment of the limb.
   - Avoid application over joints.
   - Be careful not to buckle and trap skin folds under tourniquet.
   - Again, time of application should be marked with indelible marker and particular handover to be given about a tourniquet that is applied.
2. *Direct Pressure*

   Applying direct pressure to a bleeding wound is often the first step. Place a sterile dressing over the wound and apply firm pressure. For high-velocity wounds with irregular surfaces, additional hemostatic gauze (Fig. 5.11) may be needed to pack the wound before applying pressure. While most effective on extremities or accessible wounds, *it may be ineffective in cases of severe arterial bleeding without additional measures.*

3. *Hemostatic Agents and Wound Packing*
   - For junctional hemorrhage (e.g., groin, axilla, neck) or wounds not amenable to tourniquet application: apply direct pressure to control initial bleeding, pack the wound with hemostatic gauze (Fig. 5.11) directly onto the bleeding source, maintain direct pressure for at least 3 min, and apply a pressure bandage. In the Indian context, indigenous hemostatic products (Fig. 5.12) should be evaluated for effectiveness and storage stability in extreme environments encountered in operational areas.
   - For deeper wounds:
     - *Pack gauze tightly from the deepest point outward.*

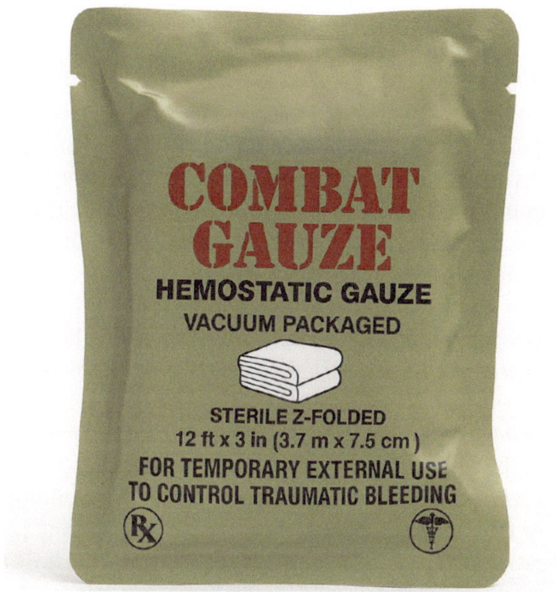

Fig. 5.11 Kaolin impregnated hemostatic gauze

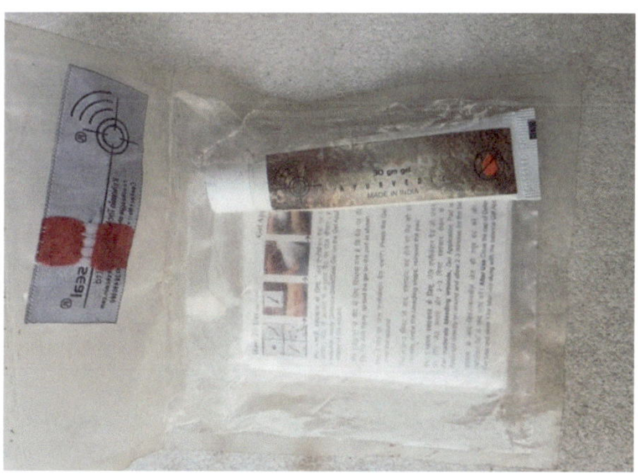

Fig. 5.12 Indian ayurvedic hemostatic ointment

   - Apply consistent pressure.
   - Then apply a pressure dressing.
 - *Non-compressible torso hemorrhage (NCTH)*: Injuries to the torso or chest cavity are challenging to control in the field. Managing NCTH focuses on rapid evacuation to a higher level of care where surgical intervention is possible.

4. *Splinting*
   - It is imperative to splint any fractured limb. Splinting decreases ongoing hemorrhage that might be concealed and pain related to the fracture site.

How Splinting Long Bones Helps in Hemorrhage Control?

A fracture of a large bone like the femur can result in significant blood loss, leading to hypovolemic shock. *Displaced fractures are dangerous because the sharp ends of the fractured bone can injure muscle tissues, nerves, and blood vessels, increasing bleeding.*

Splinting immobilizes the fractured bone, preventing further damage to surrounding tissues and reducing pain caused by movement of the sharp bone fragments. By limiting movement, splinting can help to minimize ongoing bleeding from the injured tissues and blood vessels associated with the fracture. Early splinting of long bone fractures is important to minimize further tissue damage, reduce pain, and potentially decrease bleeding.

Necessary Things to Make an Improvised Splint:

- *Two rigid objects*: Boards, poles, tree limbs, sticks, unloaded rifle, or rolled newspaper. *They should be long enough to extend beyond the joint above and below the fracture site*. For a femur fracture, one should ideally go from the groin to the foot, and the other from above the hip to the foot.
- *Padding*: Blankets, jackets, ponchos, extra clothing, shelter halves, leafy plants, or the casualty's own clothing to prevent rubbing and pressure.
- *Securing materials*: Cravats made from muslin bandages or folded material, strips of clothing, belts, pistol belts, bandoleers. *Narrow materials like wire or cord should be avoided as they can impede circulation.*

Ways to Apply a Splint and Types of Splints:

1. *General principle*: *Splint the fracture as it lies*. Do not reposition the fracture limb unless it is severely angulated and needs to be straightened to fit the splint. If straightening is needed, do it with a gentle pull.
2. *If the fracture site is not on a joint, immobilize the joint above the fracture site and the joint below the fracture site.*
3. *If a joint is fractured, apply the splint to the bone above the joint and to the bone below the joint so the joint is immobilized.*
4. *Padding* should be applied at the joints and sensitive areas to prevent local pressure.
5. *Minimize movement* of the limb until it has been splinted.

Tactical Evacuation Care (TACEVAC)

The Tactical Evacuation (TACEVAC) phase of care includes both Casualty Evacuation (CASEVAC) (evacuation with a nonmedical team and vehicle) and Medical Evacuation (MEDEVAC) (evacuation by majorly a medical team and vehicle or aircraft carrier having a red cross and no combat ability), but the principles remain consistent. *The goal of both CASEVAC and MEDEVAC is to decrease the time to damage control resuscitation and damage control surgery.* During evacuation, the focus is on maintaining circulation, airway, and breathing (CAB).

- Hemorrhage management continues with monitoring and ensuring the effectiveness of tourniquets and dressings.
- Advanced monitoring may be initiated if available.
- Reassessment of CAB—circulation, airway, and breathing
- Intravenous or intraosseous access (I-O) is established if indicated; continued fluid resuscitation is performed based on shock assessment.
- DCR protocols are adopted during resuscitation, prioritizing blood products and using warmed fluids if available.
- Tranexamic acid (TXA) should be administered early (within 3 h of injury) to help stabilize blood clots.
- Preparations are made for handoff to the next echelon of care.
- Clear communication with evacuation teams, providing critical details about the casualty's injuries, interventions, and current status (pre-evacuation briefing), is crucial.
- Documentation of interventions, such as tourniquet time and fluid volumes, ensures continuity of care.

Damage Control Resuscitation (DCR) in Tactical Combat Care

Damage Control Resuscitation (DCR) is a critical trauma management strategy developed to prevent the lethal triad of coagulopathy, acidosis, and hypothermia. Originating from military trauma medicine, DCR focuses on rapidly stabilizing a trauma casualty's physiology through minimal but life-sustaining interventions. Its relevance is particularly pronounced in Indian tactical settings—whether in the dense jungles of Chhattisgarh, mountainous terrain along the LOC, or urban warfare environments—where resource constraints, delayed evacuation, and high-velocity injuries challenge traditional resuscitation protocols.

In combat zones, providers must often make immediate decisions with minimal diagnostic support. DCR allows for timely stabilization, bridging the gap between field interventions and definitive care. Unlike standard civilian protocols, combat-adapted DCR prioritizes permissive hypotension, early hemorrhage control, and judicious fluid use. This is not merely a guideline—*it is a battle-tested doctrine that saves lives under fire!*

Evolution and Principles of DCR

The foundation of DCR was laid in the 1980s through the US naval doctrine and trauma surgery practices, but it gained momentum in battlefield applications during the Iraq and Afghanistan wars. One of the seminal contributions was by Stone et al. (1983), who emphasized abbreviated surgical intervention and rapid physiologic stabilization. Later, Rotondo and colleagues formalized the concept of "damage control laparotomy," reinforcing the interdependence of surgical control and resuscitation.

The DCR Model Emphasizes Four Overarching Principles:

1. *Early recognition of trauma-induced coagulopathy*
2. *Limiting fluid overload*
3. *Avoiding hypothermia at all costs*
4. *Promoting rapid hemorrhage control through surgical or prehospital means*

The Lethal Triad of Trauma and the Evolving Diamond of Trauma Care

The cornerstone of *Damage Control Resuscitation (DCR)* is the prevention and early reversal of the *lethal triad of trauma—hypothermia, acidosis, and coagulopathy* (Fig. 5.13). These three physiological derangements are interdependent and perpetuate a vicious cycle that rapidly leads to uncontrolled hemorrhage and death if not addressed promptly.

Hypothermia (<35 °C) is common in trauma patients due to environmental exposure, hemorrhagic shock, and resuscitation with unwarmed fluids and blood

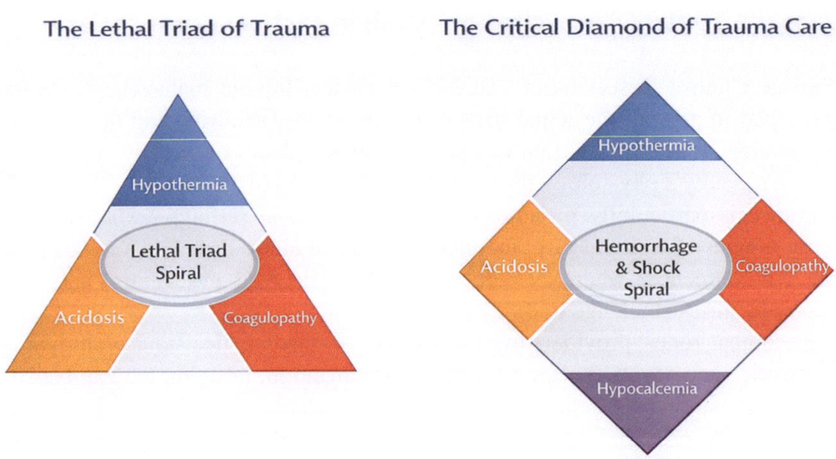

Fig. 5.13 The lethal triad of trauma and the critical diamond of trauma care

products. Hypothermia impairs platelet function and reduces the activity of clotting enzymes, thereby exacerbating bleeding.

Acidosis results from systemic hypoperfusion and anaerobic metabolism, leading to lactic acid accumulation. Metabolic acidosis depresses myocardial contractility, worsens hemodynamic instability, and directly inhibits the coagulation cascade.

Coagulopathy in trauma occurs early and is multifactorial, driven by tissue injury, shock, hypothermia, acidosis, and dilution from excessive crystalloid administration. Trauma-induced coagulopathy sets the stage for ongoing, uncontrolled hemorrhage and is a major predictor of mortality.

Contemporary trauma care recognizes that these three components rarely exist in isolation. Increasing evidence has highlighted *hypocalcemia* as an additional, critical contributor to physiological collapse during massive hemorrhage and transfusion. Citrate-containing blood products, dilutional effects, and shock-related metabolic derangements result in reduced ionized calcium levels, leading to myocardial depression and further impairment of coagulation.

This expanded understanding has given rise to the concept of the *Critical Diamond of Trauma Care*, which incorporates *hypothermia, acidosis, coagulopathy, and hypocalcemia* as four interlinked drivers of traumatic shock. Modern DCR strategies therefore aim not only to interrupt the lethal triad but also to proactively recognize and correct hypocalcemia, completing the transition from the classic triad to a more comprehensive physiological model of trauma-induced collapse.

FORCE Tactical Pearl

Each of these elements exacerbates the others. Preventing this spiral is the primary aim of tactical resuscitation.

Core Strategies of Damage Control Resuscitation

1. *Permissive Hypotension*

   In penetrating trauma without traumatic brain injury (TBI), maintaining a systolic blood pressure of 80–90 mmHg is recommended to avoid dislodging blood clots. This practice buys time until surgical hemorrhage control is possible. Higher targets (SBP >100 mmHg) are reserved for casualties with suspected TBI to preserve cerebral perfusion.
2. *Restrictive Fluid Administration*

   Overuse of crystalloids contributes to dilutional coagulopathy and increases abdominal compartment syndrome risk. Trauma guidelines now recommend restricting crystalloids to <1 L of warmed fluids, transitioning early to blood products when possible.
3. *Hemostatic Resuscitation*

   Blood product administration (whole blood or 1:1:1 ratio of PRBC:FFP:platelets) should be prioritized over crystalloids. MHP or massive hemorrhage protocols can be used in combat settings to rapidly mobilize blood to the treating medical facility. Early administration of blood products supports clot formation, restores volume, and addresses coagulopathy simultaneously. Combat Medical Treatment Facilities (CMTFs) must be equipped for rapid blood mobilization.

4. *Tranexamic Acid (TXA)*

   TXA reduces fibrinolysis and stabilizes clot formation. A 1 g bolus of TXA should be given within 3 hours of injury, followed by an infusion. Its use has shown mortality reduction in both military and civilian trauma settings.

5. *Rewarming Measures*

   Maintaining normothermia is essential. Measures include:

   - Use of foil blankets and poncho liners
   - Body-to-body warming in field conditions
   - Prewarmed IV fluids and blood
   - Heated, humidified oxygen delivery

   Even in hot climates, trauma casualties can become hypothermic due to exposure and blood loss.

6. *Early Hemorrhage Control*

   Hemostasis in the field involves tourniquets, pressure dressings, junctional devices, and hemostatic agents. Rapid control of bleeding is nonnegotiable and takes precedence over fluid resuscitation.

7. *Viscoelastic Assay (VEA)-Guided Resuscitation*

   Though rarely available in field conditions, tools like TEG or ROTEM allow precise assessment of coagulation defects and guide transfusion strategies. These are more relevant at higher facilities.

Integration of Damage Control Surgery (DCS) into DCR

In tactical trauma care, Damage Control Surgery (DCS) is not a standalone concept; *it is the surgical arm of Damage Control Resuscitation (DCR).* Together, they form a unified response aimed at stabilizing severely injured casualties through rapid physiological restoration rather than definitive anatomical repair. The phases of DCS are outlined in Table 5.2 and Fig. 5.14.

Combat Adaptations and Remote DCR

Remote DCR (RDCR) refers to DCR principles applied in austere, prehospital environments. Essential components include:

- Freeze-dried plasma or pre-stored blood products
- Field transfusion capabilities (e.g., walking blood banks)
- Early airway protection, hemorrhage control, and TXA administration

Table 5.2 Phases of DCS

Phase	Focus	Actions	Key goals
Phase 0: prehospital preparation	Early recognition	Field application of tourniquets, TXA administration, hypothermia prevention, rapid triage decisions	Slow physiological decline; prioritize rapid evacuation
Phase 1: initial operation	Hemorrhage and contamination control	Packing bleeding sites, ligating major vessels, temporary shunting, stapling bowel perforations, rapid temporary closures	Stop bleeding; prevent gross contamination; avoid lengthy definitive procedures
Phase 2: ICU resuscitative phase	Physiological restoration	Correction of hypothermia, coagulopathy, and acidosis; aggressive rewarming; guided fluid resuscitation; ventilation support	Stabilize biochemistry and hemodynamics before further surgery
Phase 3: definitive surgery	Anatomical repair	Definitive vascular anastomosis, organ repairs, orthopedic fixations	Repair injuries only after full physiological normalization

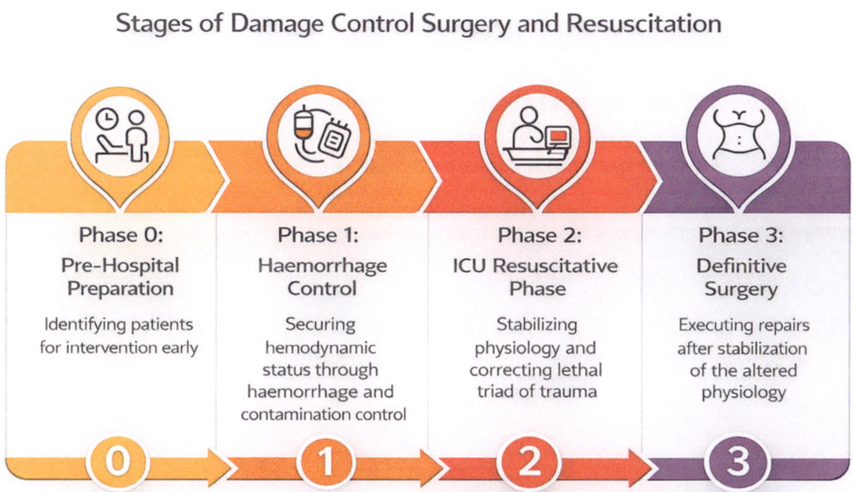

Fig. 5.14 Stages of DCS

RDCR extends the resuscitative window during long evacuations—a common scenario in Indian operations across difficult terrain or under active fire.

Identifying Candidates for DCR

Combat providers must rapidly identify casualties requiring DCR based on simple physiological indicators:

- SBP <90 mmHg
- HR >120 bpm
- pH <7.30
- Blood loss >1500 mL
- Multiple visceral or vascular injuries
- FAST-positive abdomen with poor perfusion
- GCS <8 or evidence of TBI (modifies hypotension target)

FORCE Tactical Pearl
Avoiding over-resuscitation is as critical as initiating resuscitation. Providers must continually balance interventions with clinical response and environmental limitations.

Scoring Systems to Trigger Massive Hemorrhage Protocol (MHP) and DCR

1. *Trauma-Associated Severe Hemorrhage (TASH) Score*
   Predicts massive transfusion needs using injury pattern, vitals, and lab parameters. *TASH >24 warrants DCR/MHP activation.*
2. *Assessment of Blood Consumption (ABC) Score*
   A rapid tool using systolic BP, HR, positive FAST, and penetrating mechanism. *ABC >2 is predictive of massive transfusion needs* (Fig. 5.15).

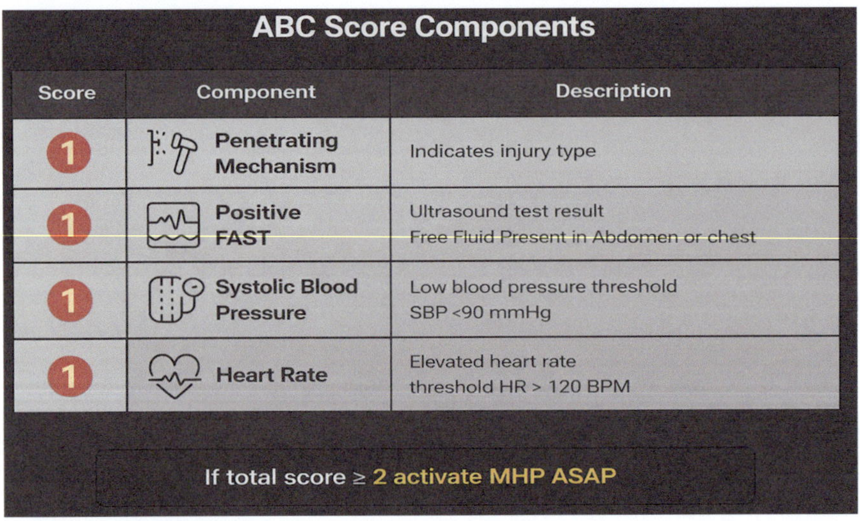

Fig. 5.15 ABC score

3. *Shock Index (SI = HR/SBP)*
SI >0.9 indicates increased mortality risk and correlates with need for aggressive resuscitation.

These scores help to activate MHP protocols even before labs are available.

In Indian combat trauma settings, a typical MHP at a Combat Medical Treatment Facility could look like as given in Table 5.3.

Situations Where Traditional DCR *Should Not Be Followed*

Although DCR principles form the backbone of trauma resuscitation, there are critical exceptions where traditional DCR practices, especially permissive hypotension, must be modified to avoid catastrophic consequences.

In casualties with *severe traumatic brain injury (TBI)*, cerebral perfusion pressure must be protected at all costs. Hypotension—even a single episode with systolic blood pressure below 100 mmHg—is associated with worsened neurological outcomes. *In such cases, the goal shifts to maintaining systolic blood pressures above 100–110 mmHg to ensure adequate brain perfusion.*

Additionally, in cases of *penetrating chest trauma* complicated by active hemothorax or tension pneumothorax, the focus must first shift to decompression and stabilization of ventilation rather than strict adherence to hypotensive protocols.

Finally, in *prolonged field care situations*, where evacuation is delayed beyond six hours, pure permissive hypotension strategies become risky. Ongoing perfusion support through careful fluid titration based on clinical markers (presence of radial pulse, mentation status, urine output) is vital to prevent insidious hypoperfusion, acidosis, and organ failure.

Table 5.3 Massive hemorrhage protocol at an Indian Combat Medical Treatment Facility

Step	Action	Details
Trigger activation	Based on scoring systems	TASH >24, ABC >2, or shock index >0.9
First blood release	Uncrossmatched O-negative or O-positive blood	2 PRBC + 2 FFP + 2 RDP
Second release (after 15 min)	Crossmatch started, if possible	Repeat 2:2:2 ratio
Third batch (after 15 min)	Forward and reverse crossmatch confirmation	Repeat 2:2:2 ratio Adjust based on lab results and ongoing assessment
Adjuncts	1 g TXA IV + calcium gluconate IV (if multiple transfusions)	Address coagulopathy and hypocalcemia
Termination	Once bleeding controlled and vital signs stabilize	Deactivate based on clinical judgement

TASH trauma-associated severe hemorrhage, *ABC* assessment of blood consumption, *PRBC* packed red blood cells, *FFP* fresh frozen plasma, *RDP* random donor platelets, *TXA* tranexamic acid

In all these situations, the core DCR principle of judicious, goal-directed resuscitation remains, but the *blood pressure targets and priorities must be individualized* based on the specific needs of the casualty.

Fresh Whole Blood (FWB) and Walking Blood Banks

Fresh Whole Blood (FWB) is unmatched in its ability to provide volume, oxygen delivery, and clotting factors in one unit. It is ideal for prehospital transfusion when component therapy is unavailable.

Walking Blood Bank (WBB)
Pre-screened, on-site personnel donate blood during emergencies. This system is invaluable in remote or prolonged field care settings, allowing immediate access to warm, fresh blood.

WBB protocols require:

- Regular pre-deployment screening for blood group and infections
- Rapid donor mobilization systems
- Field-compatible transfusion kits

Fluid Resuscitation Protocols and Damage Control Resuscitation Principles

Resuscitation fluids should be prioritized in the following order:

1. Whole blood
2. A combination of plasma, red blood cells (RBCs), and platelets in a 1:1:1 ratio
3. Plasma and RBCs in a 1:1 ratio
4. Plasma or RBCs individually
5. Prewarmed crystalloid solutions, such as Lactated Ringer's or Plasma-Lyte A
6. Hextend, which should not exceed a total volume of 1000 mL

For casualties who are not in shock, intravenous fluids are unnecessary; conscious individuals can be given oral fluids. In cases of shock, administer a *500 mL bolus of the prewarmed most critical available fluid*, and then reassess after each bolus or unit. *Continue this process until achieving a palpable radial pulse, improved mental function, or a systolic blood pressure between 80 and 90 mmHg*. For casualties with traumatic brain injury (TBI) and shock, aim to maintain a systolic blood pressure above 90 mmHg during resuscitation. *Indian forces should consider forward positioning of blood products at Battalion Aid Posts when feasible, development of walking blood bank programs, and implementation of low-titer O whole blood protocols for emergency use, along with cold chain management solutions for extreme environments.* Limited use of crystalloids (around 500 ml boluses) is preferred if blood products are unavailable, as they can dilute clotting factors and exacerbate hypothermia. Permissive hypotension aims to support perfusion without disrupting clot formation.

Intraosseous Access

In tactical settings, obtaining peripheral intravenous (IV) access can be challenging due to factors like shock, collapsed veins, or environmental conditions. When peripheral IV access is difficult or not readily achievable, intraosseous (IO) access is a rapid and effective alternative for fluid resuscitation and medication administration (Fig. 5.16). IO access allows direct entry into the bone marrow's vascular network, providing a non-collapsible route to the systemic circulation.

Indications for IO Access:

1. Difficult or impossible peripheral IV access in casualties requiring immediate fluid resuscitation or medication.
2. Hemorrhagic shock where rapid vascular access is critical.

IO Access Sites:

Several IO access sites are commonly used (Fig. 5.17):

1. *Sternal*: The manubrium (upper part of the sternum) is a preferred site in adults due to its high flow rates. Devices like the FAST1 system and the Sternal EZ-IO (Teleflex Incorporated, Los Angeles, USA) are designed for sternal access.

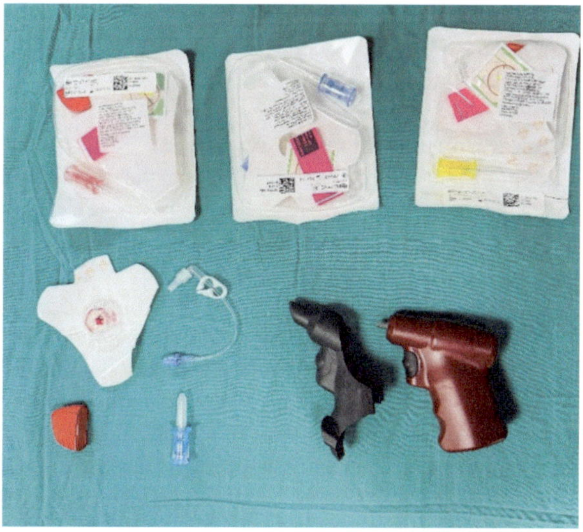

Fig. 5.16 Arrow™ EZ-IO™ intraosseous vascular access system

Fig. 5.17 Anatomical sites for IO access

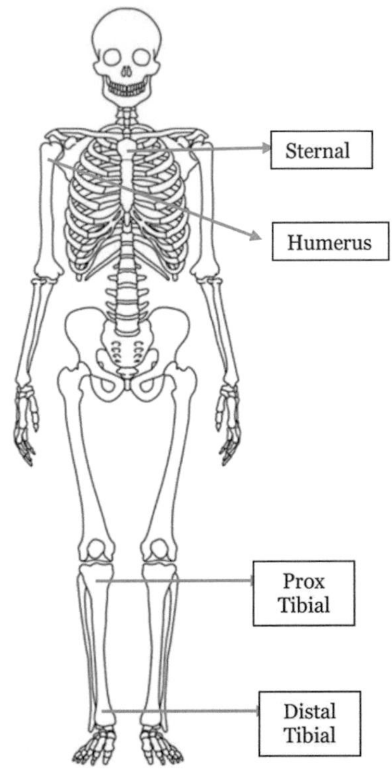

2. *Proximal tibia*: The flat bone on the anterior-medial surface of the tibia, approximately 2–3 finger widths below the patella and 1–2 finger widths medial to the tibial tuberosity, is a common site.
3. *Distal tibia*: The medial malleolus (bony prominence on the inside of the ankle) is another potential site.
4. *Proximal humerus*: The greater tubercle of the humerus can be used but requires specific training and positioning.

General Considerations for IO Access:

- Use proper technique and follow the specific instructions for the chosen IO device.
- Avoid insertion over joints, injured extremities, or extremities with significant wounds proximal to the insertion site.
- Flush the IO catheter with at least 10 ml of normal saline to displace bone marrow and ensure adequate flow. "*No flush equals no flow*."
- Infuse fluids under pressure to overcome the resistance of the bone marrow. The pressure in the medullary space is about one-third of the casualty's arterial pressure.
- Continuously reevaluate the insertion site for signs of extravasation or leakage.
- Removal of IO devices should typically be performed by medical personnel experienced in the procedure.

Pharmacological Management and Supportive Measures

- *Tranexamic acid (TXA)*: TXA, an antifibrinolytic that reduces clot breakdown, should be administered to casualties with hemorrhagic shock, major amputations, penetrating torso trauma, or evidence of severe bleeding. The dosing protocol is *1 g in 100 mL NS/LR IV over 10 min, ideally within 3 h of injury,* followed by a second dose after initial fluid resuscitation. Early TXA administration has been shown to reduce mortality.
- *Vasopressors*: Generally avoided in hemorrhagic shock due to the risk of reducing tissue perfusion.
- *Airway and breathing support*: Maintaining an open airway and adequate oxygenation is critical as respiratory compromise exacerbates shock. Ensure the airway is clear and secure it with an advanced airway device if necessary. Provide supplemental oxygen when available. Be cautious with positive pressure ventilation as it can decrease venous return and worsen shock.
- *Pain management*: A tiered approach based on casualty status is recommended. For casualties in shock, ketamine (50 mg IM/IN or 20 mg slow IV/IO) is preferred, considering ondansetron for nausea.
- *Antibiotics*: Administer antibiotics as early as possible. Moxifloxacin (oral) for those who can take oral medication and Ertapenem (IV/IM) for those who cannot. In jungle/monsoon operations, earlier antibiotic administration is particularly important due to increased infection risk.
- *Hypothermia prevention*: Hypothermia accelerates coagulopathy and worsens outcomes. Prevention measures include minimizing environmental exposure, keeping protective gear on, replacing wet clothing, using hypothermia prevention kits, blankets, and warming IV fluids when possible. These measures are particularly crucial in high-altitude areas.
- *Wound care*: At the third phase after CASEVAC all the wounds of the casualty should be diligently examined after exposing the whole torso and logrolling. All the wounds should be documented. Wounds should be cleaned and thoroughly decontaminated and dressed.
- *Monitoring and documentation*: When tactically feasible, initiate electronic monitoring of vital signs, document all interventions including tourniquet application times, record fluid administration volumes and times, and monitor for recurrence of shock.

The approach to shock and hemorrhage control evolves across the TCCC continuum—Care Under Fire, Tactical Field Care, and Tactical Evacuation—each with escalating levels of intervention and monitoring. Figure 5.18 summarizes this phased management strategy and highlights the critical priorities at each stage.

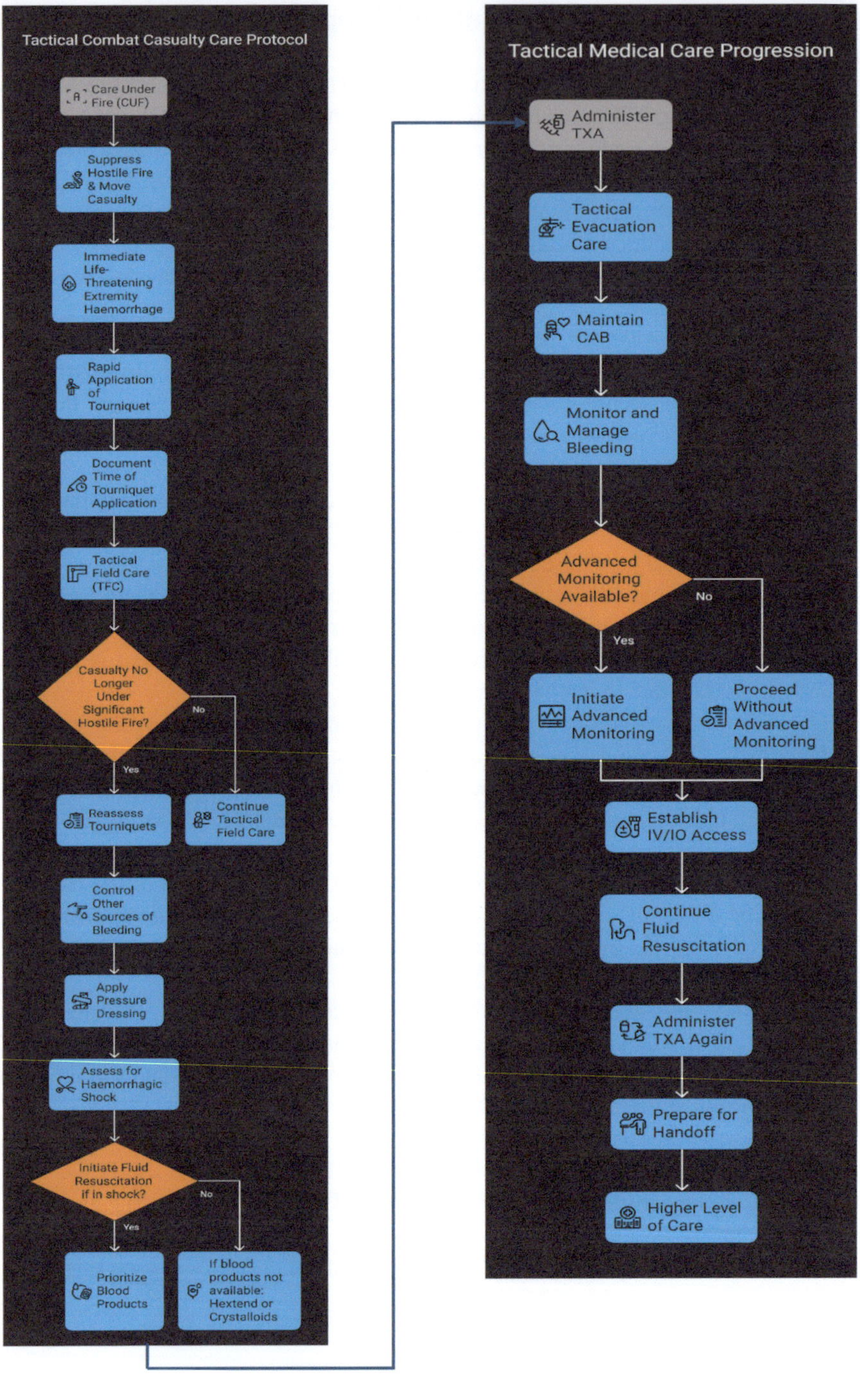

Fig. 5.18 Summary of management of shock and hemorrhage as per TCCC phases of care. (Figure illustrated using AI tools with OpenAI, ChatGPT-4, 2025)

Care After TACEVAC

All interlevel transfers in the military are primarily informed processes. Upon the arrival of a patient in shock at a base or command hospital's emergency department, a structured handoff is performed. Simultaneously, the casualty undergoes reassessment through a primary survey, adhering to the priorities of airway, breathing, circulation, disability, and exposure. An extended Focused Assessment with Sonography for Trauma (eFAST) is conducted promptly, and the adjuncts of the primary survey are repeated. Following this, at the conclusion of the primary survey and ongoing damage control resuscitation (DCR) efforts, the patient's hemodynamic parameters—blood pressure (BP), heart rate (HR), Glasgow Coma Scale (GCS), and respiratory rate (RR)—are reassessed.

Three potential outcomes may emerge from this process:

1. *Responder*: If a patient initially in shock demonstrates sustained improvement in hemodynamics following DCR, they are classified as a "responder." In such cases, a secondary survey is carried out along with further radiological investigations as needed.
2. *Nonresponder*: If a patient in severe shock fails to show hemodynamic improvement despite DCR efforts, they are deemed a "nonresponder." Nonresponders with evident sources of bleeding—such as positive findings on FAST for intra-abdominal hemorrhage, massive hemothorax, obvious pelvic fractures, penetrating torso injuries suggesting great vessel damage in the thorax or abdomen, or exsanguinating extremity vascular injuries—are candidates for Damage Control Surgery (DCS). *The primary objective of DCS is hemorrhage control.* It is essential to recognize that DCS is an integral component of DCR and can take various forms:
   - Damage control laparotomy
   - Damage control thoracotomy
   - Damage control vascular surgery
   - Damage control orthopedics
3. *Transient responder*: This group includes patients who *initially respond to resuscitation efforts but subsequently experience a decline in hemodynamic stability.* These "transient responders" require close monitoring due to their precarious condition. Once their vital parameters deteriorate again, they must be managed similarly to nonresponders.

Special Considerations for the Indian Context: Environmental and Logistical Adaptations

India's diverse operational environments present unique challenges.

- *High-altitude operations (Ladakh, Siachen)*:
  Increased risk of hypothermia accelerating coagulopathy, hypoxia exacerbating shock, and fluid management challenges due to cold-induced diuresis necessitate aggressive warming during fluid resuscitation and consideration of a lower threshold for oxygen supplementation.
- *Desert operations (Rajasthan)*:
  Preexisting dehydration complicating shock assessment and extremes of temperature affecting equipment may require *higher initial fluid volumes in known dehydration states.*
- *Jungle/monsoon operations (Northeast)*:
  Increased infection risk with *delayed wound management* and challenges in maintaining *necessitate earlier antibiotic administration and waterproof packaging for hemostatic agents.*

Implementing effective shock and hemorrhage management requires integration with existing Indian military medical echelons, training adaptations for all levels of personnel, and equipment standardization, including indigenous alternatives and temperature-controlled storage solutions.

Case Resolution

Scenario 1: Eastern Manipur—Active Combat Zone

This scenario illustrates the rapid application of Tactical Combat Casualty Care (TCCC) principles in a hostile environment. The casualty sustained a gunshot wound to the thigh with suspected torso injury. During the Care Under Fire (CUF) phase, a high and tight tourniquet was immediately applied, effectively controlling femoral bleeding. This swift action was essential to prevent exsanguination while under active fire.

However, despite initial hemorrhage control, field responders remained alert for evolving signs of shock—tachycardia, altered mentation, or weak peripheral pulses—which could indicate ongoing internal bleeding or inadequate tissue perfusion. Recognizing such indicators of hemorrhagic shock, even after tourniquet placement, is critical for timely escalation of care.

In the Tactical Field Care (TFC) phase, bleeding from the torso was managed using hemostatic gauze and compression dressings, and warmed IV fluids were initiated. The decision to administer tranexamic acid (TXA) early reflected a proactive approach to combat trauma-induced coagulopathy.

Given the absence of on-hand blood products, the team evaluated the need for transfusion using clinical parameters such as persistent hypotension, ongoing bleeding, and weak radial pulse—factors that would typically trigger early blood product use if available.

Upon entering the Tactical Evacuation Care (TACEVAC) phase, Damage Control Resuscitation (DCR) strategies were employed: permissive hypotension with a systolic BP goal of 80–90 mmHg, continued warming, and reassessment of perfusion. In scenarios where IV access may have failed, field medics would resort to oral fluids (if conscious), intraosseous access, and continuous mental status monitoring to maintain perfusion and prevent decompensation.

This protocol-driven, structured approach ensured the casualty was stabilized for definitive surgical intervention, reinforcing the importance of early intervention, ongoing reassessment, and adaptive field decision-making under fire.

Scenario 2: Siachen Glacier—Delayed Evacuation in Cold Terrain

This scenario highlights the dual threats of trauma and environment in high-altitude warfare. The casualty, following a cliff fall, presented with pelvic instability, a femoral fracture, and signs of severe hypothermia. The tactical situation demanded prolonged field care prior to evacuation.

At the scene, responders prioritized passive and active rewarming, spinal precautions, and stabilization. The application of an improvised pelvic binder was a decisive step in preventing further hemorrhage. Signs such as absent radial pulse, prolonged capillary refill, and pale extremities pointed toward internal bleeding as the likely cause of shock.

In cold environments where vascular access may be difficult, the medic must strategically prioritize TXA and fluid delivery. Warming fluids before administration and selecting intraosseous routes, if IV fails, are essential. TXA should be delivered as early as possible, ideally within 3 hours, to reduce fibrinolysis and support clot stability.

Delaying pelvic stabilization could lead to ongoing internal hemorrhage, worsening shock, and increased mortality. Early binder application and minimizing patient movement were key to damage control. Upon arrival at the forward base, DCR principles guided resuscitation with warmed fluids and surgical planning for pelvic packing or angioembolization.

This case highlights the integration of trauma management with environmental considerations. The team's ability to adapt to limited resources and prolonged care challenges ensured the casualty was stabilized for evacuation, emphasizing that survivability in austere conditions hinges on timely interventions, improvisation, and reassessment.

Key Messages

- Effective management of combat casualties begins with the immediate control of massive hemorrhage, as this is the leading preventable cause of combat fatalities. Rapid intervention is crucial even under hostile fire.
- The MARCH protocol provides a critical framework for the sequential management of life-threatening conditions, prioritizing massive hemorrhage, airway, respiration, circulation, and head injury/hypothermia in the field. This structured approach guides initial assessment and treatment.
- Tourniquet application is a primary management technique for life-threatening extremity bleeding during Care Under Fire. Proper application, "high and tight" initially, is essential for achieving hemorrhage control.
- During Tactical Field Care, reassessment and potential repositioning of tourniquets are key management steps to optimize blood flow to uninjured areas while maintaining hemorrhage control at the injury site.
- Management of non-compressible hemorrhage in junctional areas and the torso relies on techniques like direct pressure and wound packing with hemostatic agents to control bleeding when tourniquets are ineffective.
- Judicious fluid resuscitation is a critical aspect of shock management, with current principles prioritizing the early administration of blood products and whole blood when available and aiming for permissive hypotension in the absence of traumatic brain injury.
- Early administration of tranexamic acid (TXA) is a vital management intervention for casualties in hemorrhagic shock, as it helps to stabilize blood clots and reduce mortality when given within the first three hours of injury.
- *Damage Control Resuscitation is a physiologic-first approach*—designed to interrupt the lethal triad of hypothermia, acidosis, and coagulopathy through permissive hypotension, early hemostatic transfusion, TXA, and hypothermia prevention—particularly vital in austere, prehospital, and tactical environments.
- *Damage Control Surgery (DCS) is not separate but the surgical continuation of DCR,* aiming for rapid hemorrhage control and contamination limitation, progressing through defined phases from prehospital recognition to staged definitive repair after physiological stabilization.
- Combat-specific challenges demand adaptation of DCR principles, including the use of walking blood banks, viscoelastic-guided transfusion, remote DCR, and modified blood pressure targets for patients with TBI, ensuring individualized, survivable care in resource-limited and time-critical settings.
- Field recognition of shock for effective management relies on rapid assessment of clinical signs such as altered mental status and the presence of weak or absent peripheral pulses, especially in resource-limited environments.

(continued)

- Splinting of fractured limbs is an important management strategy that not only reduces pain but can also help to minimize ongoing hemorrhage associated with bone movement and tissue damage.
- Upon arrival at a higher echelon of care, a structured handoff and reassessment are crucial for guiding subsequent management, including Damage Control Resuscitation and potentially Damage Control Surgery for nonresponder.

Conclusion

Successful management of combat trauma begins with decisive, protocol-driven interventions at the point of injury. The MARCH algorithm, integrated with Tactical Combat Casualty Care (TCCC) phases, provides a reliable framework for addressing life-threatening conditions in a systematic order. Immediate hemorrhage control, especially with prompt tourniquet application—remains the cornerstone of survival in the Care Under Fire phase. Transitioning into Tactical Field Care, reassessment of bleeding, airway, respiration, and circulation ensures continued stabilization. Techniques such as wound packing, early TXA administration, judicious fluid resuscitation, and pelvic binding are critical, particularly in polytrauma and non-compressible hemorrhage. Splinting, thermal management, and field shock recognition further enhance outcomes. Upon handover, structured communication and imaging guide advanced interventions like Damage Control Resuscitation or Surgery. This chapter reinforces that timely, well-sequenced actions—guided by MARCH and grounded in tactical awareness—can transform battlefield chaos into coordinated, lifesaving care.

Bibliography

1. Achneck, Hardean E et al. "A comprehensive review of topical hemostatic agents: efficacy and recommendations for use." *Annals of surgery* vol. 251,2 (2010): 217–28. doi:https://doi.org/10.1097/SLA.0b013e3181c3bcca
2. American College of Surgeons Committee on Trauma. ATLS: Advanced Trauma Life Support. 10th ed. Chicago: American College of Surgeons; 2018. ISBN: 978-0996826235
3. Bulger, Eileen M et al. "An evidence-based prehospital guideline for external hemorrhage control: American College of Surgeons Committee on Trauma." *Prehospital emergency care* vol. 18,2 (2014): 163–73. doi:https://doi.org/10.3109/10903127.2014.896962
4. Butler, Frank K Jr. "Tactical Combat Casualty Care: Beginnings." *Wilderness & environmental medicine* vol. 28,2S (2017): S12–S17. doi:https://doi.org/10.1016/j.wem.2016.12.004
5. Clasper, J C et al. "Limb complications following pre-hospital tourniquet use." *Journal of the Royal Army Medical Corps* vol. 155,3 (2009): 200–2. doi:https://doi.org/10.1136/jramc-155-03-06
6. Cruciani, Mario et al. "The use of whole blood in traumatic bleeding: a systematic review." *Internal and emergency medicine* vol. 16,1 (2021): 209–220. doi:https://doi.org/10.1007/s11739-020-02491-0

7. Frank K. Butler, John Hagmann, E. George Butler, Tactical Combat Casualty Care in Special Operations, *Military Medicine*, Volume 161, Issue suppl_1, August 1996, Pages 3–16, https://doi.org/10.1093/milmed/161.suppl_1.3
8. Kotwal RS, Butler FK, Edgar EP, Shackelford SA, Bennett DR, Bailey JA. *Saving Lives on the Battlefield: A Joint Trauma System Review of Pre-Hospital Trauma Care in Combined Joint Operating Area – Afghanistan (CJOA-A) – Final Report.* U.S. Central Command; 2013 Jan 30. Available from: https://www.researchgate.net/publication/253336029
9. Mizobata, Yasumitsu. "Damage control resuscitation: a practical approach for severely hemorrhagic patients and its effects on trauma surgery." *Journal of intensive care* vol. 5,1 4. 20 Jan. 2017, doi:https://doi.org/10.1186/s40560-016-0197-5
10. Nielsen, J.S., Watson, J. Damage Control Resuscitation and Surgery in a Forward Combat Setting. *Curr Trauma Rep* **2**, 165–172 (2016). https://doi.org/10.1007/s40719-016-0049-8
11. Ravi, Parli R, and Bipin Puri. "Fluid resuscitation in haemorrhagic shock in combat casualties." *Disaster and military medicine* vol. 3 2. 17 Jan. 2017, doi:https://doi.org/10.1186/s40696-017-0030-2
12. Rotondo, M F et al. "'Damage control': an approach for improved survival in exsanguinating penetrating abdominal injury." *The Journal of trauma* vol. 35,3 (1993): 375–82; discussion 382–3.
13. Sauer, Samual W et al. "Saving Lives on the Battlefield (Part II) ? One Year Later A Joint Theater Trauma System and Joint Trauma System Review of Prehospital Trauma Care in Combined Joint Operations Area?Afghanistan (CJOA-A) Final Report, 30 May 2014." *Journal of special operations medicine: a peer reviewed journal for SOF medical professionals* vol. 15,2 (2015): 25–41. doi:10.55460/GI15-HVCY
14. Stewart, Sarah K et al. "Improvised tourniquets: Obsolete or obligatory?." *The journal of trauma and acute care surgery* vol. 78,1 (2015): 178–83. doi:https://doi.org/10.1097/TA.0000000000000485
15. Stone, H H et al. "Management of the major coagulopathy with onset during laparotomy." *Annals of surgery* vol. 197,5 (1983): 532–5. doi:https://doi.org/10.1097/00000658-198305000-00005
16. U.S. Army Medical Department Center and School. *Treating Fractures in the Field: Subcourse MD0533, Edition 200.* Fort Sam Houston, TX: U.S. Army Medical Department; [cited 2025 Apr 23]. Available from: http://nursing411.org/Army/MD0533.pdf

Securing Airway and Breathing in a Combat Zone

6

Priyanka Modi

Learning Objectives

- Understand the critical importance of airway and breathing management in combat settings.
- Learn rapid assessment and intervention techniques for airway compromise.
- Recognize indications for basic and advanced airway management strategies.
- Apply Tactical Combat Casualty Care (TCCC) guidelines effectively.
- Utilize POCUS for rapid diagnosis of respiratory conditions in combat trauma.

Introduction

Effective airway and breathing management in combat zones is critical for casualty survival. The unique challenges posed by the combat environment—such as harsh terrain, limited medical resources, and ongoing hostilities—demand that healthcare providers respond rapidly and decisively to prevent hypoxia and ensure adequate ventilation. This chapter outlines the best practices, techniques, and considerations for managing airway and breathing in combat trauma, emphasizing Tactical Combat Casualty Care (TCCC) guidelines.

P. Modi (✉)
The Faculty of Medicine and Health Sciences, SGT University, Gurugram, Haryana, India

N. T. Rai, S. Misra (eds.), *Frontline Operational Resuscitation and Combat Emergencies (FORCE) Manual*, https://doi.org/10.1007/978-981-92-1622-2_6

Case Scenario

A 26-year-old soldier is found unconscious approximately 15 meters from the blast epicenter following an ambush during a convoy halt. The casualty is located in semi-cover and is extracted via buddy drag under fire. Immediate threat persists during the first response; suppressive fire is required.

- *Care Under Fire (CUF):* No interventions performed except a buddy drag to cover. Bleeding noted from the face; airway compromise suspected.
- *Tactical Field Care (TFC):*

  After suppressive fire clears, a full MARCH assessment and supportive care is initiated.

  MARCH assessment:

  M—massive hemorrhage:

  Facial bleeding controlled with direct pressure and gauze. No other hemorrhage detected in limbs or junctional zones.

  A—airway:

  Blood suctioned from oropharynx. Jaw thrust applied; cervical collar placed. Mandibular fracture necessitates emergency cricothyrotomy (Fig. 6.1).

  R—respiration:

  SpO_2 improved from 32% to 93% after cricothyrotomy and bag-valve mask ventilation. Sucking chest wound sealed, needle decompression done, flail chest stabilized.

  C—circulation:

  Signs of shock: HR 140/min, BP 82/56 mmHg. IV access achieved; warmed fluids given. No pelvic or spinal injury found on log roll.

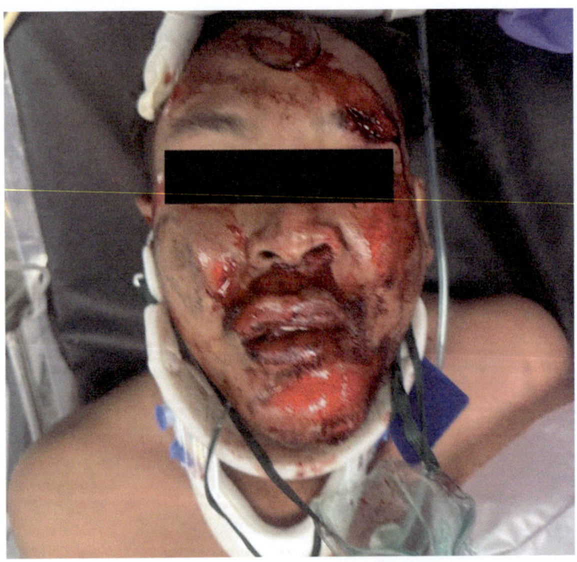

Fig. 6.1 Soldier with extensive maxillofacial injuries necessitating surgical cricothyrotomy

H—head injury/hypothermia:
GCS 9, anisocoria present. Core temperature 34 °C. Rewarming initiated with blankets and insulation.
Secondary survey:
Facial lacerations sutured. Right hand fracture splinted. Chest shows paradoxical motion; flail segment managed. Back and pelvis unremarkable.

- *Tactical Evacuation Care (TACEVAC):*
  Initial access delayed by enemy fire. Lifesaving interventions executed in limited space. Airway management prioritized amid low visibility. Patient evacuated with assisted ventilation with BVM support via cricothyrotomy, continuous monitoring, and pre-alert to surgical team via MIST handover including airway, chest trauma, and neurological alerts.

Reflective Questions

1. What early indicators in this scenario suggested the need for a surgical airway rather than basic adjuncts or endotracheal intubation?
2. How would you manage airway control in a casualty with maxillofacial trauma and ongoing facial bleeding if suction is unavailable?
3. What are the risks of inadequate ventilation through a cricothyrotomy, and how can you monitor and ensure effective oxygenation during prolonged TACEVAC?
4. When managing both airway compromise and thoracic trauma (e.g., sucking chest wound + flail chest), how do you prioritize and sequence your interventions?

Approach to Airway Management in a Combat Zone

In battlefield trauma, early recognition and immediate management of a threatened airway is critical for survival. Airway obstruction—whether from blast trauma, burns, maxillofacial injuries, or unconsciousness—is a preventable cause of death. The MARCH algorithm used in Tactical Combat Casualty Care (TCCC) prioritizes airway after massive hemorrhage, highlighting its lifesaving role. A patent airway ensures adequate oxygenation and ventilation, preventing hypoxia—a leading cause of avoidable battlefield deaths.

In the combat or trauma environment, airway compromise is a life-threatening emergency. The FORCE provider must rapidly assess, predict potential difficulty, and select the most appropriate technique to secure the airway based on the tactical situation, anatomical challenges, and available equipment.

FORCE Tactical Pearl
Airway control is not a choice—it is a responsibility. Choose the right tool, at the right time, for the right patient.

Airway Management Algorithm in Trauma/Combat Setting

1. *Assess airway patency*: Consciousness, phonation, spontaneous breathing
2. *Is the airway compromised or at risk?*
   - Yes → Proceed to airway intervention
   - No → Monitor and prepare for deterioration
3. *Is the patient breathing adequately?*
   - No → Begin with basic airway maneuvers and BMV ventilation
4. *Need for Definitive Airway?* (e.g., GCS ≤8, facial trauma, burns, massive bleeding, hypoxia despite BMV)
   - Yes → Proceed to advanced airway technique
5. *Can laryngoscopy be performed safely?*
   - Yes → Endotracheal intubation (direct or video) with RSI
   - No/failed attempts → Use supraglottic device
   - Still compromised → Surgical airway (cricothyrotomy)

Combat Indicators of a Threatened Airway

Field recognition of airway compromise relies on inspection, auscultation, and communication (Table 6.1): If the casualty can speak normally, the airway is likely intact. Silence, gurgling, or snoring may suggest partial or complete obstruction.

Typical combat signs of a threatened airway:

Table 6.1 Threatened airway in combat: field indicators and immediate actions

Cause	Field indicators	Immediate action
Soft tissue obstruction	Gurgling, snoring, unconsciousness, vomiting	Chin lift/jaw thrust, NPA/OPA insertion, lateral recovery position if safe
Maxillofacial trauma	Facial deformity, bleeding, missing teeth, inability to ventilate	Suction, NPA/OPA if possible, consider cricothyrotomy if ventilation fails
Burns/inhalation injury	Soot, singed nasal hairs, facial swelling, hoarseness	High suspicion for airway edema, early cricothyrotomy if stridor or voice change
Foreign body or fluid	Blood, vomit, loose teeth in airway	Suction, recovery position, airway adjuncts
Decreased consciousness (GCS <10)	Unresponsive, pooling secretions, tongue obstruction	Jaw thrust, NPA insertion, suction, prepare for surgical airway if needed
Suspected spinal injury	Blunt trauma, blast, motor vehicle collision, altered mental status	Manual stabilization, jaw thrust, hard collar application post-airway control

Abbreviations: OPA oropharyngeal airway, *NPA* nasopharyngeal airway, *GCS* Glasgow Coma Scale

- Snoring, gurgling, stridor
- Inability to speak, gasping, cyanosis
- Maxillofacial injuries, disrupted anatomy, active bleeding
- Burns of face/neck, singed hairs, soot in oropharynx
- Pooling secretions, vomiting, altered mental status (GCS ≤8)
- Subcutaneous emphysema, hoarseness (suggesting laryngeal injury)

Immediate Airway Interventions in the Field

In trauma management, understanding normal airway anatomy is essential. The airway is divided into the upper and lower tracts. The upper airway includes the nasal and oral cavities, pharynx, and larynx, which function as conduits for air entry. The epiglottis protects the trachea during swallowing, while the vocal cords, located within the larynx, control airflow. The lower airway comprises the trachea, bronchi, and lungs, responsible for gas exchange. Trauma may compromise these structures through swelling, bleeding, or fractures. Recognizing deviations from normal anatomy helps guide interventions like airway clearance, intubation, or surgical airway management to prevent hypoxia. Table 6.2 summarizes choosing the right airway.

Stepwise Management

1. *Airway Maneuvers*

Field providers should use manual maneuvers to open the airway in unconscious casualties. Use the jaw thrust maneuver (Fig. 6.2a) if spinal injury is suspected and the chin-lift in all others. Avoid head tilt in trauma. If foreign material like vomitus or blood is present, suction the oropharynx immediately. If spinal injury is not a concern and the casualty is vomiting, place them in the recovery position.

Table 6.2 Airway management strategies in common trauma scenarios

Scenario	Preferred technique	Backup option
GCS ≤10, no facial trauma	RSI	SGA → cricothyrotomy
Facial trauma, bleeding	Video laryngoscopy	Cricothyrotomy
Airway burns, stridor	RSI if possible	Cricothyrotomy
Failed endotracheal intubation	SGA	Cricothyrotomy
Combat setting, unconscious, no equipment	BMV + OPA/NPA	SGA → ETI
Cannot intubate, cannot ventilate	Cricothyrotomy	None

Abbreviations: RSI rapid sequence intubation, *ETI* endotracheal intubation, *SGA* supraglottic airway, *OPA* oropharyngeal airway, *NPA* nasopharyngeal airway

Spinal precaution: If the mechanism of injury suggests cervical spine trauma (e.g., falls, blast overpressure, blunt trauma, MVC), apply a hard cervical collar after airway is secured and the neck is manually stabilized. Do not delay airway management for collar placement. Cervical collars are indicated in any casualty with altered consciousness, distracting injury, or neck pain/tenderness (Fig. 6.2).

2. *Airway Adjuncts*
   - *Nasopharyngeal airway (NPA)*: This is the first-line adjunct in unconscious or semiconscious casualties. Select an appropriate size (from nostril to earlobe), lubricate with water-based gel, and gently insert with bevel toward the nasal septum (Figs. 6.3a and 6.4a). Avoid NPA in cases of suspected basilar skull fracture or major nasal trauma.
   - *Oropharyngeal airway (OPA)*: Used in unconscious casualties without gag reflex. Select proper size (corner of mouth to angle of mandible), insert upside down, and rotate 180° as it advances over the tongue (Figs. 6.3b and 6.4b). Alternatively, use a tongue depressor to avoid trauma. Improper sizing can worsen obstruction.
   - *Supraglottic airway (SGA):* SGA plays a vital role in trauma management, particularly when endotracheal intubation is difficult or delayed (Fig. 6.5). SGAs, such as the laryngeal mask airway (LMA) or I-gel, bypass the need for direct visualization of the vocal cords by providing a seal around the laryngeal inlet. They are quick to insert and effective in maintaining oxygenation and ventilation, especially in patients with difficult airways due to facial trauma, cervical spine injuries, or limited mouth opening. However, SGAs may not fully protect against aspiration, making them a temporary solution until definitive airway control is established.

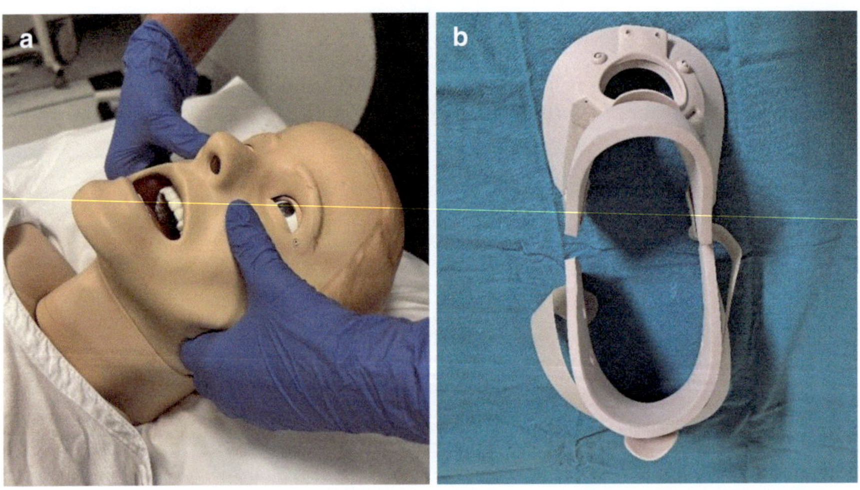

Fig. 6.2 (**a**) The jaw-thrust maneuver. (**b**) Hard cervical collar. (**c**) Applied hard cervical collar on a manikin. (**d**) Measurement of appropriate size of hard cervical collar on a manikin. (**e**) Choosing appropriate size of hard cervical collar

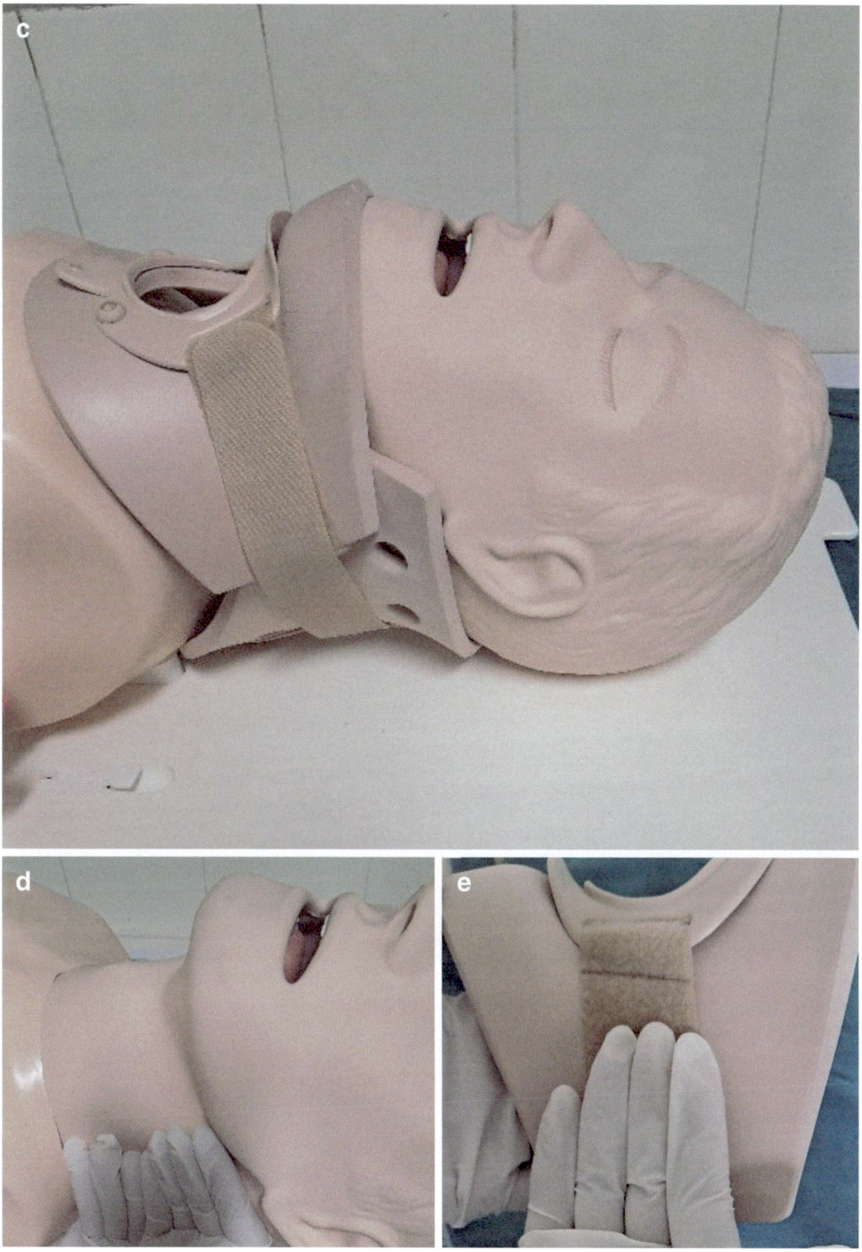

Fig. 6.2 (continued)

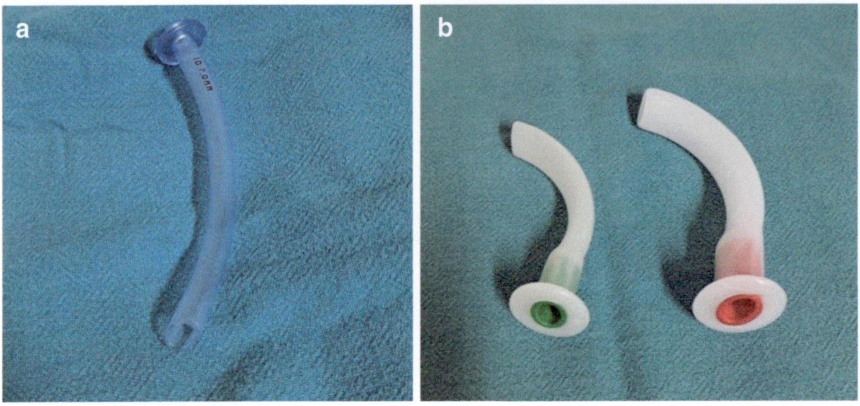

Fig. 6.3 (**a**) Nasopharyngeal airway, (**b**) oropharyngeal airway

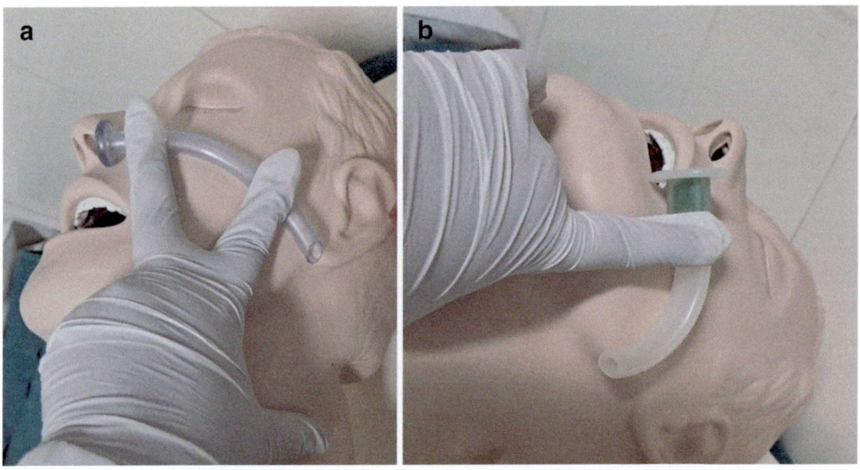

Fig. 6.4 Measurement of appropriate size of airway adjunct. (**a**) Nasopharyngeal airway, (**b**) oropharyngeal airway

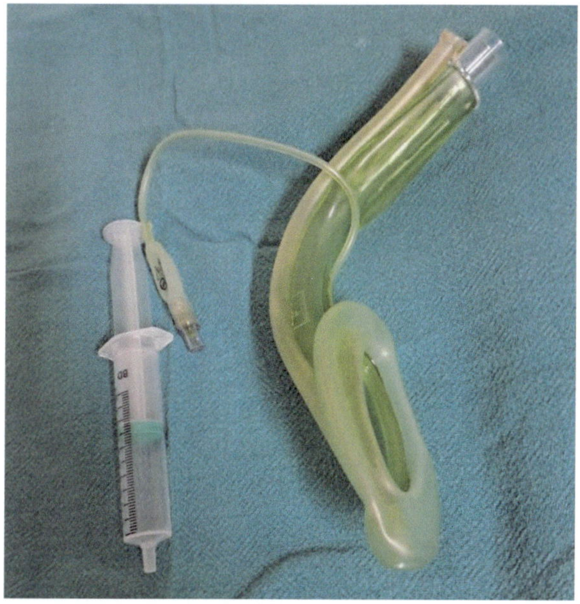

Fig. 6.5 Supraglottic airway—laryngeal mask airway

3. *Advanced Airway Techniques*

Advanced airway management is a cornerstone of trauma care. This chapter outlines the tools and techniques a FORCE provider must master—from intubation to surgical airway—and when to deploy each, especially in the heat of resuscitation.

I. *Endotracheal Intubation (ETI)*

Indications include:

- GCS ≤8
- Apnea or hypoventilation
- Severe maxillofacial trauma
- Risk of aspiration (vomiting, bleeding)
- Predicted deterioration (e.g., shock, inhalational injury)

Preparation includes:

- *Airway assessment.* Use the LEMON mnemonic:
  *L*ook externally
  *E*valuate 3-3-2 rule
  *M*allampati score
  *O*bstruction
  *N*eck mobility

- *C-spine stabilization:* Assume cervical injury in all trauma cases. Apply manual in-line stabilization (MILS) (Fig. 6.6).
- *Preoxygenation:* 100% oxygen via non-rebreather mask or BVM with PEEP valve.
- *Equipment check:* All equipment includes bag mask, Macintosh laryngoscope with different blade sizes, endotracheal tube, gum elastic bougie, syringe, oropharyngeal airway, video laryngoscope with attached standard blade—if available should be checked during preparation for intubation (Fig. 6.7).

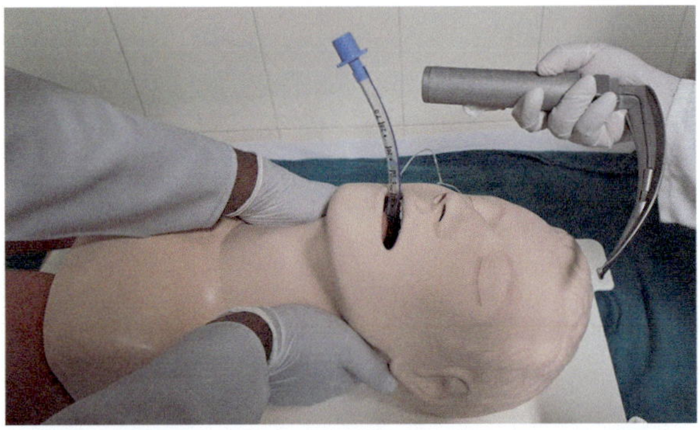

Fig. 6.6 Manual in-line stabilization during intubation from front

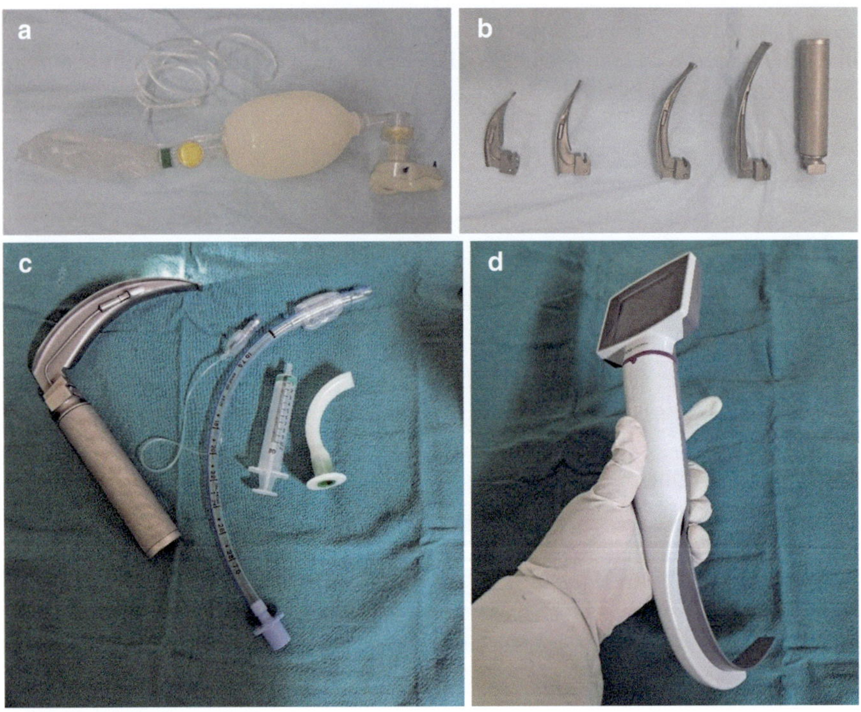

Fig. 6.7 (**a**) Bag-valve-mask device, (**b**) Macintosh laryngoscope with different blade sizes, (**c**) intubation equipment (Macintosh laryngoscope, endotracheal tube, syringe, oropharyngeal airway), (**d**) video laryngoscope with attached standard blade

Rapid Sequence Intubation (RSI)

RSI is the preferred method in trauma. It allows swift and controlled intubation while minimizing aspiration risk.

Steps:

1. *Preparation:* Gather ETT, laryngoscope, suction, capnography, BVM, and backup airway tools.
2. *Pre-treatment (when indicated):*
   - Lidocaine for suspected raised ICP
3. *Induction agents:*
   - Etomidate (0.3 mg/kg)—for hemodynamic stability
   - Ketamine (1–2 mg/kg)—ideal for hypotension or bronchospasm
4. *Paralytic agents:*
   - Succinylcholine (1.5 mg/kg)—rapid onset, short duration
   - Rocuronium (1 mg/kg)—if succinylcholine is contraindicated
5. *Cricoid pressure* (Sellick's maneuver or backward, upward, and rightward pressure *[BURP]*): Optional; apply only if it does not obstruct the view (Fig. 6.8).
6. *Intubation:* Insert ETT under vision, inflate cuff, and confirm position with:
   - End-tidal CO_2 (capnography—gold standard)
   - Bilateral chest rise
   - Equal breath sounds (5-point auscultation)

If MILS interferes, briefly ease hand pressure during intubation without cervical movement.

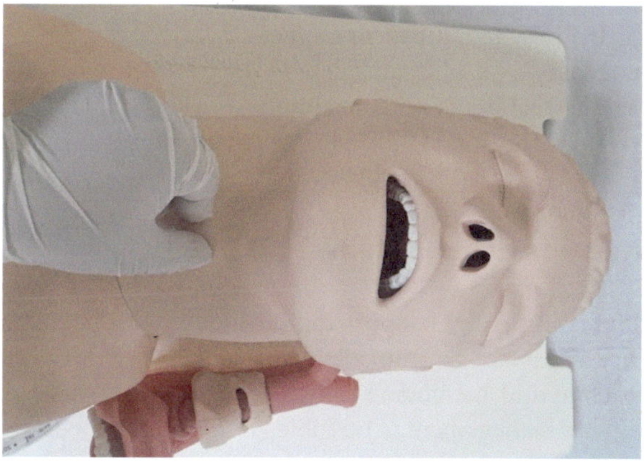

Fig. 6.8 Sellick's maneuver

Direct vs. Video Laryngoscopy

Direct laryngoscopy is preferred when:

- The provider is experienced with it
- Equipment is limited
- There is minimal blood or trauma

Video laryngoscopy is preferred when:

- A difficult airway is anticipated
- Equipment is available
- Direct laryngoscopy provides poor view

Retrograde Intubation

Rare and used only by highly trained providers when:

- There is distorted anatomy but a patent trachea
- Patient is stable, and all other options fail

II. *Needle Cricothyrotomy and Surgical Cricothyrotomy*

Absolute Indications:

- Inability to intubate or oxygenate
- Massive facial trauma
- Thermal injury with swelling
- Upper airway hemorrhage or obstruction

Needle Cricothyrotomy

It is a lifesaving, temporizing procedure used in combat settings when a definitive airway cannot be immediately secured. It involves placing a needle through the cricothyroid membrane into the trachea to provide oxygen until more advanced airway management is possible (Fig. 6.9). This buys time, converting an emergent situation into an urgent one.

The percutaneous transtracheal oxygenation (PTO) technique is executed by inserting a large-bore cannula—12 to 14 gauge for adults—through the cricothyroid membrane into the trachea, below the level of airway obstruction. Oxygen is then delivered at 15 L/min (50–60 psi), using a Y-connector or a side-port created in the tubing between the oxygen source and cannula.

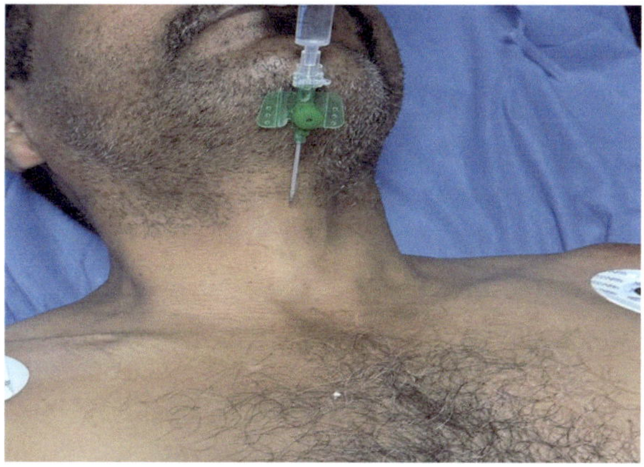

Fig. 6.9 Needle cricothyrotomy—confirmation of correct placement by checking for bubbling in saline-filled syringe

Ventilation is done via intermittent insufflation—pressing the thumb over the Y-connector or side hole for 1 s to insufflate and then releasing for 4 s to allow passive exhalation. This cycle provides oxygenation for 30–45 min, enough to stabilize and prepare for evacuation or definitive airway placement.

Important considerations in the field: *PTO is only a temporary measure.* Inadequate CO_2 clearance leads to gradual buildup, particularly dangerous in patients with head injuries. In cases of complete upper airway obstruction, such as a foreign body at the glottis, air may not escape, increasing the risk of barotrauma or tension pneumothorax. Monitor for chest rise and signs of air trapping. If no exhalation is occurring, abort the technique and reassess.

Surgical Cricothyrotomy

This emergency airway procedure involves making a skin incision through the cricothyroid membrane. The incision is then widened using a curved hemostat or the handle of a scalpel. After dilation, a small endotracheal tube (internal diameter 5–7 mm) or a tracheostomy tube (outer diameter 5–7 mm) is inserted into the trachea to establish airflow.

If an endotracheal tube is used, it must be carefully secured to prevent complications such as migration into a bronchus or accidental dislodgement.

Although percutaneous tracheostomy has emerged as a less invasive option compared to open tracheostomy, it is not suitable in acute trauma cases. The procedure requires neck hyperextension for proper placement—something that is often unsafe or impractical in trauma patients.

FORCE Tactical Pearl

Your calm head and steady hands at the airway can turn chaos into control. Master these tools—not just how to use them, but when to use them.

Approach to Breathing Management in a Combat Zone

Once the airway is secured, the next priority is ensuring adequate ventilation and oxygenation. Pulse oximetry and capnography, where available, should be used to monitor oxygen saturation and verify proper ventilation. Maintaining an oxygen saturation (SpO2) level above 90% is particularly important for casualties with traumatic brain injuries (TBI), as hypoxia can worsen secondary brain injury.

Oxygen Delivery Devices

Combat zones may lack the resources to provide continuous supplemental oxygen, but where available, high-flow oxygen should be administered to casualties with significant respiratory compromise. This is particularly crucial for patients with conditions like tension pneumothorax or blast lung, where oxygenation can be impaired despite a patent airway.

In trauma care, ensuring adequate oxygenation is critical to maintaining tissue perfusion and preventing hypoxia. Various oxygen delivery devices provide tailored oxygen support based on the patient's respiratory needs and injury severity. Selecting the appropriate device is essential to meet oxygenation needs efficiently and improve outcomes in trauma care. The various oxygen delivery devices are as follows:

Nasal Cannula

A nasal cannula delivers low-flow oxygen (1–6 L/min) and is suitable for patients with minor respiratory distress. It provides 24–44% oxygen, which may be insufficient for severe trauma cases but effective for milder hypoxia.

Simple Face Mask

The simple face mask supplies moderate oxygen levels (5–10 L/min) with 40–60% oxygen concentration. It is used for patients needing more support than a nasal cannula but not requiring high-flow oxygen (Fig. 6.10).

Non-Rebreather Mask (NRBM)

An NRB mask delivers high-flow oxygen (10–15 L/min) at nearly 100% concentration. It is indicated for patients in significant distress or with potential for hypoxia, as it ensures a high FiO2 without rebreathing expired air (Fig. 6.11).

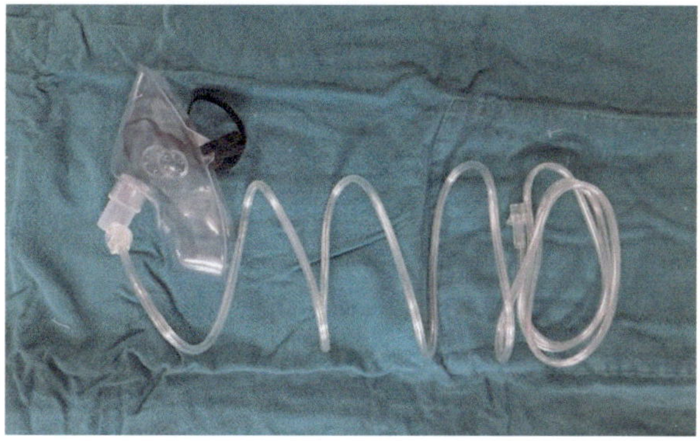

Fig. 6.10 Simple face mask

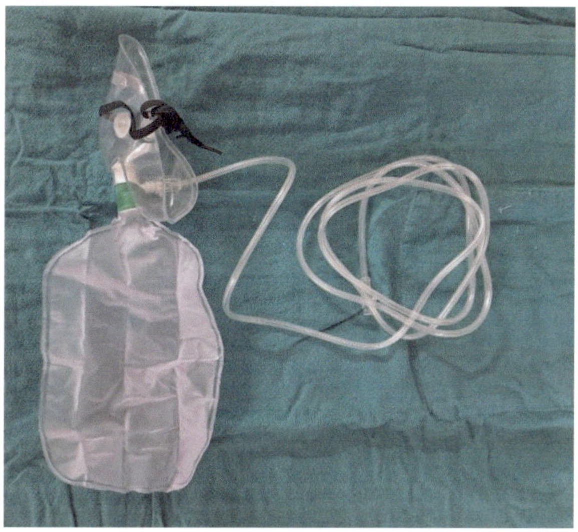

Fig. 6.11 Non-rebreather mask

Bag Valve Mask (BVM)

A BVM provides manual ventilation for unconscious or apneic patients. Delivering 100% oxygen when connected to an oxygen source, it is essential in preoxygenation, resuscitation, and when preparing for advanced airway interventions. If a casualty requires assisted ventilation, bag-valve-mask (BVM) devices can be used. Care must be taken to avoid barotrauma, especially in patients with chest injuries, as overzealous ventilation can lead to or worsen pneumothorax.

Point-of-Care Ultrasound (POCUS) for Breathing Diagnosis in Combat Zone Trauma

In combat zones, managing trauma-related respiratory conditions swiftly and accurately is vital. Point-of-Care Ultrasound (POCUS) has emerged as an invaluable tool, offering rapid, bedside assessments to diagnose and guide treatment of respiratory issues, especially in resource-limited or hostile environments.

Pneumothorax Identification

Tension pneumothorax is a life-threatening condition commonly seen in combat trauma, particularly in cases of penetrating chest injuries or blast trauma. It occurs when air becomes trapped in the pleural space, increasing intrathoracic pressure and compressing the lungs and heart.

POCUS is highly effective for detecting pneumothorax, a common consequence of blast injuries or penetrating trauma. By scanning the anterior chest with a linear or phased array transducer, providers can observe lung sliding and the presence of "B-lines" (comet-tail artifacts), both of which indicate healthy lung tissue. The absence of these signs, often replaced by a "barcode" or "stratosphere" sign on M-mode, suggests pneumothorax. Quick diagnosis of pneumothorax is critical in combat, as untreated cases may progress to life-threatening tension pneumothorax.

Hemothorax Detection

Hemothorax, another common result of chest trauma, can be detected through the rapid assessment of pleural spaces. Using the POCUS probe in the low thoracic area at the posterior axillary line, providers can identify anechoic (dark) fluid collections that indicate blood in the thoracic cavity. Early detection of hemothorax is essential to guide immediate interventions, such as chest tube placement, to prevent respiratory compromise from accumulating blood.

Pulmonary Contusion

Blunt trauma can lead to pulmonary contusions, resulting in localized alveolar damage and bleeding. POCUS can identify these areas by revealing "B-lines" that appear in focal, patchy distributions rather than the uniform patterns seen with pulmonary edema. In combat situations, this assessment allows field providers to differentiate between pulmonary contusion and other causes of respiratory distress, guiding more accurate triage and treatment.

Diaphragm Function Evaluation

In cases of suspected diaphragmatic injury or dysfunction, POCUS can evaluate diaphragm movement. By placing the probe at the subcostal or intercostal margin, providers can assess for paralysis or abnormal diaphragm motion, which may contribute to respiratory insufficiency. This assessment is particularly relevant in blast injuries where thoracoabdominal trauma may impair diaphragm function.

By leveraging POCUS in combat settings, healthcare providers can quickly assess and diagnose breathing-related injuries, supporting timely interventions that are crucial for survival. Its portability and immediate feedback make POCUS an ideal tool for the unique demands of trauma management in combat zones.

Chest Trauma

Rapid identification of life-threatening thoracic injuries is critical in the frontline management of breathing, as these conditions can lead to rapid deterioration or death if not immediately addressed. Key thoracic injuries include tension pneumothorax, massive hemothorax, open pneumothorax, flail chest, cardiac tamponade, and tracheobronchial injury. These can be recognized through clinical signs such as absent or diminished breath sounds, tracheal deviation, distended neck veins, hypotension, paradoxical chest movement, and subcutaneous emphysema. For example, tension pneumothorax typically presents with severe respiratory distress, tracheal shift, and absent breath sounds, requiring urgent needle decompression followed by chest tube insertion. An open pneumothorax (sucking chest wound) is managed with a three-sided occlusive dressing and chest drain, while massive hemothorax demands rapid chest tube placement and volume resuscitation. Flail chest, identified by paradoxical movement of a chest wall segment, necessitates pain control and ventilatory support. Cardiac tamponade, often resulting from penetrating trauma, manifests with Beck's triad (hypotension, muffled heart sounds, and distended neck veins) and may require pericardiocentesis or surgical relief. Tracheobronchial disruptions, although rare, should be suspected in cases of persistent air leak and surgical emphysema, requiring definitive airway control and surgical consultation. The prompt recognition of these injuries using a structured approach—as outlined in Table 6.3—is essential for effective frontline resuscitation and survival in combat emergencies.

Needle Decompression

The primary intervention for suspected tension pneumothorax is needle decompression. TCCC guidelines recommend using a 14-gauge, 3.25-inch needle, typically inserted at the one of the following two sites whichever is more accessible:

Table 6.3 Identification of life-threatening thoracic injuries

Condition	Key findings	Clinical indicators	Emergency management
Tension pneumothorax	Absent breath sounds, tracheal shift, distended neck veins, hypotension	Severe respiratory distress, cyanosis	Needle decompression → chest tube
Massive hemothorax	Dull percussion, hypotension, absent breath sounds	Shock, reduced chest expansion	Chest tube, fluid resuscitation
Open pneumothorax	Sucking chest wound, bubbling air, visible chest wall defect	Respiratory compromise, air movement through wound	Occlusive 3-sided dressing, chest tube
Flail chest	Paradoxical movement of chest segment	Hypoxia, severe chest pain, respiratory effort	Oxygen, splinting, pain control, assisted ventilation if needed
Cardiac tamponade	Penetrating chest injury, hypotension, muffled heart sounds, JVD	Beck's triad, PEA	Pericardiocentesis, surgical intervention
Tracheobronchial disruption	Subcutaneous emphysema, massive air leak, respiratory distress	Persistent pneumothorax despite chest tube	Secure airway, surgery, possible ECMO (if available)

Abbreviations: JVD, jugular vein distension; PEA, pulseless electrical activity; ECMO, extracorporeal membrane oxygenation

(a) Second intercostal space (ICS) at the midclavicular line on the side of the injury
(b) Fifth intercostal space in the anterior axillary line on the side of the injury

After the procedure, the casualty must be monitored closely for signs of recurrence, as the condition can redevelop during evacuation or transport.

Chest Seals

Open or "sucking" chest wounds, which allow air to enter the pleural space, must be sealed immediately with vented chest seals. These devices prevent air from being drawn into the chest cavity during inspiration while allowing it to escape during expiration, thus reducing the risk of tension pneumothorax.

Advanced Techniques in Combat Zone Breathing Management

In advanced cases where simple interventions fail, more complex techniques may be required to ensure continued ventilation.

Chest Tubes

If needle decompression fails to alleviate symptoms or if the casualty is expected to undergo a prolonged evacuation, a chest tube may be inserted to continuously drain air from the pleural cavity. This procedure requires advanced medical personnel and specialized equipment, which may not always be available in the combat setting.

Advanced Monitoring

For casualties undergoing prolonged care or evacuation, continuous monitoring of respiratory status is critical. Pulse oximeters should be used to track oxygen saturation levels, while capnography is useful for ensuring that ventilations are effective.

Tactical Considerations and Environmental Challenges

Combat zones present several challenges for airway and breathing management, including ongoing hostilities, environmental hazards, and logistical constraints. Care providers must adapt their interventions to the situation while prioritizing their own safety and that of the casualty.

Care Under Fire

During the Care Under Fire phase, the primary focus is on stopping life-threatening hemorrhage and taking cover. Airway management is typically deferred unless the casualty is unable to breathe or has an obvious airway obstruction. Once the immediate threat has subsided, more advanced interventions can be performed during Tactical Field Care.

Prolonged Field Care and Evacuation

When dealing with prolonged field care scenarios, such as delayed evacuation, maintaining a patent airway and ensuring effective breathing becomes even more critical. Combat medics must frequently reassess the casualty's airway and breathing status, especially during transport, to ensure that interventions like NPAs, chest seals, and decompression needles remain effective.

Case Resolution

This case illustrates a critically injured combat casualty with multisystem trauma, where airway and thoracic compromise posed an immediate threat to life. The soldier, found unconscious post-blast, presented with facial bleeding, a threatened airway, a sucking chest wound, flail chest, and signs of both obstructive and hypovolemic shock.

Early indicators such as blood-filled oropharynx, distorted facial anatomy, and a GCS ≤ 8 necessitated a rapid shift from basic adjuncts to a definitive airway. The decision to perform an emergency surgical cricothyrotomy was driven by the inability to ventilate using conventional methods due to facial trauma and mandibular disruption. This highlights the importance of early airway assessment and choosing the right intervention in time-critical scenarios.

In environments lacking suction, managing ongoing facial bleeding becomes a challenge. In this case, suction was fortunately available. However, if unavailable, techniques such as lateral positioning, use of gauze packing, and aggressive jaw thrust must be employed while preparing for a surgical airway.

Ventilation through the cricothyrotomy was continuously monitored, with SpO_2 rising from 32% to 93% after BVM support. The team remained vigilant for signs of inadequate ventilation or air trapping—risks that are magnified during prolonged evacuations. Monitoring chest rise, respiratory rate, and oxygen saturation was key to ensuring adequate oxygenation en route.

The casualty also had concurrent airway and thoracic injuries—a sucking chest wound and flail segment—necessitating precise prioritization. The airway was secured first, immediately followed by sealing the chest wound and performing needle decompression. Ventilatory support was initiated early to manage the flail chest and maintain oxygenation under high-stress field conditions.

In accordance with TCCC, the MARCH protocol was applied seamlessly across CUF, TFC, and TACEVAC phases. Facial bleeding was controlled, a surgical airway established, chest injuries addressed, and hypovolemic shock managed with warmed IV fluids. The patient's neurological signs (GCS 9, anisocoria) suggested possible traumatic brain injury, warranting neuroprotective ventilation strategies.

Flail chest was managed conservatively after stabilization. The distal hand fracture was splinted. Passive and active rewarming was critical, given the patient's hypothermia—a common but underestimated complicating factor in battlefield trauma that contributes to coagulopathy and poor outcomes.

The soldier was successfully evacuated with BVM ventilation via cricothyrotomy, monitored by a trauma-trained team member. A structured MIST handover ensured continuity of care, particularly regarding airway, thoracic, and neurological priorities. This case highlights the importance of training, preparation, and protocol adherence in executing lifesaving airway and breathing interventions, even in the most resource-limited, high-stakes combat environments.

Key Messages

- Airway compromise is a leading preventable cause of death in combat trauma—rapid recognition and intervention are essential for survival in resource-limited, hostile environments.
- The MARCH algorithm and TCCC framework provide a lifesaving structure for managing airway and breathing across all three phases: Care Under Fire, Tactical Field Care, and Tactical Evacuation.
- Basic airway maneuvers (jaw thrust, suctioning, NPA/OPA) are frontline tools in combat scenarios and must be second nature to every provider.
- Surgical cricothyrotomy is a critical skill in facial trauma, burns, or failed intubation—it must be practiced and performed confidently when indicated.
- Point-of-care ultrasound (POCUS) enhances thoracic injury diagnosis (pneumothorax, hemothorax, contusions) and should be incorporated into combat medic protocols when available.
- Chest seals, needle decompression, and chest tubes are cornerstone interventions for treating life-threatening thoracic trauma such as sucking chest wounds and tension pneumothorax.
- Environmental factors such as hypothermia and prolonged field care significantly impact airway and breathing outcomes—prevention and reassessment are continuous responsibilities.
- *Effective airway management begins with preparation and ends with reassessment*—team coordination, equipment readiness, and protocol adherence are nonnegotiable in saving lives under fire.

Conclusion

Airway and breathing management in the combat zone requires a combination of rapid decision-making, practical skills, and adherence to TCCC protocols. Whether addressing a blocked airway or treating a life-threatening pneumothorax, these interventions are designed to stabilize casualties and improve their chances of survival before they can reach definitive care. Providers must be well-trained in both basic and advanced techniques, remain adaptable to the ever-changing combat environment, and continuously reassess the patient's condition to ensure that lifesaving interventions remain effective throughout the continuum of care.

Bibliography

1. 17-13-tactical-casualty-combat-care-handbook-v5-may-17-distro-a.pdf [Internet]. [cited 2024 Oct 27]. Available from: https://api.army.mil/e2/c/downloads/2023/01/19/31e03488/17-13-tactical-casualty-combat-care-handbook-v5-may-17-distro-a.pdf
2. Airway Management in Prolonged Field Care [Internet]. [cited 2024 Oct 27]. Available from: https://tccc.org.ua/en/guide/airway-management-in-prolonged-field-care-pcc

3. Dye, Collin et al. "Airway Management in Prolonged Field Care." Journal of special operations medicine: a peer reviewed journal for SOF medical professionals vol. 20,3 (2020): 141–156. doi:https://doi.org/10.55460/BAF7-3BM3
4. FA-manual.pdf [Internet]. [cited 2024 Oct 27]. Available from: https://www.indianredcross.org/publications/FA-manual.pdf
5. Module 07: Airway Management in TFC [Internet]. [cited 2025 Apr 12]. Available from: https://tccc.org.ua/en/guide/module-07-airway-management-in-tfc-cmc
6. Ranger Training Brigade, U.S. Army Infantry School, U.S. Department of the Army. Ranger Handbook: U.S. Army Ranger Handbook SH 21-76. Revised Feb 2011. New York: CreateSpace Independent Publishing Platform; 2013. ISBN: 978-1304107619
7. Schoeber, Nino H C et al. "Healthcare professionals' knowledge of the systematic ABCDE approach: a cross-sectional study." BMC emergency medicine vol. 22,1 202. 12 Dec. 2022, https://doi.org/10.1186/s12873-022-00753-y
8. Thim, Troels et al. "Initial assessment and treatment with the Airway, Breathing, Circulation, Disability, Exposure (ABCDE) approach." International journal of general medicine vol. 5 (2012): 117–21. https://doi.org/10.2147/IJGM.S28478

7 Hypothermia Management in Extreme Conditions

Vrinda Lath and Freston Marc Sirur

Learning Objectives

By the end of this chapter, the reader will be able to:

- Define hypothermia and describe its pathophysiology in the tactical and wilderness settings.
- Identify key predisposing factors and preventive measures to minimize risk during operations.
- Recognize the signs and symptoms of hypothermia and classify its severity using clinical features.
- Implement immediate field care for mild, moderate, and severe hypothermia using passive and active rewarming techniques.
- Manage localized cold injuries such as frostbite, trench foot, and chilblains.
- Understand the implications of hypothermia in polytrauma and adjust field resuscitation accordingly.
- Outline best practices for safe transport and evacuation of hypothermic casualties to definitive care facilities.

V. Lath (✉) · F. M. Sirur
Department of Emergency Medicine, Kasturba Medical College, Manipal, Karnataka, India
e-mail: vrinda.latha@manipal.edu

N. T. Rai, S. Misra (eds.), *Frontline Operational Resuscitation and Combat Emergencies (FORCE) Manual*, https://doi.org/10.1007/978-981-92-1622-2_7

Introduction

Hypothermia is an often underestimated but critical threat to survival in tactical, combat, and extreme environmental operations. *Defined as a core body temperature below 35 °C (95 °F)*, hypothermia can develop rapidly or insidiously, even in relatively moderate climates when casualties are wet, immobilized, or exposed. In the combat context, hypothermia not only endangers life but can significantly degrade operational capability, as even mild cooling impairs decision-making, dexterity, and physical performance.

In austere environments—whether high-altitude bases, dense jungles with cold rain, desert night operations, or mountainous terrains—the risk of accidental hypothermia increases dramatically. Furthermore, trauma victims are particularly vulnerable: blood loss, shock, immobilization, and wet clothing accelerate heat loss, and the onset of hypothermia can exacerbate coagulopathy, acidosis, and systemic collapse—the lethal triad of trauma.

Recognizing hypothermia early, preventing its progression, and initiating appropriate field-based interventions are fundamental responsibilities of every combat medic, first responder, and team member. Hypothermia prevention must be built into mission planning, casualty evacuation drills, and tactical field care protocols. When hypothermia is allowed to develop, resuscitation efforts become significantly more complex and survival chances diminish.

This chapter provides a focused guide to understanding, preventing, identifying, and managing hypothermia in extreme conditions.

Case Scenario

During a long-range patrol in the high-altitude sector of Eastern Ladakh, a 26-year-old soldier slips off a narrow ridge and sustains a lower limb fracture. His team extricates him within 20 min, but the temperature is −10 °C with high wind chill. The casualty is found lying immobile on snow-covered ground, soaked after falling into a shallow stream.

- *Care Under Fire (CUF):*
  No enemy engagement is reported. The perimeter is confirmed secure. No immediate life-threatening bleeding detected; casualty is moved rapidly to a safe position using a manual drag technique. A thermal blanket and ground insulation are improvised using available clothing and foam mats to prevent direct exposure to the snow-covered surface.
- *Tactical Field Care (TFC):*
  Following the *MARCH sequence*:
  M—massive hemorrhage: No active bleeding noted. A rapid blood sweep confirms absence of major hemorrhage.
  A—airway: The casualty is conscious but shivering violently. Airway remains patent. Nasopharyngeal airway (NPA) kit is kept ready if mentation deteriorates.

R—respiration: Chest movement is symmetrical. Respiratory rate elevated at 28/min but no respiratory distress or chest injury.
C—circulation: Pale, weak radial pulse. Capillary refill >3 s. Immediate concern for hypothermia-induced circulatory collapse.
H—hypothermia/head injury: Core temperature estimated <35 °C. Wet clothing is immediately stripped away; the soldier is insulated using dry ponchos, space blankets, and his teammates' jackets. A hypothermia prevention kit is activated.

- *Tactical Evacuation Care (TACEVAC):*
  Evacuation is delayed by 45 min due to whiteout conditions. Continuous monitoring for mental status deterioration and hypothermia progression is performed. Warmed IV fluids are prepared for administration if signs of shock worsen.

Reflective Questions

1. How should rewarming be initiated in a field setting with limited resources?
2. When should active rewarming versus passive rewarming strategies be chosen?
3. What are the warning signs of impending cardiac instability due to hypothermia?

Understanding Hypothermia in Tactical Combat Settings

In the unforgiving terrains faced by Indian Forces—from snow-laden mountain posts at the LAC to cold jungle nights in Northeast counterinsurgency zones—*hypothermia is not just an environmental threat but a tactical killer*. Even in temperate climates, injured soldiers are highly vulnerable to hypothermia due to heat loss from exposed wounds, wet clothing, shock, and immobilization during evacuation delays.

Hypothermia is classically defined as a drop in core body temperature below 35 °C (95 °F). In trauma patients, however, even "mild" hypothermia (35–36 °C) significantly worsens mortality by impairing coagulation, amplifying acidosis, and accelerating shock progression—a deadly spiral known as the "*Trauma Triad of Death*."

In tactical environments, hypothermia must be suspected early and treated preemptively, regardless of ambient temperature or apparent weather conditions. An injured soldier lying motionless on cold ground, soaked in sweat or blood, rapidly loses body heat even at 15–20 °C air temperature—a common oversight during tropical operations.

Pathophysiology: Why Hypothermia Is Deadly in Trauma

The human body maintains a tightly regulated core temperature through metabolic heat production and regulated heat loss. Trauma disrupts this equilibrium through several mechanisms:

- *Heat loss mechanisms:*
  - *Radiation:* Loss of heat to the environment from exposed body surfaces (biggest contributor).
  - *Convection:* Wind removes the thin warm air layer surrounding the body—common at high-altitude posts.
  - *Conduction:* Direct transfer of heat to colder surfaces—lying on cold ground or wet surfaces.

    Evaporation: Loss from sweating or wet clothing—often overlooked when patients are soaked with blood or rain.
- *Heat generation impairments:*
  - Massive bleeding reduces metabolism and perfusion.
  - Shock and acidosis impair muscle shivering responses.

    Sedatives, analgesics, and head injuries blunt thermoregulatory centers.

As core temperature falls:

- Coagulation cascades fail, promoting ongoing hemorrhage.
- Cardiac conduction slows, increasing risk of lethal arrhythmias (e.g., ventricular fibrillation).
- Metabolic acidosis worsens, further reducing cellular oxygen delivery.
- Immune defenses collapse, leading to higher infection rates.

FORCE Tactical Pearl
Even a 1 °C drop can triple the chances of death in battlefield trauma.

Phases of Hypothermia and Tactical Recognition in the Field

In the combat setting, *recognizing hypothermia early—even before classic clinical signs appear—is critical.* Waiting for obvious shivering or low thermometer readings wastes precious time.

Hypothermia is classified by severity based on core body temperature and clinical features as described in Table 7.1.

Tactical Field Recognition Without Thermometers: In most Indian operational zones, field medics or buddies rarely have access to core thermometers. Therefore, *simple field cues must drive suspicion:*

- Is the casualty immobile, soaked, or exposed?
- Has bleeding been prolonged?
- Is shivering absent in a cold environment?
- Is the casualty deteriorating despite bleeding control?
- Are mental status and pulse quality worsening?

Table 7.1 Classification of hypothermia

Phase	Core temp (°C)	Clinical features	Tactical field clues
Mild	32–35 °C	Shivering, tachycardia, normal BP, mental alertness	Patient shivering actively; complains of cold but responds normally to questions
Moderate	28–32 °C	Loss of shivering, confusion, bradycardia, hypotension, slowed reaction	Casualty shivering stops; drowsy, slurred speech, struggles to follow commands
Severe	<28 °C	Unconsciousness, arrhythmias, profound bradycardia, very low BP	Unresponsive or unconscious; irregular pulse; extremely cold to touch

FORCE Tactical Pearl
Absence of shivering is a red flag—not a reassuring sign. It signals energy exhaustion and progression to moderate/severe hypothermia.

Principles of Hypothermia Prevention During Tactical Care

Preventing hypothermia must begin immediately at the point of injury and be maintained during every phase: Care Under Fire (CUF), Tactical Field Care (TFC), and Tactical Evacuation (TACEVAC).

1. Care Under Fire (CUF)

Primary focus: Suppress fire, control major bleeding, move to cover—but minimal initial hypothermia protection is still possible.

- *Quick action:* If feasible under fire, drag the casualty onto an insulating surface like a poncho, backpack, or foliage rather than cold ground.
- *Minimal exposure:* Only expose wounds necessary for tourniquet application; do not strip off clothing yet.
- *Checklist:* As soon as fire suppression and bleeding control occur, hypothermia must move up in priority.

2. Tactical Field Care (TFC)

Primary focus: Full medical assessment and stabilization while under relative cover.

- *Strip-then-wrap:* Remove wet, bloody clothing only if immediately replaceable with dry coverings or thermal blankets.
- *Insulation layers:*
  - Place an insulating layer underneath the casualty (poncho liner, foam pad, branches).
    Use body heat from other soldiers if no warming devices are available.

- *Cover head and neck:* 50% of body heat is lost through the head and neck—ensure these are covered early.
- *Minimize wind chill:* Create windbreaks with tarps, rocks, packs, or vehicles whenever possible.

3. Tactical Evacuation (TACEVAC)

Primary focus: Sustain warming measures en route and prevent deterioration.

- *Dedicated hypothermia packaging:*
  - Use hypothermia prevention kits if available (e.g., HPMK® Hypothermia Prevention and Management Kit) or improvised techniques like Burrito Wrap (Fig. 7.1).

    Reinforce insulation during loading and transport.
- *Monitor closely:*

    Reassess temperature, mental status, and peripheral perfusion every 15 min if possible.
- *Pre-warmed IV fluids:*
  - Always administer warmed fluids if available during evacuation.

    Rapid infusers or inline warmers (even makeshift ones) must be prioritized for casualties in shock.

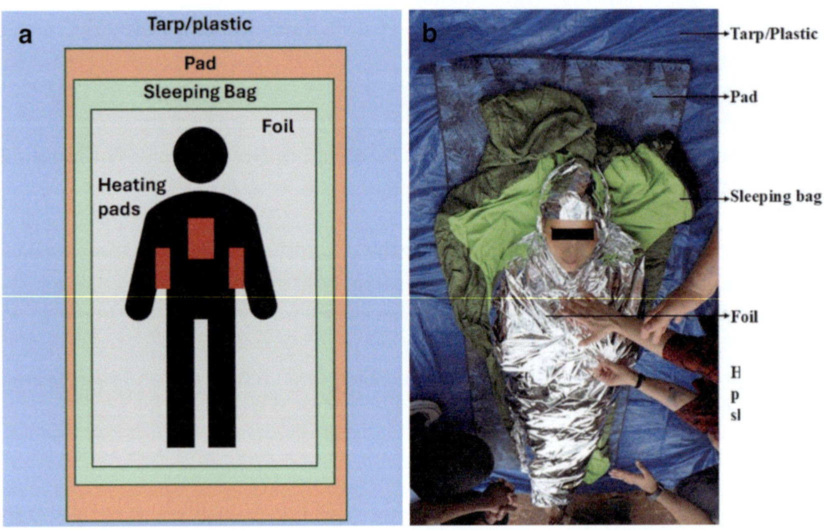

Fig. 7.1 Burrito wrap technique—improvised wrap with internal heating pads and vapor barrier

Field Management of Hypothermic Casualty Based on Severity

FORCE Tactical Pearl

In combat, you do not wait for hypothermia—you fight against it from the start!

In tactical combat environments, recognizing and stratifying hypothermia severity allows providers to apply the most appropriate interventions swiftly, maximizing survival without exhausting limited resources. Hypothermia in trauma is often *occult*—casualties may appear normothermic externally while already experiencing internal thermal loss.

Management of hypothermia in the field is outlined in Table 7.2.

Table 7.2 Field management of hypothermia

Severity	Signs	Field actions
Mild hypothermia (32–35 °C/89.6–95 °F)	Shivering (defense mechanism intact) Alert and coherent Pale, cold skin Tachypnea and tachycardia	Insulate immediately with dry layers (ponchos, blankets). Encourage voluntary shivering. Oral intake of warm, sweet fluids if awake and able (avoid caffeine/alcohol). Strip only wet clothing, preserve maximal body coverage. *Avoid rough handling to prevent arrhythmias.*
Moderate hypothermia (28–32 °C/82.4–89.6 °F)	Altered mental status (confusion, lethargy) Shivering stops (ominous) Bradycardia and slowed breathing Hypotension may develop	Aggressive external rewarming (thermal wraps, chemical heat packs on core areas). No oral intake (aspiration risk). Administer warmed, humidified oxygen if available. *Handle gently to avoid provoking lethal arrhythmias.* Recognize increased risk of ventricular fibrillation.
Severe hypothermia (<28 °C/<82.4 °F)	Unconscious, unresponsive Slow or absent pulse Severe bradycardia, hypotension Fixed dilated pupils (still salvageable) Risk of ventricular fibrillation/asystole	*Handle minimally—rough handling can cause cardiac arrest.* If cardiac arrest occurs, prioritize CPR and be prepared for multiple defibrillation attempts. *Passive external warming only—avoid aggressive rewarming.* Urgent evacuation to higher care. Continue resuscitation until warmed to confirm death ("*No one is dead until they are warm and dead*").

Advanced Warming Techniques and Field Innovations for Hypothermia Management

In prolonged field care (PFC) settings—especially under Indian operational conditions like high-altitude posts or prolonged jungle patrols—advanced field warming techniques are crucial to prevent hypothermia progression during delayed evacuation.

Even with limited resources, tactical teams can implement effective rewarming strategies:

1. Passive External Rewarming

Objective: Minimize further heat loss.

How:

- Insulate using multiple dry layers (blankets, ponchos, sleeping bags).
- Minimize exposure during reassessments.
- Shelter casualty from wind, rain, and ground conduction using tarpaulins, stretchers, and mats.

Improvised tactics:

- *Poncho liner + Mylar blanket wrap*: Reflects 80% of body heat back.
- *Buddy system*: Casualty sandwiched between two warm team members (body-to-body rewarming).
- *Dry sandbags or foam mats* underneath casualties in rocky or snow terrain.

2. Active External Rewarming

Objective: Increase the casualty's core temperature safely.

How:

- *Chemical heat packs:*
  - Apply heat packs over *axillae*, *chest*, and *groin* (*never directly on bare skin*). Regularly rotate packs to avoid burns.
- *Battery-powered or fuel-based heating blankets:*
  Carried in mountain operations by Indian Special Forces.
- *Field-expedient methods:*
  - Warm canteens wrapped in cloth placed near core areas.
  - Campfire at a safe distance to warm ambient air inside tents.
    Hot stone method: Heated stones wrapped in cloth placed around casualty (strict monitoring to prevent burns).

FORCE Tactical Pearl

In moderate-severe hypothermia, external warming must be gradual. Rapid heating of extremities can cause "afterdrop"—a dangerous sudden drop in core temperature.

3. Internal (Core) Rewarming (Hospital-Only)
These techniques are reserved for definitive care facilities:

- Warmed intravenous fluids via inline rapid warmers
- Warmed, humidified oxygen
- Peritoneal, bladder, or thoracic lavage with warm fluids in extreme cases
- Extracorporeal warming (ECMO) in surgical hospitals

Tactical Evacuation Priorities and Hypothermia Management in Mass Casualty Scenarios

In combat and disaster settings, evacuation priorities must be aligned with the threat of hypothermia, which can silently worsen outcomes—even among initially "stable" casualties.

Whether in counterinsurgency operations in Siachen, a VBIED blast in Kupwara, or a landslide in Arunachal Pradesh, *tactical field care must embed hypothermia mitigation into every evacuation decision.*

Challenges
- Limited warming equipment
- Cold, windy, or wet operational environments
- Prolonged extrication and triage delays
- High casualty-to-medic ratio

Evacuation Priorities in Hypothermia Risk

1. Highest priority for CASEVAC:
- Casualties with *moderate to severe hypothermia* (core temperature <34 °C).
- Patients with altered mental status due to cold exposure (confusion, lethargy).
- Casualties with polytrauma who are exposed to cold (even if bleeding is controlled).

> **FORCE Tactical Pearl**
> *A lightly injured but profoundly hypothermic casualty may require earlier evacuation than a more obviously wounded but normothermic one.*

2. Packaging for evacuation:
- *Layering:* Casualty wrapped in multiple insulating layers (poncho liner, dry clothing, thermal blanket).
- *Windproof and waterproof protection:* Use plastic sheeting, raincoats, or tarpaulins.

- *Horizontal evacuation:* Keep the casualty supine. *Standing worsens afterdrop and cardiovascular collapse.*
- *Minimize Handling:* Excessive movement can trigger cold-induced arrhythmias in severe hypothermia.

3. En route care:
- Continuously insulate casualty inside CASEVAC vehicle or helicopter.
- Passive rewarming continued throughout flight or ground movement.
- Warm IV fluids administered if feasible.
- Monitor airway, breathing, circulation, and mental status every 10–15 min.

Nonfreezing Cold Injuries

Nonfreezing cold injuries (NFCIs) are a significant concern for soldiers, first responders, and tactical operators exposed to wet and cold environments, even when ambient temperatures remain above freezing. Unlike frostbite, NFCIs develop due to prolonged exposure to cold, damp conditions rather than actual freezing of tissues.

Two major types of NFCI are *trench foot* and *chilblains*.

- *Trench foot* (also called immersion foot) occurs when feet are exposed to wet, cold conditions (0–15 °C) for extended periods, often without adequate drying or warming. Tissue perfusion is compromised, leading to pale, mottled skin, numbness, pain, swelling, and eventual blistering. In advanced stages, it can cause permanent nerve and vascular damage.
- *Chilblains* (pernio) are inflammatory skin lesions caused by repeated exposure to cold, nonfreezing temperatures. They present as painful, itchy, reddish-purple patches on exposed extremities like fingers, toes, ears, and nose (Fig. 7.2). Although chilblains are usually reversible, repeated episodes can lead to chronic ulceration.

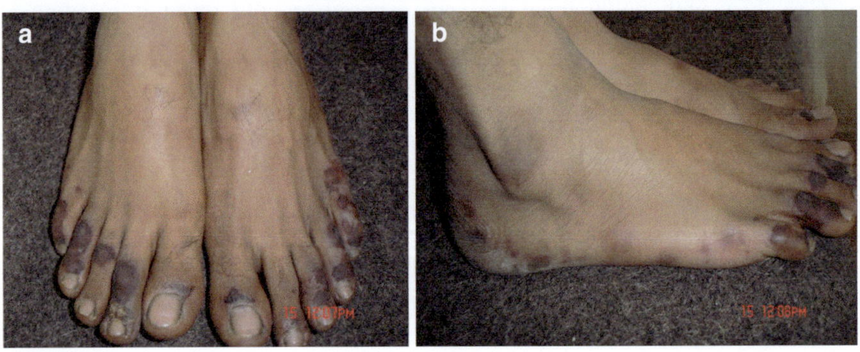

Fig. 7.2 Soldier with chilblains due to prolonged cold exposure

Field Management of Nonfreezing Injuries

- Early recognition is crucial. Check extremities regularly for color changes, numbness, or swelling during prolonged field operations.
- Move the soldier to a dry, warm environment as soon as feasible.
- *Gently rewarm the affected area at ambient temperatures—avoid direct heat or rubbing, which can worsen tissue injury.*
- Elevate affected limbs if swollen and protect against further cold exposure.
- Administer analgesics for pain relief and monitor for signs of secondary infection.

FORCE Tactical Pearl
Prevention is paramount in tactical environments: maintaining dry socks, rotating footgear, using foot powders, and enforcing regular foot inspections are vital during prolonged cold-weather deployments.

Special Operational Considerations

Combat operations across diverse terrains present unique environmental threats that significantly impact casualty care, particularly the risk of hypothermia. Often underestimated in warm or temperate climates, hypothermia can arise rapidly under specific operational conditions such as high altitude, dense jungles, or desert nights. In these austere settings, effective casualty management must go beyond injury treatment to include proactive environmental adaptation. Table 7.3 summarizes the key hypothermia threats and recommended field adaptations across three distinct combat environments frequently encountered by Indian forces—Siachen, the Northeast jungles, and the deserts of Rajasthan—each demanding tailored preventive measures for optimal survivability.

Table 7.3 Hypothermia considerations across extreme combat environments

Environment	Hypothermia threat	Field adaptation
High altitude (e.g., Siachen)	Ambient temperatures −30 °C; evaporation loss through breathing	Oxygen therapy humidified and warmed if possible; layered insulation; bivouac shelters
Jungle (e.g., Northeast)	Continuous rain, wet clothing accelerates hypothermia	Aggressive dry clothing change; plastic poncho shelters; body-to-body warming
Desert nights (e.g., Rajasthan)	Extreme daytime heat followed by freezing nighttime temperatures	Vigilant night hypothermia monitoring; shelter establishment after sundown

Case Resolution

The casualty was systematically managed in the field following MARCH algorithm. The casualty was conscious, shivering violently, with an elevated respiratory rate and pale extremities. While his airway remained patent and symmetrical chest movement ruled out thoracic injury, concern grew over hypothermia-induced circulatory compromise. Capillary refill was delayed, and his radial pulse was weak. Wet clothing was immediately stripped away, and he was insulated using dry ponchos, jackets from his team, space blankets, and materials from a hypothermia prevention kit. In this austere environment, rewarming was initiated using passive external methods, which are the first-line approach when powered devices like heating pads or forced-air warmers are unavailable. This included layered insulation, wind shielding, and body heat transfer from teammates if necessary. These methods are safe, low-risk, and effective in preventing further heat loss in mildly to moderately hypothermic patients who remain hemodynamically stable.

Active rewarming was deferred in the field due to equipment constraints. In a tactical context, passive rewarming is preferred when the patient is alert, perfusing adequately, and not in cardiovascular collapse. Active external warming, such as heat packs or external devices, becomes necessary when core temperature continues to fall, mentation worsens, or there is no improvement with passive measures. These strategies must be applied cautiously to avoid afterdrop—a phenomenon where cold peripheral blood returns to the core during rapid rewarming, worsening cardiac instability.

Throughout the 45-min evacuation delay caused by white-out conditions, the casualty's mental status was monitored closely. Though mildly confused, he remained alert, maintaining airway patency without need for a nasopharyngeal airway. With passive rewarming, his radial pulse became more palpable, and capillary refill time improved slightly, suggesting early reversal of cold-induced vasoconstriction. Warning signs of impending cardiac instability in hypothermia—such as bradycardia, hypotension, and altered consciousness—were actively monitored but did not manifest, due to early insulation and continuous reassessment.

Upon arrival at the forward surgical unit, the soldier's core temperature was confirmed at 34 °C, indicating moderate hypothermia. Under controlled conditions, active external warming was initiated using a forced-air warming system, and warmed IV fluids were administered carefully to avoid fluid overload or arrhythmias. The fractured femur was splinted and definitively stabilized without complication.

Through disciplined field care, early thermal management, and strategic rewarming decisions based on the tactical environment, the casualty avoided major complications such as ventricular arrhythmias, coagulopathy, or cardiovascular collapse. He fully recovered and returned to duty after 10 weeks of structured rehabilitation—signifying the importance of early hypothermia recognition and methodical care even in resource-constrained, extreme-weather conditions.

Key Messages

- *Hypothermia is a silent and deadly threat in trauma*—even mild cooling can worsen bleeding, shock, and mortality in tactical and wilderness settings.
- Every casualty in cold, wet, or windy environments must be assumed hypothermic unless proven otherwise, especially after trauma or prolonged exposure.
- *Prioritize* ***dry, cover,*** *and* ***insulate****—even before IV fluids or oxygen—in a cold environment.* Heat loss is fastest through conduction and evaporation.
- *Prevention of heat loss starts at the point of injury*, during Care Under Fire, and must continue aggressively through Tactical Field Care and Evacuation phases.
- *Loss of shivering signals danger*—when shivering stops, assume moderate to severe hypothermia and act immediately to prevent cardiac arrest.
- Passive insulation (dry, wrap, cover) saves lives and is achievable even with limited field resources—space blankets, ponchos, and buddy-warming techniques must be part of standard drills.
- Field responders should prioritize packaging and minimal handling of casualties to avoid precipitating cold-induced arrhythmias, especially during transport.
- Mass casualty management must integrate hypothermia control, triaging based on thermal risk and establishing warming points at casualty collection sites.

Conclusion

Hypothermia remains one of the most overlooked yet deadly threats in tactical trauma care, especially in the diverse and challenging terrains encountered by Indian forces. Combat medics and first responders must recognize that survival hinges not only on controlling hemorrhage or maintaining airways but equally on preserving core body temperature from the very first moment of injury.

By embedding hypothermia prevention into every phase of casualty care—from Care Under Fire through Tactical Evacuation—survival odds can be markedly improved. Drying, insulating, protecting against wind and cold, and cautiously rewarming are lifesaving interventions that must be second nature on the battlefield.

In extreme conditions, disciplined hypothermia management is not merely supportive care—it is definitive trauma care. Every effort to retain body heat preserves the casualty's clotting ability, cardiac stability, and overall resilience. When field teams master both the science and the art of hypothermia control, they transform high-risk environments into survivable spaces, giving wounded warriors their best chance to heal, recover, and return to life and duty.

Bibliography

1. American College of Surgeons Committee on Trauma. ATLS: Advanced Trauma Life Support. 10th ed. Chicago: American College of Surgeons; 2018. ISBN: 978-0996826235
2. Auerbach PS, Cushing TA, Harris NS. Auerbach's Wilderness Medicine. 7th ed. 2 vols. Philadelphia: Elsevier; 2016. ISBN: 9780323359429
3. Bennett, Brad L et al. "Management of Hypothermia in Tactical Combat Casualty Care: TCCC Guideline Proposed Change 20-01 (June 2020)." Journal of special operations medicine : a peer reviewed journal for SOF medical professionals vol. 20,3 (2020): 21–35. https://doi.org/10.55460/QQ9R-RR8A
4. Dow, Jennifer et al. "Wilderness Medical Society Clinical Practice Guidelines for the Out-of-Hospital Evaluation and Treatment of Accidental Hypothermia: 2019 Update." Wilderness & environmental medicine vol. 30,4S (2019): S47–S69. https://doi.org/10.1016/j.wem.2019.10.002
5. McIntosh, Scott E et al. "Wilderness Medical Society Clinical Practice Guidelines for the Prevention and Treatment of Frostbite: 2024 Update." Wilderness & environmental medicine vol. 35,2 (2024): 183–197. https://doi.org/10.1177/10806032231222359
6. Rund, Titus J. "Casualty evacuation in arctic and extreme cold environments: A paradigm shift for traumatic hypothermia management in tactical combat casualty care." International journal of circumpolar health vol. 82,1 (2023): 2196047. https://doi.org/10.1080/22423982.2023.2196047

Head and Face Trauma in Combat Settings

8

Asish Kishore

Learning Objectives

By the end of this chapter, the reader will be able to:

- Identify common mechanisms of head and facial trauma in combat scenarios.
- Conduct a rapid neurologic and facial trauma assessment using field-adapted tools like AVPU and GCS.
- Outline the initial stabilization steps for patients with TBI and craniofacial injuries in prehospital environments.
- Apply appropriate hemorrhage control strategies for scalp and facial lacerations, including use of hemostatic dressings.
- Differentiate between types of skull and facial fractures requiring urgent surgical referral or stabilization.
- Implement practical airway protection and anti-shock interventions for complex head and face trauma.
- Recognize when to initiate evacuation and advanced interventions such as neurosurgical or maxillofacial care.

A. Kishore (✉)
Department of Emergency Medicine, Kasturba Medical College, Manipal, Karnataka, India

N. T. Rai, S. Misra (eds.), *Frontline Operational Resuscitation and Combat Emergencies (FORCE) Manual*, https://doi.org/10.1007/978-981-92-1622-2_8

Introduction

In the chaos of modern warfare, head and facial trauma present some of the most formidable challenges to field medics and frontline providers. These injuries account for a substantial proportion of battlefield morbidity and mortality, often leading to airway compromise, massive hemorrhage, and devastating neurological outcomes. In combat zones, where evacuation is delayed, and imaging is unavailable, the responsibility for rapid triage, stabilization, and damage control falls squarely on the shoulders of trained tactical providers.

The spectrum of combat-related head injuries ranges from concussions and scalp lacerations to skull fractures and penetrating brain trauma. Simultaneously, facial trauma can result in airway obstruction, vision loss, cosmetic disfigurement, and functional impairments involving mastication and speech. Rapid recognition and field-based interventions, often in austere and resource-limited environments, are essential to preserve life and minimize long-term sequelae.

This chapter provides an evidence-based, combat-adapted approach to managing head and face trauma. It introduces battlefield evaluation techniques, including the AVPU and Glasgow Coma Scale, to guide neurologic assessment and outlines essential interventions such as cervical spine stabilization, hemorrhage control using advanced hemostatic agents, hypertonic saline administration, and seizure prophylaxis. Maxillofacial trauma is tackled through a structured clinical examination method, with attention to airway, vision, and structural integrity.

Case-based scenarios woven throughout the text reinforce key principles and decision-making under fire. The goal is not only to support survival but to empower providers to deliver skilled, timely care in the face of uncertainty, delay, and high stakes. In doing so, it ensures that those injured in combat receive the best possible chance at recovery—even in the harshest of conditions.

Case Scenario

During an early morning convoy movement to a forward operating base in the mountainous terrain of Arunachal Pradesh, visibility is compromised due to dense fog and poor road conditions. The unit is traveling in an armored all-terrain vehicle along a narrow, gravel-lined descent. At 0615 h, the lead vehicle skids during a downhill turn and rolls onto its side. A 29-year-old soldier, call sign *Bravo 6*, is partially ejected from the vehicle and sustains blunt head trauma after striking a rock. His helmet is dislodged on impact (Fig. 8.1). Fellow soldiers initiate spinal precautions and extricate him within minutes.

- Care Under Fire (CUF):
  No active enemy threat reported. Convoy perimeter is secured. Casualty is immediately dragged to cover and initial hemorrhage control is prioritized. Facial bleeding is controlled with field dressings while maintaining situational awareness for any secondary threats.

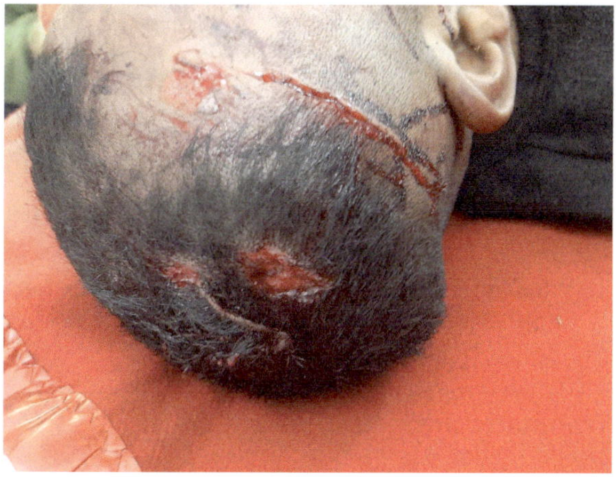

Fig. 8.1 Soldier injured after being partially ejected from a moving vehicle

- *Tactical Field Care (TFC):*
  Following the MARCH sequence:
  M—massive hemorrhage: Steady bleeding from a scalp laceration over the right parietal region is controlled using Axiostat® hemostatic gauze and Raney clips. Facial bruising and lacerations present but no involvement of major vessels.
  A—airway: Semiconscious with facial trauma and blood pooling in the oral cavity. Gurgling breath sounds present; no gag reflex. Positioned in lateral recovery to prevent aspiration. NPA inserted with minor resistance. Cricothyrotomy kit prepared in case of deterioration.
  R—respiration: Shallow breathing at 20/min. SPO_2 at 91% on room air. Chest exam shows symmetrical movement and clear breath sounds. No evidence of thoracic trauma. Head elevated to aid ventilation. No supplemental oxygen available.
  C—circulation: Radial pulse weak at 110 bpm. SBP estimated at 100 mmHg. 18G IV cannula placed; 500 ml Ringer's Lactate administered. 1 g *tranexamic acid* given IV within 30 min of injury.
  H—head injury/hypothermia: GCS: E2V2M5 = 9. Pupils unequal and sluggish (right > left). Cervical collar applied. Saline-soaked dressing placed over head wound. Mylar blanket used for thermal insulation. Facial asymmetry suggests probable mandibular fracture.
- *Tactical Evacuation Care (TACEVAC):*
  Evacuation to Level II care delayed by 60 min due to terrain and fog. En route, neuro status is monitored. A repeat GCS shows decline, prompting a second IV bolus and administration of 3% hypertonic saline. Airway patency and bleeding control are reassessed every 10–15 min.

Reflective Questions

1. After completing the MARCH assessment, what interventions should be repeated during en route monitoring, and why?
2. If signs of impending brain herniation appear (e.g., unilateral fixed pupil, decerebrate posturing), what interventions should be initiated in the field, and what are their limitations?
3. How should the airway be managed if evacuation is delayed and mandibular fracture with oral bleeding continues?
4. What clinical signs would prompt reclassification of this casualty's evacuation priority from routine to urgent surgical intervention?

Traumatic Brain Injuries in Combat

Among the most daunting injuries faced in the battlefield, traumatic brain injury (TBI) stands out for its potential to cause devastating and irreversible consequences—*often silently and insidiously*. Unlike external wounds, which are visible and often dramatic, brain injuries may be occult yet rapidly progressive, compromising not just consciousness but also breathing, circulation, and neurologic control. In the chaos of combat, where minutes matter and diagnostic tools are sparse, *the early recognition and management of TBI can spell the difference between life and death—or between recovery and lifelong disability.*

This section delves into the mechanisms, classification, and field management of TBI, equipping frontline providers with a systematic approach grounded in evidence and adapted for the austere realities of combat medicine. From understanding the impact of blunt, penetrating, and blast-related forces to recognizing subtle signs of intracranial pressure and herniation, this segment offers medics the cognitive tools and actionable steps needed to preserve brain function under fire.

Importantly, the section reinforces the MARCH-aligned principles of airway protection, prevention of hypoxia and hypotension, and timely neuroprotective interventions such as hypertonic saline, TXA, and seizure prophylaxis. Whether managing a disoriented soldier post-blast or an unconscious casualty with signs of skull trauma, this guide serves as a vital resource to navigate the clinical uncertainty of combat head injuries with tactical clarity and clinical precision.

Mechanism

Head injuries, including traumatic brain injuries (TBI), are caused by various external forces impacting the head. These forces can be direct or indirect and include:

- *Blunt force trauma*: This occurs when a nonpenetrating force, such as a blow to the head, causes injury. Examples include falls, combat injuries, and physical assaults.
- *Sharp force trauma*: This involves an object piercing the skull, such as a bullet or shrapnel, leading to brain injury.

- *Rotational or angular forces*: These forces cause shear stress to brain tissue, often seen in motor vehicle accidents or combat-related injuries where the head experiences rapid acceleration and deceleration.
- *Blast injuries*: Common in military contexts, where explosive forces cause rapid pressure changes that can damage the brain.

Diagnosis of Traumatic Brain Injury

In the FORCE framework, *early recognition of head injury in the field relies less on diagnostics and more on disciplined clinical thinking.* Two practical anchors guide this process: *history of the event* and *assessment of severity.* In austere environments—where imaging is absent and evacuation may be delayed—these elements become critical in shaping immediate decisions.

The *history of injury* is often the first and most valuable diagnostic tool available to the responder. It begins with understanding the *mechanism*, *timing*, and *operational context* of the event. Was the casualty exposed to a blast? Did they sustain a fall during movement over uneven terrain? Was there a high-velocity impact during combat or vehicular movement? Such details are not merely descriptive—they are predictive. High-energy mechanisms, rapid deceleration, or blast exposure should immediately raise concern for significant traumatic brain injury, even if the casualty is initially conscious.

Equally important are *associated features* reported at the scene: *loss of consciousness, confusion, disorientation, seizures, or abnormal behavior.* In tactical settings, where continuous monitoring is often not feasible, these early clues help determine urgency, need for evacuation, and allocation of limited resources. A seemingly "awake" victim may still be harboring a deteriorating brain injury—history helps identify that risk before clinical decline becomes obvious.

The *mechanism of injury* is broadly classified into *blunt* and *penetrating trauma*, each carrying distinct operational implications.

Blunt injuries—common in falls, blunt assault, or blast waves—often result in diffuse or evolving brain injury patterns that may deteriorate over time. These casualties require close observation, repeated neurological checks, and a low threshold for evacuation.

Penetrating injuries, on the other hand, involve direct disruption of cranial integrity by objects such as bullets, shrapnel, or fragments. These are usually obvious but carry a significantly higher risk of rapid deterioration, hemorrhage, and infection. In field conditions, they demand immediate prioritization and expedited evacuation.

From an anatomical standpoint, the distinction hinges on whether there is a *breach of the dura mater*—the brain's outer protective covering. However, in real-world scenarios, responders are rarely making this distinction anatomically. Instead, the emphasis is on *recognizing patterns*: visible skull breach, exposed brain matter, or embedded fragments should always be treated as penetrating injury until proven otherwise.

By integrating mechanism-based suspicion with focused history, responders can make rapid, experience-driven decisions—ensuring that head injuries are neither missed nor underestimated in the chaos of the operational environment.

When to Suspect Traumatic Brain Injury?

Mechanisms:

- Involvement in a vehicle blast event, collision, or rollover
- Presence within 50 meters of any blast (inside or outside)
- A direct blow to the head or witnessed loss of consciousness
- Exposure to more than one blast event
- Gunshot or shrapnel wound to head, open skull fracture, etc.

Symptoms:

H—Headaches and/or vomiting
E—Ear/Nose bleed or fluid leakage
A—Amnesia, altered consciousness, or loss of consciousness
D—Double vision or dizziness
S—Seizures or "Something feels off" (subjective sense that something is not right)
+ *Distance*: Was the individual *within 50 meters* of the blast?
Brain Imaging is required for the people with these symptoms. The aim of detection of TBI is to reduce secondary brain injury alongside deciding on the need for surgical intervention for the primary injury.

Classification of Traumatic Brain Injury

AVPU vs. *Glasgow Coma Scale (GCS)*

The classification of traumatic brain injuries is crucial for determining the appropriate medical response. The AVPU (Alert, Verbal, Pain, Unresponsive) scale and the Glasgow Coma Scale (Table 8.1) are two commonly used methods for assessing the level of consciousness in patients with head injuries.

- Equivalence and correlation between AVPU and GCS:
  - There is a clear correlation between AVPU and GCS scores. Specifically, "Alert" corresponds to a GCS of 15, "Verbal" to a GCS of 13–14, "Pain" to a GCS of 8–11, and "Unresponsive" to a GCS of 3.
    AVPU is particularly valuable for initial assessments.
- Predictive ability of GCS:
  - GCS scores are effective at predicting outcomes in head-injured patients, especially when combined with other factors such as patient age and pupillary response.

Table 8.1 Components of Glasgow Coma Scale

Eye opening (E)	
Spontaneous	4
To sound	3
To pressure	2
None	1
Non-testable	NT
Verbal response (V)	
Oriented	5
Confused	4
Words	3
Sounds	2
None	1
Non-testable	NT
Best motor response (M)	
Obeys commands	6
Localizing	5
Normal flexion	4
Abnormal flexion	3
Extension	2
None	1
Non-testable	NT

Adapted from Teasdale and Jennett [12]

Table 8.2 Severity of TBI based on GCS score

Severity	Mild	GCS 13–15
	Moderate	GCS 9–12
	Severe	GCS <8

Abbreviations: TBI traumatic brain injury, *GCS* Glasgow Coma Scale
Adapted from American College of Surgeons Committee on Trauma [11]

> The motor component of the GCS is particularly predictive and yields similar results to the total GCS score.

TBI is classified as mild, moderate, and severe based on the Glasgow Coma Scale (GCS) score as shown in Table 8.2.

After quantification of the GCS score, pupillary examination, and examination of the head and face for signs of external trauma, *a concise neurologic assessment comprising of sensory and motor examination should be performed.*

Field Management of Traumatic Brain Injury

In the operational environment, management of traumatic brain injury (TBI) begins at the point of injury and evolves dynamically with available resources, tactical constraints, and evacuation timelines. Resuscitation is not delayed for definitive diagnosis—*it is initiated alongside the primary MARCH assessment*, with a constant focus on preventing secondary brain injury.

Initial Actions in the Field

1. *Ensure scene safety and relocation*

   The victim should be moved out of immediate threat zones (active fire, unstable terrain, environmental hazards) before initiating detailed care. Tactical safety always precedes medical intervention.

2. *Assess for cervical spine injury*

   Head injury should always raise suspicion for concurrent cervical spine trauma. Spine protection must be maintained where indicated.

   The risk of significant cervical injury is low if the casualty demonstrates:

   - No neck pain or midline tenderness
   - Normal alertness and orientation
   - No evidence of intoxication
   - No focal neurological deficits (e.g., weakness, numbness, tingling)
   - No distracting injuries

   If any of these are present, *assume instability and maintain spinal precautions* using available methods (manual stabilization, improvised supports).

Management of Moderate to Severe TBI

(Defined operationally as an injured soldier unable to follow commands with evidence of head trauma or high-risk mechanism such as blast or blunt impact)

3. *Prevent hypoxia and hypotension—the two killers of TBI*

   (a) *Optimize oxygenation*

   Maintain oxygen saturation above 90–95%.

   - Initiate basic airway maneuvers (jaw thrust, airway adjuncts if available).
   - If oxygenation remains inadequate, *exclude reversible causes such as tension pneumothorax or ongoing hemorrhage.*
   - Consider advanced airway placement if feasible and within skill capability.

   (b) *Maintain adequate perfusion*

   Prevent hypotension by targeting systolic blood pressure ≥*100–110 mmHg.*

   - In suspected hemorrhagic shock → prioritize *blood or plasma resuscitation.*
   - If no evidence of bleeding → cautious crystalloid bolus (up to 1 L).

FORCE Tactical Pearl

Even a single episode of hypoxia or hypotension significantly worsens outcomes in TBI—these must be aggressively avoided.

Recognition and Management of Raised Intracranial Pressure (Herniation)

4. *Identify early signs of herniation*

   Suspect in cases of:

   - Progressive decline in consciousness
   - Unequal or fixed dilated pupils
   - Abnormal posturing

   Management (only if evacuation to definitive care is ongoing):

   - Administer hypertonic saline:
     - 3% or 5% saline (250 mL) *or* 23.4% saline (30 mL) via slow IV/IO over ~10 min

       May repeat once after 20 min if no response.
   - Monitor infusion site closely; stop if extravasation occurs.
   - Elevate head end to ~30° if not in shock and tactically feasible.
   - Controlled hyperventilation (if capnography available): target $EtCO_2$ ~ 32–38 mmHg.

Adjunctive Medical Management

5. *Tranexamic acid (TXA)*

   Administer 1 g IV/IO as early as possible (within 3 h of injury) in suspected polytrauma or hemorrhagic risk.
6. *Analgesia and sedation*

   Pain control should be balanced with preservation of airway reflexes and neurological assessment.

   - Use agents judiciously (e.g., fentanyl, ketamine, NSAIDs depending on context).
   - Document baseline mental status using *AVPU* before administration.
   - Ensure weapon safety/disarmament after administering sedating agents.

> **FORCE Tactical Pearl**
> Oversedation in TBI can mask deterioration—frequent reassessment is essential.

7. *Antiemetics*

   Administer ondansetron (4 mg ODT/IV/IM) as required to prevent vomiting and aspiration risk.
8. *Seizure management and prophylaxis*

   - In victims with GCS <10 or witnessed seizures → initiate anticonvulsant therapy.
   - Example: Levetiracetam 1 g IV over ~20 min.

Definitive Priority

9. *Evacuation to higher care*

   All moderate to severe TBIs require urgent transfer to a facility with neuroimaging and neurosurgical capability.

   During transport, continuous reassessment of airway, breathing, circulation, and neurological status is critical.

Scalp Lacerations

Scalp lacerations are a common injury that can lead to significant blood loss, potentially resulting in hypovolemic shock. Effective and rapid control of bleeding is crucial in managing these injuries. Various techniques and methods have been studied to achieve quick and effective hemostasis in scalp lacerations.

- *Raney clips*
  Raney clips are effective in controlling hemorrhage from severe scalp lacerations, providing rapid hemostasis and stabilizing patients with significant blood loss.
- *Hair apposition technique (HAT):*
  The hair apposition technique (HAT) using tissue adhesive is a viable method for closing scalp lacerations, offering benefits such as shorter procedure times, less pain, fewer complications, and minimum equipments.
- *Axiostat® hemostatic dressing*
  Axiostat® chitosan-based hemostatic dressing significantly reduces time to achieve hemostasis and blood loss compared to conventional cotton gauze. It is effective in pre-hospital settings and does not cause side effects like tissue loss or rebleeding [4].
- *iTClamp*
  The iTClamp is effective in controlling bleeding from craniomaxillofacial injuries, including scalp lacerations, in pre-hospital environments. It offers an alternative to direct pressure and packing, providing adequate hemorrhage control in most cases.

General Wound Management Principles

- Effective management of scalp lacerations includes disinfecting the surrounding skin, infiltrating local anesthetics for pain control, and employing various closure techniques such as sutures, staples, and tissue adhesives. For strongly bleeding lacerations, incorporating the epicranial aponeurosis into the hemostasis is recommended.

FORCE Tactical Pearl
"Think Beyond the Bleed" Scalp and facial injuries may appear deceptively dramatic, but the underlying risk of intracranial injury should always be considered—especially if GCS <13, pupils are abnormal, or mechanism suggests blast/blunt force. Control visible bleeding aggressively, but never stop reassessing for signs of herniation or neurologic decline.

Skull Fracture

In the field, a skull fracture necessitates evacuation. These fractures can be open or closed, linear or stellate, and may occur in either the skull vault or base. Skull fractures have a high risk of associated intracranial injury. Fractures with depression deeper than the skull's thickness may require surgical elevation, but this should not be attempted in the field. *Any exposed brain tissue should be covered promptly with the cleanest covering available, ideally moistened with a crystalloid solution.* Loose bone or brain fragments should not be moved. If a broad-spectrum antibiotic is accessible, it should be given. Once the wound is attended to and any other injuries are stabilized, rapid evacuation is essential.

- *CT imaging for skull base fractures:*
  CT scans are essential for diagnosing and planning the management of skull base fractures. They help identify complications such as cerebrospinal fluid (CSF) leaks, encephalocele, meningitis, and cranial nerve injuries, which are critical for determining the need for surgical intervention.
- *Surgical management of depressed skull fractures:*
  Depressed skull fractures often require surgical intervention, especially when there is a depression deeper than the skull's thickness. Factors such as motor deficits, low Glasgow Coma Scale (GCS) scores, pneumocephalus, and prolonged hospital stays are predictors of unfavorable outcomes.
- *Management of bone fragments in compound depressed skull fractures:*
  In cases of compound depressed skull fractures, primary bone fragment replacement after decontamination is a safe option if performed within 72 h of trauma.

Penetrating Head Injuries

In the wilderness, most penetrating head injuries are caused by gunshot wounds, though knives and arrows can also penetrate the skull. These injuries are typically severe and require immediate and appropriate medical intervention to improve outcomes (Fig. 8.2). *Over 60% of individuals with gunshot wounds to the head do not survive long enough to reach a medical facility.* Tangential wounds or low velocity

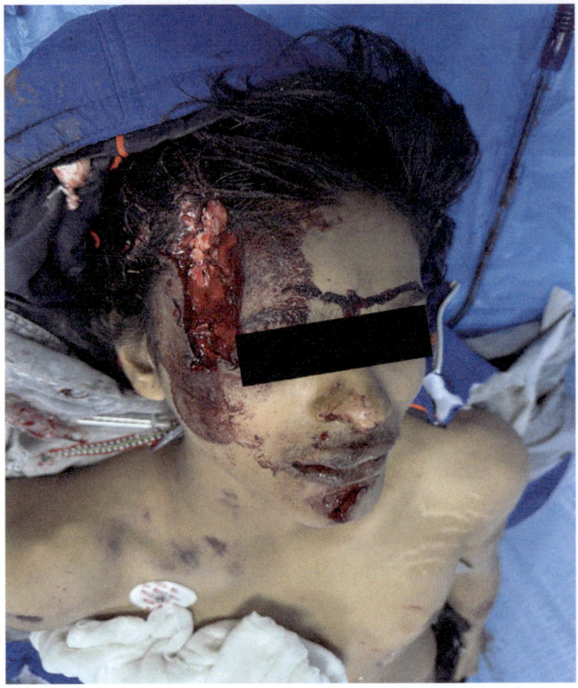

Fig. 8.2 Soldier with penetrating head injury with brain matter exposed

injuries may not be life threatening and would only require antibiotics with local debridement of the wound. If the skull has been penetrated, the patient should receive antibiotics and a tetanus shot, like the treatment for an open skull fracture. *In the uncommon case where a projectile remains embedded in the skull, it should not be removed.* If the projectile's length complicates immobilization or transport, *the excess may be carefully trimmed, provided this can be done without moving the part lodged within the skull.*

Face Trauma

Facial trauma remains a significant clinical challenge in combat zones, commonly arising from blunt force injuries, vehicular accidents, and training mishaps. These injuries may range from superficial lacerations to complex maxillofacial fractures and soft tissue avulsions (Fig. 8.3). Prompt assessment and early field management are essential to preserve airway patency, maintain functional integrity, reduce pain, and prevent secondary infections.

Initial Patient Assessment—Functional Screening Questions

- *Vision:* "Can you see clearly in both eyes?"
- *Sensation:* "Do you feel any numbness or tingling in your face or lips?"
- *Bite:* "Does your bite feel normal? Are you able to chew or close your mouth comfortably?"

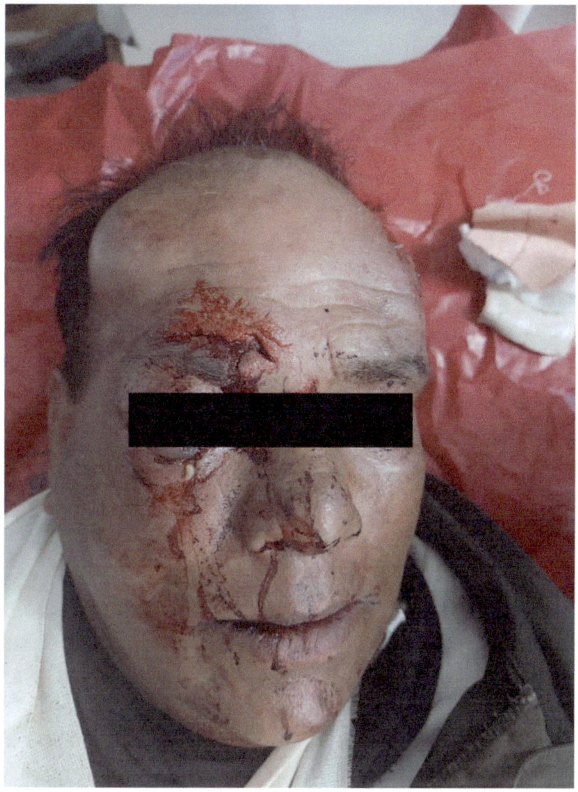

Fig. 8.3 Civilian with facial trauma due to fall from a moving vehicle

Visual Inspection

- *Frontal view:* Look for asymmetry, deformity, or swelling.
- *Lateral view:* Observe for midface flattening or malar depression—possible indicators of zygomatic complex fracture.
- *Periorbital area:* Assess for ecchymosis ("raccoon eyes"), hyphema, or subconjunctival hemorrhage.
- *Nasal and otic areas:* Check for bleeding, bruising, or cerebrospinal fluid (CSF) leak.

Focused Physical Examination

- *Palpation:* Gently examine for bony step-offs, crepitus, tenderness, or abnormal mobility.
- *Nasal septum and ears:* Assess for hematoma, obstruction, bleeding, or pain.
- *Jaw function:* Instruct the casualty to bite down—check for occlusal misalignment or trismus.
- *Oral cavity:* Look for swelling, lacerations, avulsed or displaced teeth.

Active Bleeding Management

If arterial or persistent bleeding is observed:

1. *Direct pressure:*
   - Apply sterile gauze or a hemostatic dressing (e.g., QuikClot® Combat Gauze) over the bleeding point.
   - Maintain firm, uninterrupted pressure for several minutes.
   - Use gloved hands or elastic compression bandages if gauze is unavailable.
2. *Hemostatic gauze:*
   - Pack deep wounds with hemostatic gauze.
   - Maintain pressure for at least 3 min post-application.

FORCE Tactical Pearl
Facial bleeding can rapidly compromise the airway—always prioritize airway positioning (e.g., *lateral recovery*), *active suctioning, and be prepared to establish a surgical airway if bleeding obstructs ventilation.*

Avulsed Teeth

In battlefield environments, the management of avulsed teeth poses unique challenges due to delayed evacuation, limited access to dental specialists, and the absence of ideal storage media. However, the timely preservation of the avulsed tooth—particularly the periodontal ligament (PDL) cells on the root surface—can significantly improve the chances of successful reimplantation at higher levels of care.

The viability of PDL cells is critical for preventing root resorption and ankylosis. To preserve these cells, the tooth must be stored in a medium that maintains their vitality, clonogenic potential, and mitogenic activity. *In austere military settings, the choice of storage media must balance biologic efficacy with availability in the field.*

Recommended Storage Media

- *Milk:*
  Among all field-accessible options, pasteurized whole milk remains the most practical and effective medium due to its compatibility with PDL cells and widespread availability through field rations or local civilian supplies. It can preserve cellular viability for several hours.
- *Normal saline or sterile IV fluids (e.g., Ringer's lactate):*
  While less ideal than milk, sterile IV solutions available in field medic kits can serve as temporary storage media when milk is not accessible.
- *Saliva (buccal vestibule):*
  In the absence of sterile options, placing the tooth in the casualty's own cheek pouch (buccal vestibule) is a reasonable alternative. It helps maintain moisture and temperature, although risk of contamination is higher.
- *Propolis and coconut water:*

These are less commonly available in combat zones but may be considered in rural or tropical deployments where local resources permit.

Practical Considerations in the Field

- *Do not store in dry conditions or tap water*
  These environments damage the root surface and compromise cell viability.
- *Tooth rescue kits (e.g., Save-A-Tooth®)*
  Though ideal, such commercial kits are rarely available in forward-deployed units. If included in dental modules of combat medic bags, they offer nutrient-rich media that preserve avulsed teeth for up to 24 h.
- *Immediate action*
  The tooth should not be scrubbed or allowed to dry. Gently rinse off debris with saline and place it in the chosen medium as soon as possible. Evacuate the patient to dental or maxillofacial care within 1–2 h whenever feasible.

Nasal Bleeds

Epistaxis, or nosebleed, is a common combat casualty care concern that can range from self-limiting bleeds to profuse hemorrhage capable of compromising the airway and operational performance. In field environments, effective, rapid control of nasal bleeding is vital—both for casualty stabilization and continued mission success.

1. Direct Nasal Pressure (First-Line Intervention)

- *How to perform:*
  Instruct the casualty (or do it yourself) to firmly pinch the soft part of the nostrils (below the bony bridge) for 10–15 min without releasing.
  Position the head slightly forward to prevent blood from flowing down the throat and triggering nausea or aspiration.
- Simple, equipment-free, and effective in most mild-to-moderate cases.

2. Chemical Cautery (Trained Personnel Only)

- *When to use:*
  If bleeding persists after pressure and the bleeding point is visible, trained providers can apply *silver nitrate* to cauterize the site. Risk of mucosal injury and septal perforation.

3. Hemostatic Agents and Tranexamic Acid (TXA)

- *Thrombogenic gels and foams:* Products like Gelfoam®, Surgicel®, and FloSeal® can be applied directly to visible bleeding areas inside the nostril. They promote clotting and are bioabsorbable, requiring no removal.

- *TXA application:* Crushed tranexamic acid tablets or TXA-soaked gauze can also be packed into the nostril. This is particularly useful in moderate-to-severe epistaxis.

4. Anterior Epistaxis Devices and Expandable Tampons

- *Function:*
  These pre-formed devices expand inside the nasal cavity, exerting consistent pressure against bleeding vessels.
- *Field use:*
  Insert gently into the nostril and allow the device to expand (some versions inflate with air or expand with fluid). They are fast, effective, and ideal for tactical medicine kits.
- Avoid saline inflation, especially with Rapid Rhino® devices—if ruptured, saline may be aspirated.

5. Nasal Packing (Anterior and Posterior)

- *Purpose:*
  Used when anterior devices are ineffective or unavailable. Anterior packing addresses most bleeds (Fig. 8.4); posterior packing is for more severe, high-flow cases.
- *Materials:*

  Sterile gauze, specialized nasal sponges, or balloon tamponade systems. Posterior packs often require more training to place and should be monitored closely due to discomfort and airway risk.

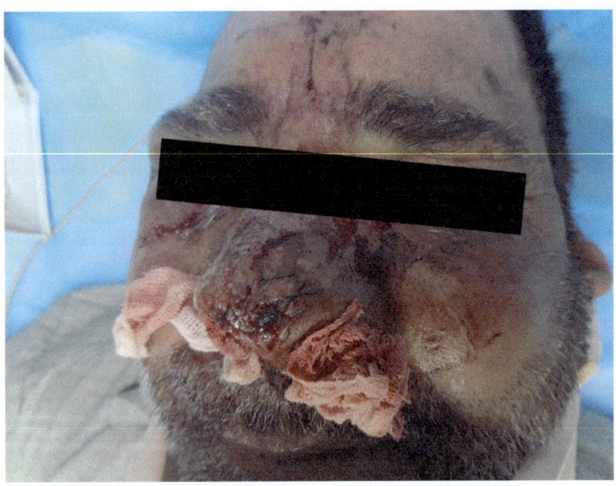

Fig. 8.4 Bilateral anterior nasal packing done for a civilian with bilateral nasal bleeding

Jaw Fractures

Mandible fractures are the second most common facial fracture after nasal fractures. Assaults, motor vehicle crashes, and falls are the most reported mechanisms. Recognizing key signs early is essential for effective prehospital care.

Clinical Presentation

Patients may present with jaw pain, especially during movement, swelling and bruising around the jaw, difficulty opening the mouth (trismus), problems with biting or chewing (malocclusion), and visible jaw deformity (Fig. 8.5).

Prehospital Management

- *Airway and bleeding control*: Ensure the airway remains open and manage bleeding with direct pressure; use hemostatic agents if available. Be alert for potential airway compromise, especially with severe swelling and tongue fall back due to bilateral body of jawbone fractures.
- *Immobilization*: Stabilize the neck with a cervical collar and consider using a mandibular support, such as a Barton bandage, to reduce movement and pain.
- *Pain control and transport*: Administer pain relief as per protocol and arrange rapid transport for higher levels of care.

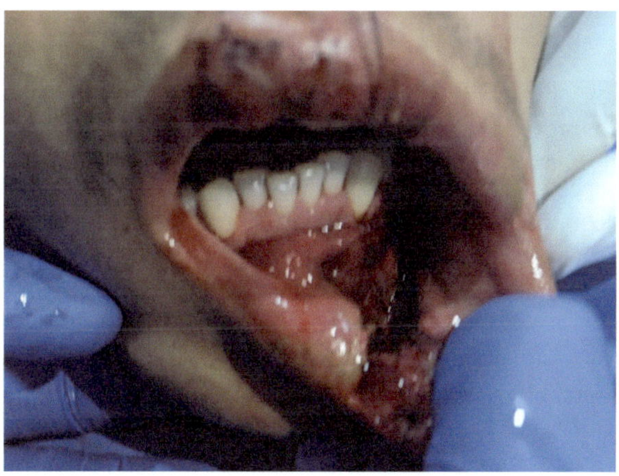

Fig. 8.5 Soldier with mandibular fracture with injury to the lower lip

Case Resolution

Bravo 6 was promptly stabilized on site using the MARCH framework, with initial priorities focused on controlling scalp hemorrhage, securing a compromised airway, and initiating neuroprotective measures. His airway was maintained in a lateral recovery position, a nasopharyngeal airway was inserted with caution, and suctioning was performed to clear pooled blood from the oral cavity. Given the suspected mandibular fracture, preparations were made for a potential surgical airway if deterioration occurred. Repeat neurological assessments were planned at 10–15-min intervals, with close attention to changes in pupil size, motor response, and level of consciousness.

Evacuation to a Level II care facility was initiated within 75 min. During transit, Bravo 6 remained hemodynamically stable; however, a decline in neurological status was noted, with his GCS dropping from 9 to 7. This prompted a second bolus of IV fluids and administration of 3% hypertonic saline over 10 min, followed by a saline flush. Head elevation was continued to promote venous drainage, and careful monitoring for signs of impending herniation—such as unilateral pupil dilation or posturing—was conducted. In anticipation of worsening airway compromise due to mandibular instability and ongoing oral bleeding, surgical cricothyrotomy equipment was kept ready, though not immediately required.

On arrival at the field hospital, CT imaging revealed a right temporal epidural hematoma, a linear parietal skull fracture, and bilateral mandibular fractures. The casualty underwent burr-hole decompression and mandibular fixation under controlled conditions. Early administration of tranexamic acid within the golden hour, maintenance of cerebral perfusion pressure, and timely neuroprotective strategies likely contributed to limiting secondary brain injury.

By the sixth day post-injury, Bravo 6 had regained full consciousness (GCS 15), was maintaining his own airway, and had begun oral intake with assistance. He was later airlifted to a higher center for neurorehabilitation and further maxillofacial care. This case signifies the critical importance of continuous airway management, repeated neurologic assessment during evacuation, and rapid recognition of signs requiring escalation to urgent surgical intervention. It highlights the effectiveness of structured field protocols and adaptive interventions in improving outcomes from severe head and facial trauma in combat settings.

Key Messages

- Head and face trauma are common and potentially life-threatening injuries in combat scenarios, requiring rapid field recognition and stabilization.
- The MARCH algorithm offers a structured, lifesaving approach to prioritize care in austere and tactical environments.
- Early identification of traumatic brain injury (TBI) using AVPU or GCS, along with timely neuroprotective interventions, is critical in minimizing secondary brain injury.

(continued)

- Scalp lacerations and facial wounds can lead to significant hemorrhage; hemostatic agents and pressure techniques are essential tools in the field.
- Airway compromise due to maxillofacial trauma must be anticipated—preemptive positioning, suctioning, and surgical airway readiness are key.
- Facial fractures, avulsed teeth, and epistaxis require targeted assessment and adaptable management using available field resources.
- Decision-making regarding evacuation and surgical referral hinges on continuous reassessment and tactical feasibility.

Conclusion

In combat medicine, the successful management of head and face trauma hinges on the ability to make rapid, informed decisions in resource-limited and high-stress conditions. This chapter outlines an evidence-informed, combat-adapted framework to assess and stabilize these injuries, prioritizing airway management, hemorrhage control, and neurologic assessment. By applying structured protocols such as MARCH and leveraging innovations in prehospital care—like hemostatic dressings, hypertonic saline, and tranexamic acid—frontline providers can significantly improve outcomes for injured personnel. Additionally, attention to practical field strategies for managing avulsed teeth, nasal bleeds, and jaw fractures ensures comprehensive care beyond lifesaving interventions. Combat providers equipped with this knowledge will not only save lives but also preserve critical function and quality of life for soldiers under fire. This chapter aims to empower providers with tactical clarity, procedural competence, and clinical foresight when every minute—and every decision—matters most.

Bibliography

1. Auerbach PS, Cushing TA, Harris NS. Auerbach's Wilderness Medicine. 7th ed. 2 vols. Philadelphia: Elsevier; 2016. ISBN: 9780323359429
2. Butler, Frank K Jr et al. "Tactical combat casualty care 2007: evolving concepts and battlefield experience." *Military medicine* vol. 172,11 Suppl (2007): 1–19. https://doi.org/10.7205/milmed.172.supplement_1.1
3. Carney, Nancy et al. "Guidelines for the Management of Severe Traumatic Brain Injury, Fourth Edition." *Neurosurgery* vol. 80,1 (2017): 6–15. https://doi.org/10.1227/NEU.0000000000001432
4. Feliciano DV, Mattox KL, Moore EE. *Trauma*. 9th ed. New York: McGraw Hill Medical; 2020. ISBN: 978-1260143355
5. Kucik, Corry J, and Timothy Clenney. "Management of epistaxis." *American family physician* vol. 71,2 (2005): 305–11
6. Menon, David K et al. "Position statement: definition of traumatic brain injury." *Archives of physical medicine and rehabilitation* vol. 91,11 (2010): 1637–40. https://doi.org/10.1016/j.apmr.2010.05.017
7. Shackford SR, Kahl JE, Calvo RY, Kozar RA, Haugen CE, Kaups KL, Willey M, Tibbs BM, Mutto SM, Rizzo AG, Lormel CS, Shackford MC, Burlew CC, Moore EE, Cogbill TH, Kallies

KJ, Haan JM, Ward J (2014). Gunshot wounds and blast injuries to the face are associated with significant morbidity and mortality: Results of an 11-year multi-institutional study of 720 patients. J Trauma Acute Care Surg; 76(2): 347–352
8. Taylor, Christopher A et al. "Traumatic Brain Injury-Related Emergency Department Visits, Hospitalizations, and Deaths - United States, 2007 and 2013." *Morbidity and mortality weekly report. Surveillance summaries (Washington, D.C. : 2002)* vol. 66,9 1–16. 17 Mar. 2017, https://doi.org/10.15585/mmwr.ss6609a1
9. Tintinalli JE, Ma OJ, Yealy DM, et al. *Tintinalli's Emergency Medicine: A Comprehensive Study Guide*. 9th ed. New York: McGraw-Hill Education; 2019. ISBN: 978-1405296434.
10. Villwock, Jennifer A, and Kristin Jones. "Recent trends in epistaxis management in the United States: 2008-2010." *JAMA otolaryngology-- head & neck surgery* vol. 139,12 (2013): 1279–84. https://doi.org/10.1001/jamaoto.2013.5220
11. American College of Surgeons Committee on Trauma. ATLS: Advanced Trauma Life Support. 10th ed. Chicago: American College of Surgeons; 2018. ISBN: 978-0996826235
12. Teasdale, G., & Jennett, B. (1974). Assessment of coma and impaired consciousness: a practical scale. *The lancet*, *304*(7872), 81–84

Spinal Injuries: Preservation of Combat Mobility

9

Jyothiswaroop Bhaskararayuni

Learning Objectives
Upon completing this chapter, the reader will be able to:

- Recognize the tactical and clinical implications of spinal injuries in combat environments.
- Apply the MARCH framework and FORCE principles in assessing potential spinal trauma.
- Differentiate between various types and mechanisms of spinal cord injury and understand their implications on neurological function.
- Implement field-adapted stabilization and spinal motion restriction techniques using standard or improvised tools.
- Execute safe and efficient evacuation protocols for casualties with suspected spinal trauma while minimizing further harm.
- Understand the principles of definitive care, rehabilitation, and criteria guiding return-to-duty decisions for injured combatants.

Introduction

In the unforgiving terrain of the battlefield, where seconds determine survival, spinal injuries present one of the most complex and high-stakes challenges for frontline medics and tactical care providers. These injuries not only compromise the physical function of the soldier but can significantly disrupt operational momentum,

J. Bhaskararayuni (✉)
Department of Emergency Medicine, AIIMS, New Delhi, India

N. T. Rai, S. Misra (eds.), *Frontline Operational Resuscitation and Combat Emergencies (FORCE) Manual*, https://doi.org/10.1007/978-981-92-1622-2_9

impacting mission continuity and morale. *A single lapse in spinal care—be it during assessment, stabilization, or transport—can result in irreversible neurological damage, making rapid and precise intervention imperative.*

Combat-related spinal trauma is unique. Unlike civilian cases, military injuries often occur in hostile, resource-limited environments where the luxury of advanced diagnostics or immediate evacuation may not be available. High-velocity projectiles, blast forces, vehicle rollovers, and falls from elevation—common in both counterinsurgency and high-altitude operations—impose distinct biomechanical forces on the spine, resulting in flexion, extension, compression, and rotational injuries. These injuries may present with subtle signs but carry devastating long-term implications.

This chapter aims to equip combat medical providers with a comprehensive, field-adapted approach to spinal injury recognition, classification, stabilization, and evacuation, grounded in combat principles and the realities of austere military medicine. It emphasizes the dual imperatives of preserving neurological integrity and enabling timely casualty extraction under fire.

Case Scenario

During late evening hours at a remote high-altitude forward operating base in the Eastern Himalayas, a 30-year-old male soldier falls approximately 5 meters from a snow-covered ledge while responding to a perimeter alert. He lands heavily on his back and head against frozen terrain. His helmet is dislodged on impact. Teammates find him lying supine, awake but disoriented. The terrain is icy, ambient temperature is below freezing, and extraction is expected to be delayed by at least 90 min due to weather and elevation.

- *Care Under Fire (CUF):*
  No enemy engagement is reported. The perimeter is confirmed secure. The casualty is carefully moved to a sheltered position using improvised spinal precautions, avoiding torsion or flexion of the spine. A thermal blanket and ground insulation are improvised using available clothing and foam mats to prevent direct exposure to the snow-covered surface.
- *Tactical Field Care (TFC):*
  Following the MARCH sequence:
  M—massive hemorrhage: No external bleeding detected. A full-body blood sweep is negative. No signs of internal bleeding appreciated on rapid abdominal or pelvic examination.
  A—airway: The airway is patent. The casualty is spontaneously breathing and converses with rescuers, though mildly confused. A nasopharyngeal airway is prepared but not inserted.
  R—respiration: Respiratory rate is elevated at 28/min and shallow. No signs of chest trauma or asymmetry. Lung auscultation (if feasible) is equal bilaterally. Casualty reports difficulty in breathing but no pain on inspiration.

C—circulation: Blood pressure is low at 80/62 mmHg. Heart rate is bradycardic at 48 bpm. Skin is pale and cold to touch. Capillary refill is delayed. No peripheral pulses palpable at the dorsalis pedis. IV access is attempted but challenging due to peripheral vasoconstriction and cold-induced vasospasm.

H—head injury/hypothermia: GCS is 15. The casualty recalls the fall but was reportedly unconscious briefly. He now complains of severe back pain and an inability to move or feel both legs. Upper limbs are moving normally. He reports tingling in his fingers. Lower limbs are flaccid. Rectal tone is diminished. Core temperature is 34 °C, indicating mild hypothermia. A high suspicion of spinal cord injury is raised. Cervical spine is stabilized using a rolled towel collar and manual in-line stabilization due to lack of a hard collar.

- *Tactical Evacuation Care (TACEVAC):*
  Evacuation is delayed by 90 min due to snow, wind chill, and terrain limitations. Passive rewarming is continued using multiple thermal layers and body insulation. The casualty is secured on a rigid stretcher improvised with skis and sleeping mats, ensuring spinal alignment. Neurological status, respiratory effort, and perfusion are monitored every 10–15 min. Core temperature is reassessed periodically using skin thermometers and passive warming techniques. Bradycardia and hypotension are treated as spinal shock until ruled otherwise. Cervical immobilization is maintained throughout transport.

Reflective Questions

1. How can spinal motion restriction be maintained in freezing conditions with limited equipment?
2. How would you clinically distinguish spinal shock from neurogenic and hypovolemic shock in this patient?
3. When should cervical spine injury be suspected in such settings, and how can immobilization be implemented using improvised field resources?

Mechanisms of Spinal Injuries

Understanding the mechanisms behind spinal injuries is essential to predict potential neurological damage, choose the appropriate intervention, and plan for safe extraction. In combat settings, where blunt force, blast exposure, and ballistic trauma frequently occur, these injuries are rarely isolated and often form part of a larger polytrauma picture.

Combat-related spinal trauma can result from a wide array of high-energy events. Each mechanism carries distinct implications for the spine, with some resulting in subtle internal damage despite minimal external findings.

- *Blunt trauma:*
  Typically caused by falls from height (e.g., into bunkers, down slopes, or during aerial insertions), vehicle rollovers, or impact with debris. This mechanism can cause compression fractures, ligament tears, and spinal cord contusions—often without external bleeding or deformity.

- *Penetrating trauma:*
  Gunshot wounds or shrapnel injuries may damage the vertebral column or transect the spinal cord directly. Unlike blunt injuries, the extent of neurological impairment often correlates more predictably with the anatomical site of entry.
- *Blast injuries:*
  Result from shock waves, body displacement, or secondary projectile impacts. These injuries may include vertebral burst fractures or dislocations from sudden axial loading. Blast waves can also cause indirect trauma via violent flexion or extension movements of the spine.
- *Combined mechanisms:*
  In real combat scenarios, it is not uncommon for a soldier to experience multiple simultaneous forces (e.g., a fall followed by blunt impact and torsion), complicating diagnosis and increasing the risk of unstable spinal injuries.

Recognizing the mechanism of injury (MOI) enables providers to anticipate underlying pathology, apply appropriate spinal motion restriction, and prioritize imaging and surgical evaluation once definitive care is available.

Based on Mechanics of Spine Injury

Combat spinal injuries can be further classified based on the mechanical forces involved. This classification helps understand the likely pattern of injury, predicts instability, and guides immediate management.

1. *Flexion injuries:*
   - Result from forward bending of the spine, such as falling head-first or sudden deceleration in a vehicle.
   - Common injuries: wedge compression fractures, anterior subluxation.
   - Risk: vertebral body compromise and potential ligament rupture.
2. *Extension injuries:*
   - Occur when the spine is forcefully bent backward, often seen in blast wave recoil or when landing supine on a hard surface.
   - Common injuries: hangman's fracture, posterior element disruption.
   - May initially appear stable but pose a high risk for delayed neurological decline.
3. *Axial loading (vertical compression):*
   - A vertical force applied through the spine, such as landing on the feet or buttocks after a fall.
   - Common injuries: burst fractures, especially in the lumbar spine.
   - Complications: spinal canal compromise from bone fragments.
4. *Rotational injuries:*
   - Caused by twisting forces, often in conjunction with flexion or lateral bending.
   - Common injuries: fracture-dislocations, ligamentous instability.
   - Often associated with neurological deficits due to spinal cord torsion.

5. *Distraction injuries:*
   - Occur when opposing forces pull the spine apart—e.g., in high-speed ejection injuries or limb entrapment scenarios.
   - Common injuries: transverse ligament rupture, unstable vertebral separation.

Spinal Cord Injury Classifications

Spinal cord injuries (SCIs) in combat scenarios range in severity and functional impact. Rapid identification and classification guide both field care and the urgency of evacuation.

1. Complete Spinal Cord Injury
- *Definition:* Total loss of motor and sensory function below the level of injury.
- *Presentation:* Flaccid paralysis, loss of reflexes, urinary retention, and absent pain response.
- *Prognosis:* Poor; long-term disability likely unless surgical decompression is prompt.

2. Incomplete Spinal Cord Injury
- *Definition:* Partial preservation of sensory and/or motor function below the injury level.
- *Presentation:* Patchy deficits, asymmetrical limb weakness, retained sacral sensation.
- *Prognosis:* Variable; often responsive to surgical and rehabilitative interventions.

3. Spine Fracture with Intact Neurological Function
- *Definition:* Vertebral injury without neurological compromise.
- *Significance:* Stability of the fracture determines management; can deteriorate without protection or during rough evacuation.

Levels of Spinal Injury

Spinal trauma must also be classified by the level of the vertebral column affected. The neurological impact and field management differ significantly between levels.

Cervical Spine Injuries (C1–C7)
- *Risks:* Immediate life threats due to compromised airway and breathing.
- *Common outcomes:* Quadriplegia, diaphragmatic paralysis (C3–C5 level involvement).
- *Combat implication:* Urgent airway protection and cervical immobilization are priorities.

Thoracic Spine Injuries (T1–T12)

- *Risks:* Autonomic dysreflexia, compromised thoracic cage stability.
- *Common outcomes:* Paraplegia below the level of injury, risk of neurogenic shock.
- *Combat implication:* Requires ongoing monitoring for vital instability and early decompression if indicated.

Lumbosacral Spine Injuries (L1–S5)

- *Risks:* Cauda equina or conus medullaris syndromes.
- *Common outcomes:* Flaccid lower limb weakness, bladder/bowel dysfunction.
- *Combat implication:* Though not immediately life-threatening, these injuries severely affect long-term mobility and operational fitness.

Based on Structures Involved

Beyond the vertebral level and mechanism, spinal injuries may affect different anatomical structures:

- *Fractures:* Involving vertebral body, lamina, pedicles—risk of instability and spinal cord impingement.
- *Ligamentous injuries:* Disruption of anterior or posterior longitudinal ligaments predisposes to vertebral displacement.
- *Spinal cord contusion or transection:* Often irreversible; requires immediate stabilization.
- *Nerve root damage:* Affects motor and sensory distribution of specific dermatomes—critical for field-level neurological mapping.

Common Spinal Cord Syndromes in Combat Care

1. *Central cord syndrome:*
   - Greater impairment in upper limbs than lower limbs; often hyperextension injury.
   - Relevant in blast recoil or backward falls with headstrike.
2. *Anterior cord syndrome:*
   - Motor and pain/temperature loss with preserved touch/proprioception.
   - Ischemic cause or direct anterior compression.
3. *Brown-Séquard syndrome:*
   - Ipsilateral motor loss + contralateral pain/temp loss.
   - Suggests penetrating trauma or lateral force impact.
4. *Posterior cord syndrome:*
   - Rare; preserved motor function but impaired coordination and balance.
   - May go undetected in field without detailed neurologic testing.

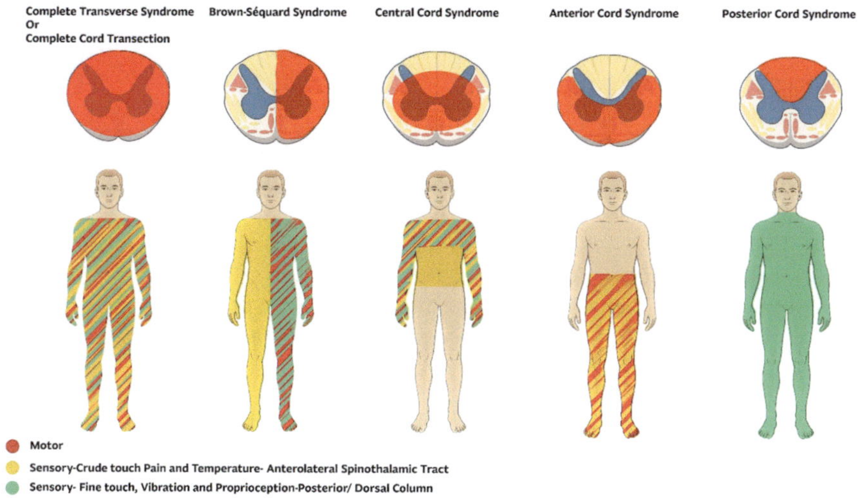

Fig. 9.1 Spinal cord syndromes

5. *Conus medullaris syndrome:*
   - Mixed upper/lower motor signs with early bowel/bladder dysfunction.
   - Typically seen in lumbar burst fractures or central disc herniation.
6. *Cauda equina syndrome:*
   - Saddle anesthesia, urinary retention, flaccid lower limb paralysis.
   - Surgical emergency—rapid identification critical (Fig. 9.1).

Approach to Spinal Injuries in Combat

In a combat zone, managing spinal injuries requires balancing lifesaving interventions with the imperative to minimize further neurologic damage. Spinal trauma often coexists with polytrauma, shock, and airway compromise, requiring providers to make swift, informed decisions under fire.

1. Scene Safety and Tactical Considerations
Before approaching the casualty:

- *Assess the environment:* Is the area still under active fire or threat of secondary explosives?
- *Ensure cover and concealment:* Attempt to secure a position that offers ballistic protection for the provider and casualty.
- *Tactical triage:* Prioritize life-threatening conditions first but remain vigilant for signs of spinal injury.

If urgent extraction is needed, *move the casualty with minimal spinal manipulation*, using manual in-line stabilization or improvised litter drags to preserve alignment.

2. Primary Assessment—MARCH Protocol

The MARCH algorithm remains the foundational trauma triage tool, with spinal injury considerations layered into each step:

- *M—massive hemorrhage:*
  Control external bleeding using tourniquets, pressure dressings, or hemostatic agents. *Do not delay hemorrhage control for spinal immobilization—stopping exsanguination takes precedence.*
- *A—airway:*
  Suspect cervical spine injury in any casualty with blunt trauma, blast exposure, or fall.
  - Maintain manual in-line stabilization (MILS) during airway maneuvers.
  - Avoid hyperextension or head tilt–chin lift. *Prefer jaw thrust* when opening the airway.
    If airway compromise persists, be prepared for surgical cricothyrotomy with spinal precautions.
- *R—respiration:*
  High cervical injuries may result in diaphragmatic paralysis (C3–C5).
  - Observe for shallow breathing, use of accessory muscles, or paradoxical movement.
  - Apply chest seals or perform needle decompression as needed, without compromising spinal alignment.
    Oxygen (if available) should be administered early.
- *C—circulation:*
  Monitor for neurogenic shock in cases of spinal trauma—signs include hypotension with bradycardia and warm extremities.
  - Initiate permissive hypotension in the absence of major hemorrhage.
  - Administer warmed fluids and TXA within the first hour if polytrauma is suspected.
    Prepare for vasopressor support in cases of suspected high spinal cord injury.
- *H—head injury/hypothermia:*
  Maintain normothermia to prevent coagulopathy and worsening of neurological outcomes.
  - Use hypothermia prevention kits, reflective blankets, and body-to-body warming where necessary.
    Monitor GCS and pupil responses continuously—decline may signal deteriorating spinal or intracranial injury.

3. Spinal Precautions: Stabilization in a Tactical Environment
Spinal motion restriction (SMR) is the preferred term over immobilization, as complete motion elimination is rarely feasible in the field. In combat settings:
Manual in-line stabilization (MILS):

- Performed immediately upon suspicion of spinal trauma.
- One provider maintains cervical spine alignment while others manage airway, bleeding, and prepare for movement.

Improvised stabilization techniques:

- *Improvised C-collars:* Use rolled towels, cravats, or jackets secured with cloth strips.
- *Backboard slternatives:* Rifles (with safety on), rigid branches, or sturdy panels tied together with belts or stretcher straps can serve as makeshift spine boards.

4. Tactical Positioning and Movement
When the casualty must be moved under fire:

- Use the drag-rescue method with the head and torso in line as much as possible.
- Once in a safe zone, reassess and re-stabilize with better equipment or materials.
- Avoid log rolls unless essential, and always use minimum providers trained in spine-safe handling.

5. Tactical Field Care for Spinal Trauma
Once immediate threats are neutralized:

- *Perform a focused neurological exam:*
  - Check motor function (grip strength, foot movement).
  - Assess sensory levels (pinprick, light touch).
    Monitor for priapism, urinary retention, or flaccid paralysis—indicators of spinal cord involvement.
- *Reassess vitals frequently:*
  - Include single breath count and monitor oxygen saturation if available.
    Watch for trends that might signal evolving cord injury or neurogenic shock.
- *Document using the MIST format:*
  - *M*echanism of injury
  - *I*njuries identified
  - *S*igns (vitals, GCS)
    *T*reatment provided

6. Tactical Evacuation Care
During CASEVAC or MEDEVAC:

- Ensure spinal alignment is maintained throughout movement—use scoop stretchers, vacuum mattresses, or improvised splints.
- Continue monitoring airway, breathing, circulation, and neurologic function.
- Prepare for in-flight deterioration, especially in high spinal cord injuries. Airway control should be secured before lift-off if in doubt.
- Document all interventions and changes in status. Clear communication with receiving facility is crucial—include suspected spinal level and MOI.

7. Special Considerations in Combat Spinal Injury Management

- *Environmental stressors:*
  Cold, altitude, and terrain can mask signs of spinal trauma and complicate stabilization.
- *Delayed evacuation:*
  Prolonged field care may necessitate ongoing spinal support, analgesia (preferably ketamine for hemodynamic neutrality), bladder monitoring, and pressure sore prevention.
- *Limited manpower:*
  Providers may be alone—prioritize airway, bleeding, and simple SMR techniques over full immobilization if time or threat level precludes full spinal precautions.

Types of Injuries and Management

Combat-related spinal injuries often result from high-energy mechanisms such as falls, blast exposure, or vehicle rollovers. These injuries may range from stable fractures to complete spinal cord transection and must be rapidly identified and managed in the field.

1. Vertebral fractures
Fractures vary in severity and mechanism:

- *Compression fractures* are common in axial loading injuries, such as falls or parachute landings, and may remain neurologically intact (Fig. 9.2).
- *Burst fractures* involve vertebral body explosion with fragment displacement into the spinal canal, often requiring urgent stabilization.
- *Chance fractures* (flexion-distraction injuries) occur in high-force horizontal trauma and may be associated with intra-abdominal injuries.

Fig. 9.2 Civilian with axial loading injury to thoracolumbar spine with deformity

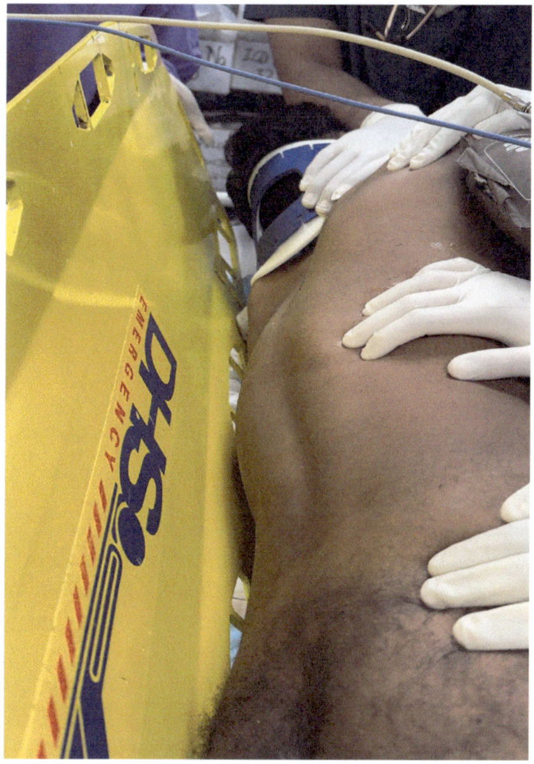

Management: Prioritize spinal motion restriction (SMR), monitor for neurological changes, administer analgesia, and prepare for evacuation. Avoid unnecessary manipulation.

2. Spinal cord injuries (SCIs)
SCIs are classified as:

- *Complete*: Total loss of motor and sensory function below the injury level. Prognosis is guarded.
- *Incomplete*: Partial function preserved—common patterns include:
  - *Central cord syndrome* (greater upper limb weakness)
  - *Anterior cord syndrome* (loss of motor and pain/temperature with preserved proprioception)
    Brown-Séquard syndrome (hemisection deficits)

Management: Provide oxygenation, maintain spinal alignment, monitor perfusion, and document using the ASIA chart. Evacuate promptly for definitive imaging and surgical consideration.

3. Spinal shock and neurogenic shock

- *Spinal shock*: Transient loss of reflexes and flaccid paralysis below the lesion. Can last days
- *Neurogenic shock*: Results from disruption of sympathetic outflow, presenting with hypotension and bradycardia (especially in cervical or upper thoracic injuries)

Management: Administer warmed fluids cautiously. Vasopressors (e.g., norepinephrine) may be necessary. Maintain oxygen delivery and normothermia.

Field Pain Management

Pain control aids in patient comfort and reduces involuntary movements that can exacerbate spinal injury.

- Ketamine is the preferred analgesic in tactical care (0.1–0.3 mg/kg IV), preserving airway reflexes and cardiovascular stability.
- Fentanyl (IN or IV) may be used with airway monitoring.
- NSAIDs and paracetamol are effective adjuncts for milder pain or maintenance therapy.

Antibiotics for Penetrating Injuries

If vertebral injury is associated with open wounds or suspected contamination:

- Administer ceftriaxone 1–2 g IV/IM.
- Add metronidazole if abdominal structures are involved.
- Consider clindamycin + ciprofloxacin in penicillin-allergic patients.

FORCE Tactical Pearl

In all cases, the field provider must reassess frequently, ensure spinal alignment is maintained, and prepare the casualty for transfer with a clear report of findings and interventions provided. Early recognition, tactical restraint in handling, and prompt evacuation form the pillars of spinal trauma management in combat zones.

Transportation of Spinal Injury Casualties in Tactical Settings

Once a spinal injury is suspected or confirmed, evacuation becomes a priority, but it must be done without aggravating the injury. *Poor transport decisions can turn a stable fracture into a cord-compromising lesion.* In combat environments, providers must weigh the urgency of extraction against the risk of further spinal insult, all while operating with limited equipment and under threat.

Principles of Safe Transport in Spinal Trauma

1. *Preserve spinal alignment:*
   Maintain head, neck, and torso in a straight line throughout movement and transfer.
2. *Minimize unnecessary motion:*
   Avoid repeated log rolls, head turning, or repositioning unless absolutely necessary.
3. *Protect vital functions:*
   Prioritize airway and hemodynamic stability, even if ideal SMR cannot be achieved initially.
4. *Reassess often:*
   Every movement phase should be followed by a neuro check and reassessment of vitals.

Tactical Spine Motion Restriction (SMR)

The goal in the field is motion restriction, not full immobilization. This allows for effective casualty care even when conventional tools (e.g., spine boards or collars) are unavailable.

Indications for SMR in the Field

- High-energy MOI (fall >1.5 meters, blast, vehicle rollover)
- Neurological symptoms (numbness, tingling, weakness)
- Midline spine tenderness
- Altered mental status or GCS <15
- Distracting injuries masking spine symptoms
- Intoxicated or uncooperative casualty

Improvised SMR Techniques

1. *Cervical collar alternatives:*
   - Rolled towels/jackets secured with bandages or tape
   - SAM splints shaped into a cervical support (Fig. 9.3)
   - Tactical neck gaiters + internal stiffening (rifle sling, thin branch)
2. *Improvised backboards:*
   - Long rifle (cleared and on safe), wooden planks, metal panels
   - Secure with belts, ropes, cravats, or strips of uniform
3. *Padding and stabilization:*
   - Use soft materials (jackets, blankets, packs) to pad voids
   - Prevent movement inside the transport platform

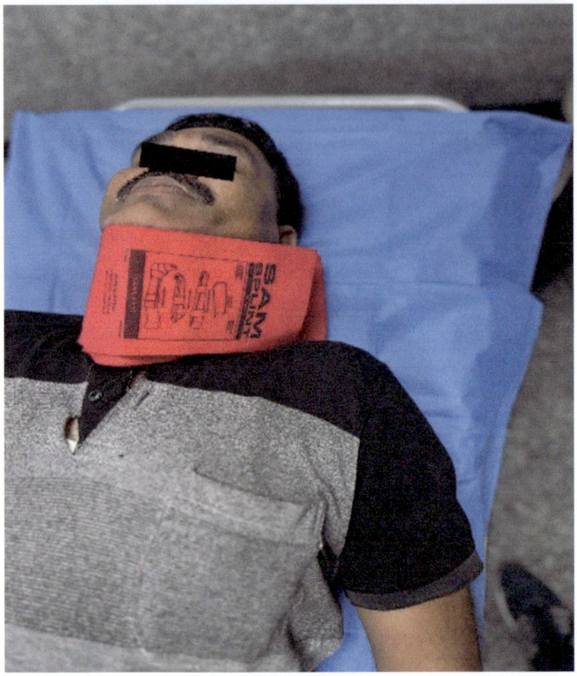

Fig. 9.3 Soldier with SAM splint used as an improvised cervical collar

Common Transport Platforms

1. Scoop Stretcher

- Best for confined spaces
- Minimal spine movement during placement
- *Procedure:* Disassemble, slide under patient, reassemble, then strap, and lift

2. Vacuum Mattress

- Conforms to body shape and offers excellent stabilization
- Ideal for rough terrain or air evacuation
- Use hand pump to evacuate air after positioning

3. Spine Board

- Traditional option; useful but uncomfortable for prolonged transport
- Best used in short extraction phases followed by vacuum or soft platform transfer
- Monitor for pressure sores, respiratory compromise, and reassess at every phase

4. KED (Kendrick Extrication Device)

- Designed for seated casualty extraction (Fig. 9.4)
- Especially useful in vehicle rollovers or cockpit extrications

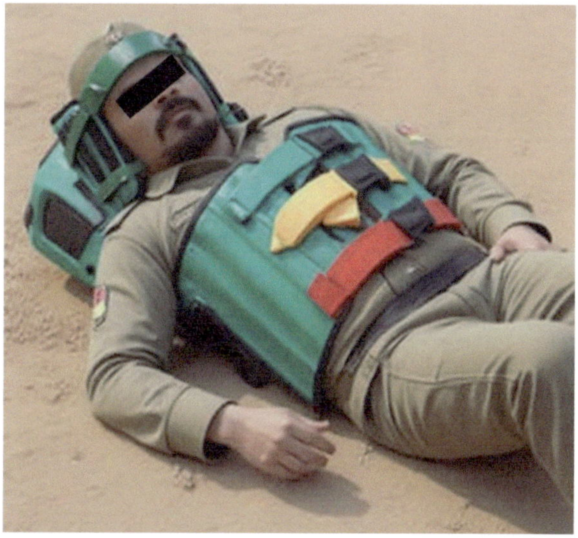

Fig. 9.4 Application of Kendrick extrication device on a soldier

5. Lateral Transfer Via Slide Board

- Reduces friction during bed-to-bed or surface transitions
- Requires coordinated movement to maintain alignment

Manual Handling Techniques (*When No Equipment Is Available*)

Even without formal gear, trained personnel can safely move a casualty using coordinated techniques:

Four-person lift:

- One at head, one at torso, one at hips, one at legs
- Lift simultaneously, maintaining alignment

Two-person carry:

- One stabilizes head and shoulders
- Second lifts pelvis and legs in line with torso

Cradle lift (for narrow terrain):

- One provider supports upper body with neck in line
- Second provider carries lower limbs, keeping spine flat

Log toll (if absolutely necessary)

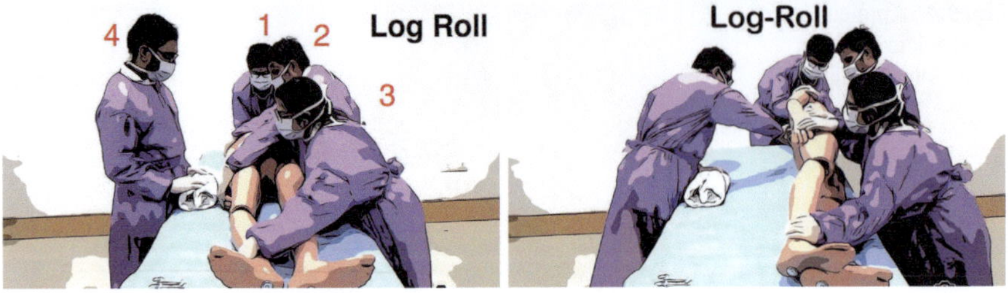

Fig. 9.5 Log roll technique

- Used only to assess the back or transfer to a rigid surface
- Minimum 3–4 personnel
- One stabilizes head/neck and leads count
- Others support shoulders, hips, and legs—roll as a single unit (Fig. 9.5)

Tactical Evacuation Considerations

- *CASEVAC vs. MEDEVAC:*
  CASEVAC (nonmedical platforms) may require extra stabilization prep. MEDEVAC platforms may allow more advanced care en route.
- *Movement in altitude or rough terrain:*
  Use padded litters, lash downs, and continuous reassessment of vitals. High altitude reduces perfusion and affects spinal cord autoregulation—use oxygen and warmth generously.
- *Prolonged field care scenarios:*

  When evacuation is delayed:
  - Reassess neuro function every 2–4 h
  - Monitor for signs of pressure injury
  - Keep the spine padded and aligned
    Adjust position slightly every few hours (with SMR maintained) to prevent complications

Risks and Complications of Transport

Prolonged SMR and improper transport may lead to:

- Pressure sores (especially on backboard)
- Respiratory compromise (in thoracic or high cervical injuries)
- Neuro deterioration due to spinal instability
- Pain and agitation, increasing movement and risk

Field Actions:

- Limit time on hard surfaces (<2 h if possible)
- Use padded supports or switch to vacuum devices at earliest opportunity
- Continue analgesia with ketamine or NSAIDs

Definitive Care

Once a spinal injury casualty reaches a higher-level facility, the focus shifts from field stabilization to detailed diagnosis, decompression, and rehabilitation. However, *the continuum of care remains tightly linked to the quality of field interventions.* The timely application of SMR, hemodynamic support, neuroprotection, and tactical evacuation decisions made earlier can directly influence long-term outcomes. Key management steps have been summarized in Table 9.1.

1. Tertiary Assessment
On arrival to a higher facility:

- Conduct a complete secondary survey, including reassessment of:
  - Airway, breathing, circulation
  - Neurologic status (ASIA charting)
    Vital sign trends from field notes
- Utilize MIST (mechanism, injuries, signs, treatment) data from prehospital phase

2. Imaging and Diagnostics
Depending on resource availability, perform:

Table 9.1 Summary of management of spinal injuries at definitive care facility

Aspect	Details
Initial assessment	Initial MARCH assessment, evaluate for spinal injury.
Immobilization	Use rigid cervical collars and spinal boards to prevent further injury.
Neurologic exam	Conduct thorough neurologic exams to assess the extent of spinal cord damage.
Radiographic assessment	Utilize X-rays, CT scans, and MRIs to identify fractures and spinal cord injuries.
Transport considerations	Ensure proper immobilization during transport.
Medical management	Administer medications to reduce inflammation and manage pain.
Surgical intervention	If necessary to stabilize the spine in unstable fractures to prevent further damage.
Rehabilitation	Implement physical therapy to maintain mobility and strength.
Return to duty	Assess the soldier's ability to return to duty based on recovery and functional capabilities.

- Lateral cervical spine X-ray (minimum in suspected cervical injuries)
- e-FAST to exclude internal bleeding
- Noncontrast CT scan—the gold standard for detecting spinal fractures
- MRI (if available) for assessing soft tissue, spinal cord edema, and ligamentous injury

3. Surgical Decision-Making
Surgery is considered based on:

- Spinal instability
- Cord compression
- Open fractures
- Progressive neurological deficits
  Surgical procedures may include:

- Decompression laminectomy
- Internal fixation using rods, screws
- Realignment and vertebral fusion
- Repair of dural tears and nerve roots

4. Neurocritical Care and Monitoring
Postoperative care includes:

- Ventilatory support, especially in high cervical injuries
- Vasopressors for maintaining spinal cord perfusion
- Bladder and bowel care
- Deep vein thrombosis (DVT) prophylaxis
- Steroid protocols (institution-dependent)

5. Rehabilitation Phase
Recovery often spans weeks to months and includes:

- Early passive range of motion exercises
- Physical and occupational therapy
- Assistive devices (braces, wheelchairs)
- Neurological reconditioning
- Psychiatric and psychological support for PTSD or adjustment disorders

Case Resolution

The soldier who sustained a fall from a 5-meter ledge at a high-altitude post was rapidly assessed and stabilized in the field. Despite sub-zero temperatures and limited equipment, spinal motion restriction was effectively maintained using improvised techniques: a rolled towel cervical collar, manual in-line stabilization, and insulation layers beneath and around the casualty to prevent spinal torsion during movement. A rigid makeshift stretcher fashioned from skis and sleeping mats was used to ensure spinal alignment throughout transport.

During Tactical Field Care, a focused neurologic exam revealed flaccid paralysis of the lower limbs with preserved upper limb function, diminished rectal tone, and tingling in the fingers—suggestive of a cervical spinal cord injury, likely above the T1 level. Cervical spine injury was immediately suspected due to the high-energy axial fall mechanism, the helmet being dislodged on impact, and the presence of neurological deficits, even though no gross deformity was noted. Immobilization was initiated early and maintained throughout.

The casualty's bradycardia (HR 48 bpm) and hypotension (BP 80/62 mmHg) were managed as neurogenic shock, rather than hypovolemic shock, due to the absence of external bleeding, warm extremities initially turning cold due to ambient exposure, and the presence of neurologic findings consistent with high spinal cord injury. Cautious fluid resuscitation with warm crystalloids was initiated, avoiding excessive volumes that could worsen hypotension from vasodilation. Passive rewarming strategies were continued using layered clothing, ponchos, and body heat transfer.

Throughout the 90-min evacuation, continuous monitoring was performed. Vitals were reassessed every 15 min, neurological status was monitored for deterioration, and spinal alignment was vigilantly preserved during transport across difficult terrain.

Upon arrival at a tertiary care facility, CT and MRI confirmed a burst fracture at the C6 vertebra with partial spinal cord compression. The casualty underwent anterior cervical decompression and fusion within the first 24 h. Early recognition of neurogenic shock, spinal immobilization, and field-based neuroprotection played a pivotal role in minimizing secondary injury.

Over the following weeks, the soldier began to show partial return of lower limb strength, particularly in proximal muscle groups. He was enrolled in a comprehensive neurorehabilitation program. By 6 months post-injury, he had regained enough function to return to active noncombat duty with assistive mobility support.

This case highlights the vital role of early spinal injury suspicion, the effective use of improvised immobilization techniques in austere environments, and the importance of differentiating spinal shock from other forms of shock. Tactical discipline in evacuation and neuroprotective strategies were instrumental in achieving long-term functional recovery and survival.

Key Messages

- Spinal trauma must always be suspected in falls, blasts, rollovers, or blunt trauma—even in the absence of visible injury.
- Spinal motion restriction (SMR), not immobilization, is the goal in combat care. Improvised tools often make the difference.
- Neurologic examination and reassessment should be ongoing. Sudden changes signal deterioration.
- Neurogenic shock presents with bradycardia and warm extremities—differentiate from hypovolemic shock and treat accordingly.
- Evacuation timing and technique are crucial. Poor handling may worsen otherwise reversible injuries.
- Ketamine is the analgesic of choice for spinal trauma in the field—maintains airway reflexes and perfusion.
- Combat providers are often the first and only line of defense in spinal cord preservation. Skill, confidence, and creativity save lives.

Conclusion

Spinal injuries on the battlefield are among the most catastrophic yet preventable causes of long-term disability. The tactical provider's ability to recognize spinal compromise early, apply motion-restricting strategies using limited resources, and plan for safe evacuation is critical to mission success and casualty survival. The unique stressors of combat—hostile terrain, environmental extremes, and delayed evacuation—demand that spinal care be improvised, disciplined, and protocol-driven.

Preserving combat mobility begins not in the hospital but in the field—at the moment of impact. Every minute counts. *Every movement matters.* And every trained provider is a force multiplier when they choose caution over haste, precision over panic, and readiness over routine.

Bibliography

1. American College of Surgeons Committee on Trauma. ATLS: Advanced Trauma Life Support. 10th ed. Chicago: American College of Surgeons; 2018. ISBN: 978-0996826235
2. Army U.S. Tactical Combat Casualty Care Handbook. Version 5. Morrisville (NC): Lulu Press Inc.; 2017. 130 p. ISBN: 9781678198312.
3. Auerbach PS, Cushing TA, Harris NS. Auerbach's Wilderness Medicine. 7th ed. 2 vols. Philadelphia: Elsevier; 2016. ISBN: 9780323359429
4. Bernstock, Joshua D et al. "Characteristics of combat-related spine injuries: a review of recent literature." *Military medicine* vol. 180,5 (2015): 503–12. https://doi.org/10.7205/MILMED-D-14-00215
5. Butler, Frank K Jr. "Tactical Combat Casualty Care: Beginnings." Wilderness & environmental medicine vol. 28,2S (2017): S12–S17. https://doi.org/10.1016/j.wem.2016.12.004

6. Connor, D et al. "Pre-hospital spinal immobilisation: an initial consensus statement." *Emergency medicine journal : EMJ* vol. 30,12 (2013): 1067–9. https://doi.org/10.1136/emermed-2013-203207
7. Furlan, Julio C et al. "Epidemiology of War-Related Spinal Cord Injury Among Combatants: A Systematic Review." *Global spine journal* vol. 9,5 (2019): 545–558. https://doi.org/10.1177/2192568218776914
8. Hawkins, Seth C et al. "Wilderness Medical Society Clinical Practice Guidelines for Spinal Cord Protection: 2024 Update." *Wilderness & environmental medicine* vol. 35,1_suppl (2024): 78S–93S. https://doi.org/10.1177/10806032241227232
9. Roberts, Timothy T et al. "Classifications In Brief: American Spinal Injury Association (ASIA) Impairment Scale." *Clinical orthopaedics and related research* vol. 475,5 (2017): 1499–1504. https://doi.org/10.1007/s11999-016-5133-4
10. Strauss, Rachel et al. "Evaluating the Tactical Combat Casualty Care principles in civilian and military settings: systematic review, knowledge gap analysis and recommendations for future research." *Trauma surgery & acute care open* vol. 6,1 e000773. 19 Oct. 2021, https://doi.org/10.1136/tsaco-2021-000773
11. Zong, Zhao-Wen et al. "Chinese expert consensus on the treatment of modern combat-related spinal injuries." *Military Medical Research* vol. 6,1 6. 20 Feb. 2019, https://doi.org/10.1186/s40779-019-0196-7

Thoracic Trauma in the Field

10

Dinesh Gora

Learning Objectives

- Identify and describe the types of thoracic trauma commonly seen in combat scenarios.
- Assess clinical signs and symptoms associated with penetrating and blunt thoracic injuries.
- Understand immediate field management strategies and when to prioritize evacuation.
- Outline advanced treatment options and the role of surgical intervention in severe cases.

Introduction

Thoracic trauma, involving injuries to the chest and its vital organs, is a frequent and often fatal occurrence in combat zones. In such settings, soldiers face unique risks of high-velocity penetrating trauma from gunfire and shrapnel as well as blunt trauma from explosions and vehicular accidents. These injuries pose a serious threat to life due to the chest's vital contents, including the heart, lungs, and major blood vessels. Immediate and effective management is crucial to survival, particularly given the limitations of the combat environment.

D. Gora (✉)
Department of Trauma Surgery and Critical Care, SMS Medical College and Hospital, Jaipur, Rajasthan, India

N. T. Rai, S. Misra (eds.), *Frontline Operational Resuscitation and Combat Emergencies (FORCE) Manual*, https://doi.org/10.1007/978-981-92-1622-2_10

Combat thoracic injuries can be broadly divided into *two categories: penetrating injuries and blunt injuries*. Penetrating injuries, such as those caused by bullets or shrapnel, often result in pneumothorax (air in the pleural cavity), hemothorax (blood in the pleural cavity), or potentially fatal damage to the heart or major vessels. Bullets and fragments from explosions can create extensive tissue damage by forming temporary cavities that disrupt surrounding structures. Blunt injuries, on the other hand, are common in blast events and vehicle-related incidents, causing rib fractures, pulmonary contusions, or a condition known as "blast lung" from shockwaves that damage lung tissue. Both types of injuries require swift recognition and intervention.

The combat field presents unique challenges for managing thoracic trauma. Medical personnel often have limited resources and are required to make rapid assessments in dangerous, sometimes austere, conditions. Traditional diagnostic tools, like X-rays or CT scans, are unavailable, requiring providers to rely on clinical skills and portable tools like ultrasound for fast diagnosis. Combat situations can also delay evacuation, so medics and field surgeons must be prepared to manage life-threatening chest injuries in the field. Given these constraints, specific training in Combat Casualty Care (CCC) has become essential. TCCC principles emphasize immediate interventions, like massive hemorrhage control, airway management, chest decompression and hypothermia prevention, to prevent death on the battlefield.

Efficient evacuation is another critical factor in survival for soldiers with thoracic trauma. Rapid transport to a facility with surgical capabilities is ideal, but logistical or environmental challenges may delay evacuation. In such cases, providers focus on stabilizing patients in the field to prevent deterioration. Tactical evacuation protocols prioritize the most severe cases, with thoracic trauma often receiving top priority due to the high risk of rapid health decline.

Advancements in combat medicine, such as portable ultrasound and vented chest seals, have improved field management of thoracic injuries. Portable ultrasound, for instance, allows detection of internal bleeding and pneumothorax, guiding timely interventions. Modern chest seals and hemostatic agents also enhance hemorrhage control and prevent complications, even in non-sterile environments. These innovations, alongside skilled assessment and combat protocols, have significantly improved outcomes for soldiers with thoracic trauma.

Effective management of thoracic trauma in combat demands a deep understanding of injury mechanisms, rapid assessment skills, and the ability to provide immediate, lifesaving care. This chapter explores these aspects, equipping medical personnel with the knowledge to handle one of the most challenging injury types on the battlefield.

Case Scenarios

Case Scenario 1: Penetrating Thoracic Injury During Firefight

During a close-quarter firefight in a forested border sector, a 27-year-old infantry soldier sustains a gunshot wound to the left chest. He is found conscious but visibly in pain and in respiratory distress. Entry and exit wounds are noted along the midaxillary line. Subcutaneous emphysema is palpable, and breath sounds are significantly diminished on the affected side. Respiration is rapid and shallow, and the heart rate is elevated.

- *Care Under Fire (CUF):*
  Under active engagement, initial hemorrhage control is applied using direct pressure and temporary dressings. The soldier is moved to cover once suppressive fire allows. No gross external bleeding is present. A non-vented chest seal is applied to the wound to manage suspected open pneumothorax and minimize air entrainment.
- *Tactical Field Care (TFC):*
  Following the MARCH sequence:
  M—massive hemorrhage: No active external bleeding. Wounds sealed with non-vented occlusive dressing. No signs of hemothorax at this stage.
  A—airway: Airway remains patent. Casualty is alert and speaking in short sentences due to breathlessness.
  R—respiration: Respiratory rate is 32/min, labored, with decreased breath sounds on the left. Subcutaneous emphysema is spreading. SPO_2 is dropping. Suspected developing tension pneumothorax prompts needle decompression at the 2nd intercostal space, midclavicular line, relieving pressure and improving ventilation.
  C—circulation: Tachycardia present but no hypotension. Capillary refill is borderline.
  H—head injury/hypothermia: No signs of head trauma. The casualty is covered with a blanket to prevent hypothermia in anticipation of shock onset.
- *Tactical Evacuation Care (TACEVAC):*
  With improved breathing post-decompression, the casualty is stabilized for TACEVAC. En route, monitoring continues for recurrence of tension symptoms. On arrival at the field surgical post, a chest tube is inserted. Imaging confirms a moderate hemopneumothorax. The patient stabilizes and is transferred to a higher care facility for further management.

Reflective Questions

1. What are the critical field indicators that differentiate a simple pneumothorax from a developing tension pneumothorax in a combat casualty?
2. What are the tactical and physiological considerations behind the initial use of a non-vented chest seal, and under what conditions should it be converted to an open seal or followed by needle decompression?

3. What factors—clinical, logistical, and tactical—should guide the decision to initiate TACEVAC after field stabilization of penetrating chest trauma?

Case Scenario 2: Blunt Thoracic Trauma from Roadside Blast

During a routine patrol near a conflict-prone border area, a 32-year-old soldier is thrown several meters following a roadside IED blast, landing on his left side. He is conscious and alert but complains of severe chest pain and dyspnea. No open wounds are visible, but abrasions and bruising are noted over the left hemithorax. Breathing is labored, and oxygen saturation is low on pulse oximetry. Rib fractures and pulmonary contusion are suspected based on mechanism and clinical findings (Fig. 10.1).

- *Care Under Fire (CUF):*
  The blast scene is cleared of secondary threats. Casualty is retrieved safely from the blast radius using a fireman's carry. Hemorrhage control is not required.
- *Tactical Field Care (TFC):*
  Following the MARCH sequence:
  M—massive hemorrhage: No external bleeding identified. Thoracic sweep reveals no penetrating trauma.
  A—airway: Airway is intact. No oropharyngeal bleeding or tracheal deviation observed.
  R—respiration: Respiratory rate is 26/min with grunting. Abrasions and tenderness over the left ribs suggest rib fractures. Breath sounds are decreased but bilateral. Pulse oximeter shows SpO_2 of 88% on room air. Supplemental oxygen is administered, and IV analgesia initiated to reduce splinting and improve ventilation.

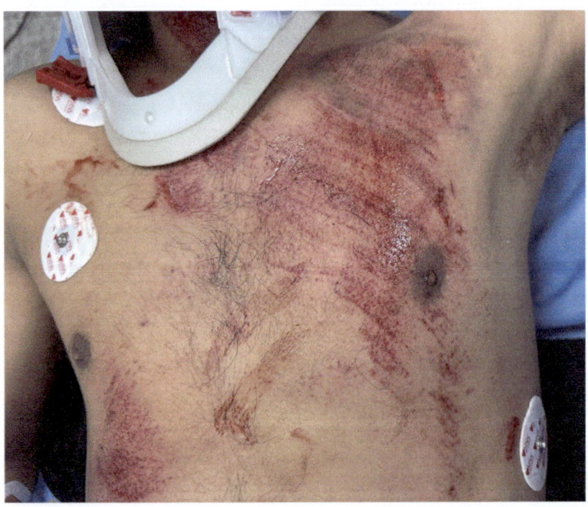

Fig. 10.1 Soldier with extensive chest abrasions following IED blast

C—circulation: BP and pulse are within normal range. Skin is warm but pale. No signs of internal bleeding.

H—head injury/hypothermia: No head injury evident. The casualty is protected from cold exposure due to extended field stay.

- *Tactical Evacuation Care (TACEVAC):*
  Evacuation is delayed due to terrain constraints. The medic provides ongoing monitoring—tracking respiratory rate, chest rise, SpO_2, and level of distress. The patient is positioned to reduce pain and optimize lung expansion. Over the next few hours, breathing stabilizes. At the field hospital, imaging confirms multiple left rib fractures with associated lung contusion, but no surgical intervention is required. Supportive care results in full recovery.

Reflective Questions

1. How do rib fractures compromise ventilation and oxygenation in a field setting, and what are the implications for functional capacity during evacuation delays?
2. Which clinical signs should heighten suspicion for pulmonary contusion in the absence of imaging, and how can field medics differentiate it from other causes of dyspnea?
3. Why is timely and adequate pain control a cornerstone of blunt chest injury management, and what are the tactical implications of undertreated pain in such casualties?
4. In resource-limited environments without access to imaging, how should field providers monitor and respond to potential respiratory decompensation in blunt thoracic trauma?

Anatomy of the Thoracic Cavity

The thoracic cavity is a complex anatomical space protected by the rib cage and containing vital organs crucial to life, including the heart and lungs. Understanding the anatomy is fundamental for diagnosing and managing thoracic trauma, particularly in the high stakes combat environment.

- *Thoracic skeleton*: The rib cage consists of 12 pairs of ribs, the sternum, and the thoracic vertebrae. The first through seventh ribs (true ribs) attach directly to the sternum, while the eighth through tenth (false ribs) connect via cartilage, and the eleventh and twelfth (floating ribs) are only attached to the spine. This structure protects the chest organs from injury, although it can fracture under significant force, potentially injuring underlying structures.
- *Diaphragm*: The diaphragm is the primary muscle of respiration, forming the lower boundary of the thoracic cavity. It is innervated by the phrenic nerve, and injury here can impede respiration, causing respiratory distress. Diaphragmatic injury can also lead to herniation, where abdominal organs enter the chest cavity.
- *Lungs*: The lungs are situated on either side of the heart and function in gas exchange. Each lung is divided into lobes (three in the right lung and two in the

left), with alveoli serving as the primary sites for oxygen and carbon dioxide exchange. The lungs are encapsulated by the pleura, a double-layered membrane with a pleural cavity in between, which contains fluid to reduce friction during lung expansion.
- *Heart and great vessels*: The heart lies centrally in the thoracic cavity, slightly tilted to the left, within the pericardial sac. Key vessels include the aorta, pulmonary arteries, and veins, and the vena cava. The proximity of these vessels to the lungs and ribs makes them susceptible to damage in penetrating or blunt trauma, leading to catastrophic hemorrhage if compromised.
- *Mediastinum*: This central compartment houses the heart, trachea, esophagus, and major vessels. Injuries here are often fatal, given the mediastinum's dense concentration of critical structures. It also provides a pathway for rapid spread of infections or air, as seen in cases of pneumomediastinum.

Mechanisms of Thoracic Trauma in Combat

Thoracic trauma in combat settings can be classified into two main types: penetrating and blunt trauma. Each mechanism presents distinct patterns of injury and management challenges due to the unique conditions of the battlefield.

- *Penetrating trauma*: High-velocity weapons like firearms and explosive devices are primary sources of penetrating injuries in combat. Bullets and shrapnel from explosions can cause extensive tissue disruption, often damaging multiple structures in the thoracic cavity. The energy transfer from high-velocity projectiles can create a temporary cavity, disrupting surrounding tissues beyond the direct path of injury.
- *Blunt trauma*: Blast waves, vehicular collisions, or falls in combat scenarios lead to blunt thoracic trauma. The force from a blast wave can cause rapid compression of the chest, leading to pulmonary contusion, rib fractures, and even rupture of the aorta. Crush injuries or concussive forces from explosions can result in complex injuries, including contusions and non-penetrating organ damage.

Types of Thoracic Injuries

(a) *Penetrating injuries*

Penetrating injuries in the thorax are typically caused by gunfire, shrapnel, or other high-velocity fragments.

1. *Pneumothorax*: When air enters the pleural cavity through a penetrating wound, the lung can collapse partially or fully (simple pneumothorax). In a tension pneumothorax, air becomes trapped in the chest, compressing the lung and shifting the mediastinum, which compromises cardiac function. Rapid needle decompression is required to prevent fatal cardiopulmonary collapse.

2. *Hemothorax*: Penetrating trauma can damage vessels, causing blood accumulation in the pleural cavity, leading to decreased lung expansion and potential hypovolemic shock. Hemothorax requires immediate evacuation of blood via chest tube to restore lung capacity and stabilize the patient.
3. *Cardiac tamponade*: Blood or fluid accumulating in the pericardium restricts heart function, impairing cardiac output and leading to obstructive shock. This condition is life-threatening, requiring pericardiocentesis or surgical intervention to relieve pressure.
4. *Open chest wounds*: An open pneumothorax, or "sucking chest wound," allows air into the pleural cavity, creating a pathway for air in and out of the chest. It prevents lung expansion, necessitating immediate application of an occlusive dressing or chest seal to maintain negative pressure within the thoracic cavity.

(b) *Blunt injuries*

Blunt thoracic injuries can result from impacts, blasts, or deceleration forces and include:

1. *Rib fractures*: Broken ribs impair respiratory function due to pain and structural instability. Multiple fractures (flail chest) create a segment that moves independently of the chest wall, often resulting in inadequate ventilation.
2. *Pulmonary contusion*: A pulmonary contusion results from alveolar-capillary membrane damage due to blunt trauma, leading to bleeding and edema within the lung parenchyma. This limits oxygenation and often worsens over time, making oxygen support critical.
3. *Blast lung*: A specific pattern from blast exposure, blast lung involves alveolar rupture, hemorrhage, and potential air embolism. Symptoms can be delayed, and oxygen therapy is necessary to manage hypoxia and prevent further injury.
4. *Diaphragmatic rupture*: Blunt trauma to the lower chest can tear the diaphragm, allowing abdominal organs to herniate into the thorax. This injury requires surgical repair but may be initially managed with respiratory support.

Clinical Assessment and Diagnosis

Effective management of thoracic trauma begins with a structured clinical assessment using the *MARCH approach* (massive hemorrhage, airway, respiration, circulation, and hypothermia prevention). Combat providers are trained to rapidly identify and prioritize life-threatening injuries.

1. *Primary survey*: Identifying immediate threats such as airway obstruction, tension pneumothorax, or cardiac tamponade. Techniques include visual inspection for open wounds, auscultation for breath sounds, and palpation for subcutaneous emphysema or rib instability.

2. *Secondary survey*: Conducted if the patient is stable, it includes a comprehensive examination to detect less obvious injuries. Field ultrasound (e.g., FAST scan) can assist in identifying hemothorax or pneumothorax.
3. *Diagnostic tools*: In the combat field, imaging options are limited, so reliance on clinical findings and portable tools like ultrasound is essential. Hypotension, tachypnea, and diminished breath sounds are critical indicators of severe injury requiring immediate action.

Field Management and Treatment Options

Initial field management aims to stabilize the patient, control bleeding, and prevent deterioration until evacuation. Key interventions include:

1. *Airway management*: Ensuring a patent airway is paramount. Basic airway adjuncts (e.g., oropharyngeal or nasopharyngeal airways) and, when trained personnel are available, advanced airway management (e.g., endotracheal intubation) may be required.
2. *Hemorrhage control*: External bleeding from chest wounds can be controlled with direct pressure, dressings, and, if necessary, tourniquets on limbs. Hemostatic agents are valuable tools in combat for controlling bleeding in noncompressible areas.
3. *Chest seals and needle decompression*: Open chest wounds are covered with vented chest seals to prevent air from entering the pleural space, minimizing pneumothorax risk. For tension pneumothorax, needle decompression in the second intercostal space at midclavicular line or in the fifth intercostal space at anterior axillary line (whichever is more accessible) releases trapped air and stabilizes breathing.

FORCE Tactical Pearl

"When breath sounds vanish, don't wait—decompress." In a combat casualty with unilateral chest trauma and signs of respiratory compromise (dyspnea, subcutaneous emphysema, hypoxia), assume tension pneumothorax and perform needle decompression promptly. Delayed intervention can lead to cardiac arrest from obstructive shock.

4. *Pain management*: Pain relief is essential for reducing hypoventilation due to rib fractures. In the field, analgesics are used, but they must be carefully managed to avoid respiratory depression.

FORCE Tactical Pearl

"Broken ribs break more than bones—they break breath." Rib fractures impair ventilation through pain-driven splinting. Early, adequate analgesia is not optional—it prevents hypoventilation, atelectasis, and field deterioration, especially when evacuation is delayed.

5. *Oxygen support and monitoring*: Portable oxygen systems provide supplemental oxygen to patients with hypoxia from pulmonary contusions or blast lung, while continuous monitoring ensures stability before evacuation.

Advanced Treatment and Surgical Interventions

Once the patient is transported to a higher level of care, advanced treatments and surgical interventions are performed as necessary:

1. *Tube thoracostomy (chest tube)*: For hemothorax or pneumothorax, insertion of a chest tube allows drainage of blood or air, re-expanding the lung and relieving respiratory distress.
2. *Thoracotomy*: In extreme cases, a thoracotomy (surgical opening of the chest) is necessary, particularly in cases of cardiac tamponade or massive hemorrhage. Although rarely performed in the field, it may be a lifesaving procedure in a well-equipped combat hospital.
3. *Damage control resuscitation (DCR)*: Aimed at controlling bleeding, DCR involves the use of blood products, minimizing crystalloid fluids, and achieving permissive hypotension to prevent further blood loss until surgical control is achieved. Combat providers trained in DCR principles can effectively manage bleeding and improve outcomes.
4. *Pericardiocentesis*: For cardiac tamponade, a needle is inserted into the pericardial sac to drain blood and relieve pressure on the heart. This procedure requires skill but can stabilize patients until they reach a surgical facility.
5. *Diaphragmatic repair*: Diaphragmatic ruptures from blunt trauma allow abdominal contents to move into the chest, requiring surgical intervention to reposition organs and repair the diaphragm.
6. *Evacuation and continuity of care*: Field stabilization efforts aim to bridge the gap to surgical care. Timely evacuation to a forward surgical team or combat support hospital is critical, as prolonged care in the field can lead to worsening complications. Triage during evacuation prioritizes patients with thoracic injuries due to their potential for rapid decline.

Case Resolution

Case 1: Penetrating Thoracic Injury

The 27-year-old infantry soldier who sustained a gunshot wound to the left chest during a close-quarter firefight was assessed and stabilized under hostile conditions. On initial examination, he presented with rapid, shallow breathing, decreased breath sounds on the injured side, and palpable subcutaneous emphysema—findings that suggested a developing tension pneumothorax. These field signs were pivotal in distinguishing it from a simple pneumothorax. Although his airway remained patent and he was alert, his worsening respiratory distress and dropping oxygen saturation demanded immediate intervention.

A non-vented chest seal was initially applied over the thoracic wound to prevent air from being drawn into the pleural space during inspiration, a key step in managing open pneumothorax in dusty, austere environments where vented seals may clog or malfunction. However, as signs of progressive intrathoracic pressure emerged—labored breathing, rising subcutaneous air, and decreasing SpO_2—the medic promptly performed needle decompression at the second intercostal space in the midclavicular line. This maneuver relieved trapped air, allowed partial lung re-expansion, and significantly improved the soldier's ventilation.

The decision to initiate tactical evacuation (TACEVAC) was guided by several factors: the likelihood of ongoing intrathoracic injury, the risk of recurrent tension physiology, and the need for definitive surgical management. Although the soldier stabilized after decompression, field care was continued during evacuation, with constant monitoring for signs of respiratory deterioration. At the field surgical unit, a chest tube was inserted, and imaging confirmed a moderate hemopneumothorax. His condition remained stable, and he was later transferred to a higher echelon of care. This case demonstrated how timely recognition of life-threatening thoracic pathology, appropriate use of non-vented chest seals, and effective decompression can prevent fatal outcomes—even in the chaos of combat.

Case 2: Blunt Thoracic Trauma

In a separate incident, a 32-year-old soldier was thrown several meters by a roadside IED blast and landed forcefully on his left side. Despite the absence of penetrating wounds, he complained of chest pain and dyspnea. Clinical assessment revealed bruising and tenderness over the left thorax, decreased breath sounds, and an SpO_2 of 88% on room air. These findings prompted field suspicion of rib fractures with underlying pulmonary contusion, based on both the mechanism and physical signs.

Rib fractures can severely impair ventilation in the field by causing pain-driven splinting, which reduces tidal volume and promotes hypoventilation. This increases the risk of atelectasis, retained secretions, and subsequent pneumonia—especially in scenarios where evacuation may be delayed. In this case, timely analgesia was initiated, relieving pain and enabling deeper breathing and more effective coughing, which are crucial for preventing secondary pulmonary complications. Supplemental oxygen was also administered to support oxygenation during the initial phase of care.

Though imaging was not immediately available, the medic monitored for signs of respiratory decompensation—increasing respiratory rate, falling oxygen saturation, and altered sensorium—through ongoing clinical assessment. Over the following hours, the casualty's respiratory status remained stable. Upon delayed arrival at the field hospital, imaging confirmed multiple left-sided rib fractures with an associated pulmonary contusion. No surgical intervention was required, and with continued supportive care, the soldier made a full recovery.

This case reinforced the importance of maintaining a high index of suspicion for internal thoracic injury in blunt trauma, even in the absence of external wounds. Early pain control, careful monitoring, and supportive interventions such as oxygen therapy played a decisive role in ensuring a favorable outcome. In remote combat environments without imaging, continuous clinical evaluation remains the cornerstone of decision-making and patient safety.

Key Messages

- Thoracic trauma is a common, potentially fatal injury in combat zones, often resulting from high-velocity penetrating wounds (bullets, shrapnel) and blunt trauma (explosions, vehicle accidents).
- The thoracic cavity houses critical organs such as the lungs, heart, major blood vessels, and diaphragm, all protected by the rib cage but vulnerable to combat-related injuries that can quickly lead to life-threatening conditions.
- Combat-related thoracic injuries are generally classified as either penetrating injuries, which can cause pneumothorax, hemothorax, or cardiac tamponade, or blunt injuries, which may result in rib fractures, pulmonary contusions, blast lung, or diaphragmatic rupture.
- Effective assessment in the field involves rapid identification of life-threatening injuries, often using the ABCDE approach (airway, breathing, circulation, disability, exposure) and, when available, portable ultrasound for detecting pneumothorax or hemothorax.
- Field management focuses on stabilizing patients before evacuation, with interventions like airway management, hemorrhage control, pain relief, and oxygen support; critical skills include applying chest seals, performing needle decompression for pneumothorax, and monitoring for complications.
- Advanced treatments, provided after evacuation, include inserting chest tubes for pneumothorax or hemothorax, thoracotomy for massive hemorrhage, pericardiocentesis for cardiac tamponade, and surgical repair for diaphragmatic injuries, with damage control resuscitation (DCR) protocols used to stabilize patients with severe blood loss.
- Innovations like portable ultrasound, vented chest seals, and hemostatic agents have improved field care and outcomes for thoracic injuries, with Tactical Combat Casualty Care (TCCC) training emphasizing the critical steps for survival on the battlefield.

Conclusion

Thoracic trauma remains one of the most lethal combat injuries, demanding swift, skilled, and protocol-driven management in the field. Whether caused by penetrating projectiles or blunt forces from blasts and impacts, chest injuries compromise vital respiratory and circulatory functions, often within minutes. This chapter highlights the importance of structured assessment using the MARCH algorithm to prioritize interventions—ranging from airway support and needle decompression to chest sealing and hypothermia prevention. The incorporation of innovations such as portable ultrasound, vented chest seals, and advanced hemostatic agents has significantly improved survival rates in austere environments. Yet the foundation of effective care lies in clinical vigilance, timely decision-making, and continuous reassessment during tactical evacuation. By mastering these principles, combat medics and frontline providers can dramatically reduce preventable deaths and stabilize casualties until definitive surgical care is available.

Bibliography

1. Holcomb, John B et al. "Causes of death in U.S. Special Operations Forces in the global war on terrorism: 2001-2004." *Annals of surgery* vol. 245,6 (2007): 986–91. https://doi.org/10.1097/01.sla.0000259433.03754.98
2. Eastridge, Brian J et al. "Death on the battlefield (2001–2011): implications for the future of combat casualty care." *The journal of trauma and acute care surgery* vol. 73,6 Suppl 5 (2012): S431–7. https://doi.org/10.1097/TA.0b013e3182755dcc
3. Mabry, Robert, and John G McManus. "Prehospital advances in the management of severe penetrating trauma." *Critical care medicine* vol. 36,7 Suppl (2008): S258–66. https://doi.org/10.1097/CCM.0b013e31817da674
4. Butler, F K Jr et al. "Tactical combat casualty care in special operations." *Military medicine* vol. 161 Suppl (1996): 3–16. https://doi.org/10.1007/978-3-319-56780-8_1
5. Shorr, R M et al. "Blunt thoracic trauma. Analysis of 515 patients." *Annals of surgery* vol. 206,2 (1987): 200–5. https://doi.org/10.1097/00000658-198708000-00013
6. Rhee, Peter et al. "Searching for the optimal resuscitation method: recommendations for the initial fluid resuscitation of combat casualties." *The Journal of trauma* vol. 54,5 Suppl (2003): S52–62. https://doi.org/10.1097/01.TA.0000064507.80390.10
7. Cap, Andrew P et al. "Damage Control Resuscitation." *Military medicine* vol. 183,suppl_2 (2018): 36–43. https://doi.org/10.1093/milmed/usy112
8. Feliciano DV, Mattox KL, Moore EE. *Trauma*. 9th ed. New York: McGraw Hill Medical; 2020. ISBN: 978-1260143355

11 Tactical Management of Abdominal and Pelvic Trauma

Amit Priyadarshi

Learning Objectives

By the end of this chapter, the reader will be able to:

- Identify key mechanisms of abdominal and pelvic trauma in combat and civilian trauma settings.
- Rapidly assess and triage patients using clinical signs and tactical algorithms.
- Implement field-based damage control resuscitation and hemorrhage control strategies.
- Determine indications for surgical intervention, including exploratory laparotomy, pelvic packing, and angioembolization.
- Apply tactical principles to stabilize patients during prolonged field care and facilitate safe evacuation.

Introduction

Abdominal and pelvic trauma represent some of the most complex and lethal injury patterns encountered in combat casualty care. These injuries, frequently caused by high-energy blasts, gunfire, and blunt trauma, can result in catastrophic hemorrhage, hollow viscus perforation, or multi-organ dysfunction. Unlike civilian settings, care in combat is often delivered under fire, without advanced imaging, and with delayed access to surgical teams. The ability of medics and field physicians to

A. Priyadarshi (✉)
Department of Trauma and Emergency Medicine, AIIMS, Bhopal, Madhya Pradesh, India

N. T. Rai, S. Misra (eds.), *Frontline Operational Resuscitation and Combat Emergencies (FORCE) Manual*, https://doi.org/10.1007/978-981-92-1622-2_11

recognize life-threatening signs and apply damage control principles at the point of injury is critical to improving survival.

Combat-related abdominal and pelvic trauma demands a dynamic approach grounded in Tactical Combat Casualty Care (TCCC) and the MARCH assessment framework. Field providers must rapidly identify signs of internal bleeding, airway compromise, pelvic instability, and hypoperfusion without relying on diagnostics like CT or X-ray. Instead, management is directed by clinical findings, mechanism of injury, and changes in patient response.

Hemorrhagic shock from pelvic fractures or intra-abdominal bleeding remains a leading cause of preventable battlefield deaths. Early interventions, such as tourniquets, pelvic binders, and tranexamic acid (TXA), alongside resuscitative strategies like permissive hypotension and warm blood products, are essential components of field-level damage control resuscitation (DCR). *The timely recognition of abdominal distension, seatbelt sign, absent bowel sounds, or scrotal bruising may be the only clues pointing toward a life-threatening bleed.*

This chapter explores the tactical management of abdominal and pelvic trauma through combat-relevant mechanisms, field-based assessment strategies, and resuscitative interventions. Anchored in real-world case application, it empowers field providers to act decisively, triage confidently, and bridge the gap until surgical care becomes available.

Case Scenario

During a dismounted foot patrol in the insurgency-affected foothills of Eastern Manipur, a 26-year-old infantry soldier is caught in the blast radius of an improvised explosive device (IED). Thrown several meters into a low stone wall, he is found moaning and semiconscious with multiple visible injuries. The area remains only partially secure, with hostile activity ongoing. No blood bank, imaging, or surgical support is available at the forward post. Evacuation is delayed by 60–90 min due to terrain and tactical limitations. A trained combat medic is the highest responder on site.

- *Care Under Fire (CUF)*
  Suppressive fire is maintained while the casualty is dragged to cover using a two-man carry. A rapid blood sweep reveals profuse bleeding from the right thigh. A tourniquet is applied immediately under fire. No further care is provided until the threat is suppressed.
- *Tactical Field Care (TFC)*
  Following the *MARCH sequence*:
  M—Massive Hemorrhage: Severe arterial bleeding from the right thigh is controlled with a high femoral tourniquet. Pelvic instability is noted on gentle compression; a pelvic binder is applied. No external abdominal hemorrhage seen, but signs suggest internal bleeding.
  A—Airway: Casualty is moaning with gurgling sounds—suggestive of partial airway obstruction. Oropharyngeal blood is suctioned, and a nasopharyngeal

airway (NPA) is inserted to maintain airway patency. He remains semiconscious.

R—Respiration: Respiratory rate is 30/min; right-sided breath sounds are diminished. Needle decompression is performed at the fifth intercostal space, anterior axillary line, with partial improvement in oxygenation and effort.

C—Circulation: Extremities are pale and cool. Radial pulse is faint. Heart rate is 138/min. Damage control resuscitation (DCR) initiated: warm crystalloid administered judiciously, followed by whole blood. TXA (1 g IV) is given within 30 min of injury.

H—Head Injury/Hypothermia: GCS is 9 (E3V2M4); pupils sluggish but equal. Presumed mild-to-moderate traumatic brain injury (TBI). Hypothermia prevention includes insulating layers and thermal wraps.

Secondary Survey:

- Lower abdominal bruising and distension without bowel sounds.
- Scrotal swelling and perineal ecchymosis, suggestive of pelvic trauma. No per rectal bleeding, but ongoing tenderness and instability on pelvic assessment (Fig. 11.1).

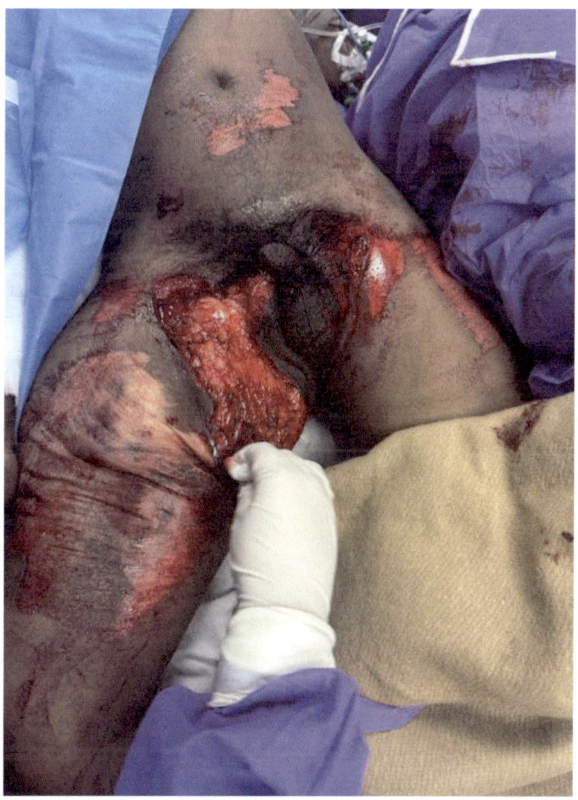

Fig. 11.1 Soldier with degloving injury over the right thigh and pelvic area due to IED blast

- *Tactical Evacuation Care (TACEVAC)*
  Evacuation is pending due to ongoing operations and difficult terrain. The casualty is monitored every 15 min for:
  - Mental status changes.
  - Signs of expanding abdominal girth.
  - Respiratory compromise.
    Hemodynamic stability.

The medic continues DCR, maintains a SBP of 110 mmHg, prioritizes blood products over crystalloids, and prepares for potential repeat needle decompression if respiratory signs worsen. Airway, circulation, and neurologic status are reassessed consistently. Coordination for aerial medevac is initiated as soon as airspace is secure.

Reflective Questions

1. What clinical signs made you suspect a pelvic fracture in the absence of radiologic imaging, and how does this influence field stabilization priorities?
2. Why is the application of a pelvic binder crucial in the prehospital phase, and what are the risks of improper placement or delayed use in suspected pelvic fractures?
3. In a resource-limited setting, how can you differentiate between abdominal distension due to internal hemorrhage and that caused by gastric dilation or bowel injury?
4. How do signs like perineal ecchymosis, scrotal swelling, and absent bowel sounds inform your working diagnosis and priorities for damage control resuscitation?
5. What are the field indicators for converting permissive hypotension to more aggressive resuscitation?

Mechanism of Injury

Understanding the *mechanism of injury (MOI)* is essential for anticipating the type and severity of trauma in a combat casualty. In the field, where diagnostics like ultrasound, X-ray, or CT scans are often unavailable, MOI becomes a key clinical tool for guiding immediate management and triage.

Blast Injuries

Blast trauma in the battlefield results in a complex interplay of multiple injury mechanisms. The four categories of blast-related injuries include primary, secondary, tertiary, and quaternary. Primary blast injuries are caused by the pressure wave and primarily affect air-filled organs, such as the lungs, intestines, and middle ear. These injuries can lead to pulmonary barotrauma, bowel perforation, and tympanic membrane rupture—sometimes with delayed presentation.

Secondary blast injuries arise from shrapnel and explosive debris. These are the most common battlefield injuries and typically result in penetrating wounds to the torso, abdomen, and extremities. Tertiary blast injuries occur when the casualty is physically displaced by the blast wind and impacts a solid surface. This often leads to blunt trauma, such as pelvic fractures, spinal injuries, and traumatic brain injury. Quaternary injuries include burns, crush injuries, inhalation injuries, and exposure to chemical contaminants.

Importantly, casualties close to the blast epicenter often experience a combination of all four types.

FORCE Tactical Pearl

Up to 50% of gluteal and perineal blast injuries involve deep pelvic, bowel, or rectal damage, often requiring surgical intervention.

Penetrating Trauma

Penetrating injuries in combat most commonly result from high-velocity rifle bullets; from fragmentation devices, such as IEDs and grenades; and, less frequently, from impalement or stab wounds. These injuries cause damage not only along the projectile path but also through temporary cavitation and fragmentation, making internal injury patterns unpredictable.

Combat statistics show that the small bowel is the most frequently injured organ in projectile trauma (50%), followed by the colon (40%), liver (30%), major abdominal vessels (25%), and diaphragm (20%). The extent of injury depends heavily on the projectile's velocity, angle of entry, fragmentation behavior, and proximity. Injuries caused by shotgun blasts or IED fragments within 3 m often result in catastrophic organ disruption and evisceration.

Suspicion should be high when:

- There is any penetrating wound between the nipple line and pubic symphysis.
- There is evisceration or exposed bowel.
- Vitals are unstable without obvious external bleeding.
- The patient has both abdominal and thoracic symptoms (indicating diaphragmatic involvement).

Combat field management includes the following:

- Apply occlusive dressings for any abdominal penetration.
- If evisceration is present, *cover—not replace*—bowel to preserve tissue integrity and prevent further contamination.
- Resuscitate per TCCC protocols (MARCH).
- Start broad-spectrum antibiotics if available.
- Elevate the head and shoulders slightly to minimize abdominal tension.

- Prioritize surgical evacuation—laparotomy is often needed even in stable patients due to risk of delayed perforation, sepsis, or bleeding.

FORCE Tactical Pearl
Any penetrating injury between the nipples and the pubic symphysis should be treated as potential abdominal trauma until proven otherwise.

Blunt Trauma

Blunt abdominal trauma is frequently seen in combat scenarios involving vehicle rollovers, falls from elevated terrain, or blast-induced body displacement. These injuries often affect solid organs, such as the liver and spleen, as well as the mesentery and retroperitoneum. Blunt trauma is particularly insidious because it can present with minimal external signs but still cause life-threatening internal bleeding.

Liver lacerations occur in approximately 40–45% of such injuries, followed closely by splenic rupture (35–40%), renal injuries (10–20%), and small bowel injuries (3–5%). Hollow viscus injuries, while less common, are particularly dangerous when diagnosis is delayed. *Mortality rises sharply when perforations go unnoticed for over 6 h, often progressing to fecal peritonitis and sepsis.*

Subtle clues, such as abdominal distension, guarding, diminished bowel sounds, and referred shoulder pain (Kehr's sign), should raise suspicion. Even in cases where vital signs appear stable, internal bleeding must be ruled out through repeated physical assessment and ongoing monitoring.

Field management priorities:

- Initiate *damage control resuscitation:* early TXA, blood products, and permissive hypotension.
- Monitor for progressive abdominal distension or worsening vitals.
- Avoid oral intake and minimize unnecessary movement.
- If evisceration is present, *cover exposed bowel with sterile, moist gauze; do not attempt to reinsert.*
- Prepare for urgent evacuation to surgical care.

FORCE Tactical Pearl
Delay in diagnosing hollow viscus injury beyond 6 h significantly increases mortality due to peritonitis and sepsis.

Pelvic Fractures

Pelvic trauma accounts for roughly 10% of all blunt trauma in combat environments and is a leading cause of non-compressible torso hemorrhage. These injuries often result from blast effects, motorcycle crashes, structural collapses, or falls from height. Fractures may be categorized into open-book (anteroposterior), lateral compression, or vertical shear types, each with unique bleeding risks and associated injuries.

Open-book fractures, commonly seen in blast trauma, lead to widening of the pelvic ring and extensive venous bleeding. Lateral compression injuries are frequently associated with vehicle crashes and can damage the bladder and urethra. Vertical shear injuries, often seen in high falls, involve displacement of the pelvis vertically, disrupting sacroiliac joints and associated vasculature.

Mortality in closed pelvic fractures with shock ranges from 10% to 42%, while open pelvic fractures can have a mortality rate as high as 50%. *Signs such as scrotal swelling, perineal bruising, leg length discrepancy, and blood at the urethral meatus should alert providers to possible pelvic disruption.*

In the field, once a pelvic fracture is suspected, manipulation should cease immediately to avoid exacerbating hemorrhage. *A pelvic binder should be applied firmly over the greater trochanters—not the iliac crests—to reduce bleeding and stabilize the fracture prior to evacuation or surgical intervention.*

> **FORCE Tactical Pearl**
> *Once a pelvic fracture is suspected, do not repeat compression. Apply a pelvic binder promptly over the greater trochanters, not the iliac crests.*

Clinical Assessment

Timely and accurate clinical assessment is the cornerstone of trauma care—especially in combat environments where access to imaging, laboratory support, and specialist consultation is often delayed or entirely unavailable. In these settings, the provider's ability to integrate mechanism of injury with structured clinical examination can determine survival. Tactical Combat Casualty Care (TCCC) recommends using the MARCH framework as the initial step in triage and stabilization, with ABCDE principles layered in as operational tempo allows.

M—Massive Hemorrhage

Hemorrhage remains the leading cause of preventable death on the battlefield. The first and most urgent task is to identify and control life-threatening external bleeding. For abdominal and pelvic trauma, the challenge lies in non-compressible hemorrhage, where bleeding is internal and not immediately visible.

In these cases, providers must think beyond extremity wounds. Pale skin, a thready pulse, rapid heart rate, altered mental status, and cool extremities may all suggest internal bleeding. Gentle palpation of the abdomen and pelvis can yield critical information: *if the pelvic ring feels unstable or if the abdomen is distended and firm, internal hemorrhage should be assumed.* In the absence of visible bleeding, these signs must prompt immediate interventions, such as pelvic binder application, volume-conserving resuscitation, and preparations for rapid evacuation.

Tourniquets should be rechecked for proper placement and pressure, especially when applied under fire. Bleeding from groin or buttock injuries may require wound packing with hemostatic agents and firm pressure, particularly when junctional tourniquets are unavailable.

A—Airway

In abdominal and pelvic trauma, airway compromise may be secondary to altered mental status, traumatic brain injury, or associated thoracic injuries, such as flail chest or diaphragmatic rupture. An unconscious or a semiconscious patient with a Glasgow Coma Score (GCS) of <8 requires airway protection.

Simple steps—such as suctioning of the oropharynx, insertion of a nasopharyngeal or oropharyngeal airway, and patient positioning—can maintain patency until definitive airway control is achieved. Facial trauma, cervical spine injury, or vomitus must all be considered when selecting the appropriate airway technique.

In cases where intubation is not feasible due to equipment limitations or anatomical distortion, cricothyrotomy should be considered early, particularly if the casualty shows signs of progressive hypoxia or airway obstruction.

R—Respiration

Assessment of breathing is essential in every casualty with thoracoabdominal or pelvic trauma. Inspection should begin with exposure of the chest and upper abdomen to evaluate for symmetry of movement, use of accessory muscles, bruising, or penetrating wounds.

Auscultation—if time and conditions allow—should confirm bilateral breath sounds. Absent or diminished breath sounds on one side, especially following blast or penetrating injury, suggest pneumothorax or hemothorax. In such cases, needle decompression should be promptly performed at the fifth intercostal space, anterior axillary line, or second intercostal space at the mid-clavicular line (whichever feasible). Chest seals may be applied to sucking chest wounds.

Blunt trauma to the lower ribs should raise suspicion for associated splenic or hepatic injury. Lower rib fractures on the left side often accompany splenic rupture; on the right, they may suggest liver laceration. Both scenarios should increase the index of suspicion for internal bleeding.

C—Circulation

Circulatory assessment in the field focuses on identifying signs of shock and directing resuscitation accordingly. Vital signs, including pulse rate, pulse quality, blood pressure (if measurable), and mental status, should be evaluated repeatedly.

Tactile signs, such as a weak radial pulse, cold limbs, delayed capillary refill, and altered mentation, may be the only available indicators of poor perfusion in the absence of monitoring equipment.

In pelvic trauma, especially when instability is noted, providers should assume active retroperitoneal bleeding. Prompt application of a pelvic binder reduces pelvic volume and promotes clot formation. If intravenous or intraosseous access is available, resuscitation should follow the *principles of damage control resuscitation (DCR): early administration of blood or whole blood, limited crystalloid use, permissive hypotension (target systolic BP of 80–90 mmHg), and early TXA administration (within 3 h of injury).*

Abdominal trauma with hypotension and a distended abdomen is a surgical emergency. Continued bleeding may lead to rapid cardiovascular collapse. In these cases, rapid packaging and evacuation take precedence over any prolonged field interventions.

H—Head Injury/Hypothermia

Although this chapter focuses on abdominal and pelvic trauma, assessment of neurologic status is essential. Blunt trauma patients may have concurrent traumatic brain injury, especially following blast exposure or falls. Assess GCS, pupillary response, and limb movement.

If the patient is confused, drowsy, or nonverbal without apparent cause, traumatic brain injury or hypoperfusion should be suspected. This affects resuscitation strategies—*permissive hypotension should be avoided in TBI cases.*

Hypothermia is a silent killer in trauma, exacerbating coagulopathy and acidosis. Even in desert or temperate zones, casualties can become hypothermic quickly due to shock, exposure, and evaporation. Use hypothermia prevention kits, wrap the casualty in layers, insulate from the ground, and warm fluids whenever possible.

Integration of Assessment into Field Practice

In the combat zone, assessments must be prioritized based on the tactical environment, available personnel, and time. The MARCH framework allows providers to rapidly identify and treat life-threatening conditions in order of urgency. Once stabilized, a more detailed secondary survey—including a full head-to-toe examination, reassessment of vital signs, and monitoring trends over time—can be performed.

Importantly, every assessment should be dynamic and repeated frequently, especially in prolonged field care scenarios. A stable casualty can decompensate without warning. *Vigilance, pattern recognition, and protocol adherence are what separate a positive outcome from a preventable fatality in battlefield trauma.*

Focused Abdominal Exam

Key signs of concern:

- Abdominal distension or rigidity.
- Seatbelt sign or flank bruising (Fig. 11.2).
- Rebound tenderness, involuntary guarding.
- Absent bowel sounds.
- Pain out of proportion to findings.

These findings suggest solid organ rupture, mesenteric tear, or perforation.

> **FORCE Tactical Pearl**
> *The absence of peritoneal signs does not rule out injury—reassess frequently.*

Pelvic Exam

Gently assess for instability; apply pelvic binder if suspected.
Check for:
Perineal bruising.
Hematuria.

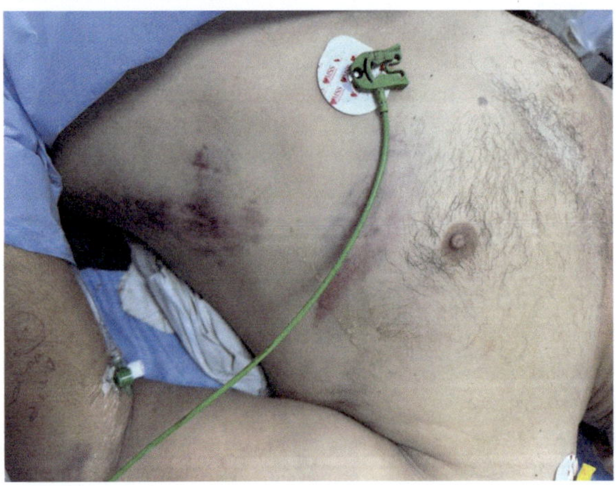

Fig. 11.2 Bruising of the abdominal wall suggestive of solid organ injury in a soldier

Rectal bleeding.
Scrotal swelling.

Do not insert urinary catheters if urethral trauma is suspected.

Management Strategies in Combat Settings

In resource-limited combat environments, managing abdominal and pelvic trauma revolves around *early hemorrhage control, damage control resuscitation (DCR), and prioritized evacuation planning*. The goal is to stabilize casualties long enough to enable survival until surgical care is available.

1. *Hemorrhage Control*
   - *Tourniquets*: For extremity wounds, apply high and tight. Document time.
   - *Pelvic binders*: Apply over greater trochanters (not iliac crests) in cases of suspected pelvic instability. Improves hemodynamics and limits bleeding volume.
   - *Hemostatic dressings*: Used for junctional wounds (groin/perineum) where tourniquets are not effective.
   - *Direct pressure + packing*: Critical for low-pressure sites and when binders are ineffective.
2. *Damage Control Resuscitation (DCR)*

> **FORCE Tactical Pearl**
> *Pelvic instability + hypotension + no obvious limb bleed = assume internal pelvic hemorrhage, until proven otherwise.*

DCR prioritizes the following:

- *Permissive hypotension*: Maintain SBP 80–90 mmHg unless TBI is suspected.
- *Early TXA*: 1 g IV within 3 h of injury, followed by a second dose as needed.
- *Balanced blood transfusion*: Whole blood preferred. If unavailable, 1:1:1 (RBC/plasma/platelets) is ideal.
- *Minimize crystalloids*: Excess fluids worsen dilutional coagulopathy and hypothermia.

In prolonged field care, warmed fluids, IO access, and resuscitative warming blankets are essential adjuncts.

3. *Prolonged Field Monitoring*
   If evacuation is delayed (>1 h), follow the *prolonged casualty care (PCC) model*:

- Reassess vitals and mental status every 15 min.
- Monitor abdominal girth and tension.
- Reevaluate airway and breathing (consider repeat decompression if worsening).

4. *Decision to Evacuate*

   Evacuation must not be delayed if:
   - Abdominal distension increases.
   - Consciousness deteriorates (esp. with TBI).
   - Shock does not respond to fluids.
   - Signs of peritonitis emerge.

Tactical triage should balance the need for surgical care with real-time threat assessment and platform availability.

Damage Control Approach

When immediate surgical repair is not possible—the damage control (DC) approach becomes lifesaving. This involves *abbreviated surgery and staged resuscitation focused on the lethal triad of trauma: hypothermia, acidosis, and coagulopathy.*

Phase I: Damage Control Surgery

Objectives

- *Stop the bleeding:*
  - *Pelvic packing*: Blunt pelvic trauma often causes venous plexus bleeding; pre-peritoneal gauze packing can tamponade bleeding.

    Ligate/clamp major vessels: Control arterial hemorrhage rapidly.
- *Control contamination:*
  - Staple or suture injured bowel.
  - Debride necrotic tissue.

    Drain biliary/pancreatic leaks.
- *Temporary closure:*

  Use VAC dressings, towel clips, or sterile sheets to loosely approximate abdominal walls.

> **FORCE Tactical Pearl**
>
> *Do not attempt definitive repair in unstable patients. Time in OR should be under 60 min.*

Phase II: Intensive Resuscitation

Done in higher facilities:

- Active rewarming (fluid warmers, Bair huggers).
- Lab-guided correction of coagulopathy (TEG/ROTEM).
- Monitor base deficit, lactate, and urine output.

Phase III: Definitive Surgery

- Return to OR within 48 h if stable.
- Remove packing, and perform organ repair, anastomosis, or definitive hemorrhage control.
- Aim for fascial closure if tissue permits; otherwise plan staged closure.

Organ-Specific Injuries

Combat trauma involving the abdomen often presents as polyvisceral injury, with damage affecting multiple organs simultaneously. In battlefield conditions—where imaging, surgical teams, and specialist support may be delayed—identifying likely injury patterns based on the mechanism of injury and physical signs becomes essential. Each organ has unique vulnerabilities and implications for field care, resuscitation priorities, and surgical urgency.

Liver Injuries

The liver is the most frequently injured solid organ in both blunt and penetrating abdominal trauma, *accounting for nearly 30–45% of cases in combat settings*. Due to its large size and rich vascular supply, hepatic trauma can result in significant blood loss.

Field recognition typically includes right upper quadrant tenderness, abdominal distension, hypotension, and signs of hypoperfusion. Referred right shoulder pain (Kehr's sign) may also occur due to diaphragmatic irritation.

In the absence of imaging, progressive abdominal firmness or tachycardia unresponsive to resuscitation should raise suspicion. FAST (if available) can help detect perihepatic fluid collections. For penetrating trauma, injury trajectory is crucial—any right-sided wound below the costal margin must be assumed to involve the liver.

Field Management
- Initiate resuscitation following DCR principles: TXA, blood products, and minimal crystalloids.
- Avoid unnecessary palpation of the abdomen.
- Prioritize early surgical evacuation if instability persists.

Splenic Injuries

The spleen is the second most common solid organ injured in abdominal trauma and is particularly vulnerable in left-sided rib fractures, falls, or deceleration injuries.

Clues to splenic injury include left upper quadrant pain, left-sided lower rib tenderness, or referred pain to the left shoulder. In battlefield scenarios, this diagnosis often relies on clinical suspicion and vital sign trends, as direct visualization is rarely possible.

Delayed rupture of the spleen is also a known risk, and casualties may initially appear stable before suddenly decompensating.

Field Management

- Monitor for hypotension, worsening pain, or increasing abdominal girth.
- Consider splenic trauma in any left thoracoabdominal mechanism.
- Plan for urgent evacuation if the patient is deteriorating despite fluids.

Hollow Viscus Injuries

Injuries to the stomach, small intestine, or colon are notoriously difficult to detect in the field but carry a high risk of morbidity and mortality due to contamination, peritonitis, and sepsis. These injuries may occur from blast overpressure, direct penetration, or blunt force.

Patients may initially appear stable but will often develop diffuse abdominal pain, guarding, and progressive distension over time. The absence of bowel sounds or rebound tenderness may be late signs. In settings where a FAST exam reveals free intraperitoneal fluid without evidence of solid organ injury, a hollow viscus injury should be suspected.

Clinical Clues

- Seatbelt sign, abdominal bruising, or visible evisceration.
- Peritonitis: rigidity, pain with movement, and involuntary guarding.
- Shock that progresses despite control of external hemorrhage.

Field Management

- Avoid oral intake.
- Begin broad-spectrum antibiotics if available.
- Expedite surgical evacuation; definitive management requires laparotomy and repair.
- Continue reassessment every 15–20 min.

Diaphragmatic Injury

The diaphragm can be injured in blunt or penetrating trauma that crosses the lower thoracic border. Left-sided injuries are more common due to the protective effect of the liver on the right. These injuries can lead to herniation of abdominal contents into the chest, impairing both respiratory and cardiac functions.

In the field, suspicion arises from:

- Abdominal trauma with concurrent dyspnea or decreased breath sounds.
- Bowel sounds heard in the chest.
- Worsening hypoxia without a clear pulmonary source.

If imaging is unavailable, consider the possibility of diaphragmatic rupture in any casualty with thoracoabdominal trauma, respiratory distress, and abnormal chest examination findings.

Field Management

- Treat for tension pneumothorax if suspected.
- Avoid positive pressure ventilation unless airway is secured.
- Urgent evacuation required for surgical correction.

Renal and Genitourinary Trauma

Kidney injuries may result from blunt trauma to the flank or deceleration injuries, while bladder and urethral injuries are often associated with pelvic fractures or perineal blast injuries.

Signs of renal trauma include flank bruising, hematuria, and lower rib tenderness. In contrast, blood at the urethral meatus, inability to void, or scrotal hematoma may suggest urethral or bladder disruption.

Combat Considerations

- Do not insert a Foley catheter if urethral injury is suspected.
- A suprapubic catheter may be required, but only by trained personnel.
- Associated rectal or vaginal injuries must be suspected in open pelvic fractures.

Field Management

- Focus on hemorrhage control and pelvic stabilization.
- Minimize manipulation of the genitalia.
- Initiate antibiotics early if perineal or rectal wounds are present.

Multi-organ Injuries

In many combat scenarios, it is not a question of which organ is injured—*but how many*? Polytrauma involving combinations of solid organ lacerations, hollow viscus perforation, and pelvic disruption is common after blasts and high-energy impacts.

Field providers must prioritize:

- Hemorrhage control (pelvic binder, fluids, TXA).
- Airway and respiratory support.
- Early identification of abdominal contamination and peritonitis.
- Triage decisions for urgent surgical intervention.

Casualties presenting with hypotension, abdominal bruising, pelvic instability, and altered mentation should be presumed to have multi-organ injury and managed aggressively from the start.

In such scenarios, the threshold for emergency laparotomy is guided by clinical and operational indicators, such as ongoing hypotension, evidence of peritoneal signs, or imaging suggestive of intra-abdominal catastrophe—criteria depicted in Table 11.1.

At a combat medical treatment facility (CMTF), trauma care is escalated based on injury mechanism—blunt versus penetrating trauma. As outlined in Fig. 11.3, blunt trauma is assessed using Focused Assessment with Sonography in Trauma (FAST) to detect free fluid, guiding resuscitation and decision-making. Penetrating injuries (Fig. 11.4), particularly those involving the torso or abdomen, are rapidly triaged for surgical intervention.

Table 11.1 Indications for exploratory laparotomy

	Blunt injury	Penetrating injury
Absolute	Anterior abdominal injury with hypotension Abdominal wall disruption Peritonitis Free air under the diaphragm on chest radiograph Positive FAST or DPL in hemodynamically unstable patient CT-diagnosed injury requiring surgery	Injury to the abdomen, back, and flank with hypotension Abdominal tenderness GI evisceration High suspicion for transabdominal trajectory after gunshot wound CT-diagnosed injury requiring surgery
Relative	Positive FAST or DPL in hemodynamically stable patient Solid visceral injury in stable patient Hemoperitoneum on CT without clear source	Positive local wound exploration after stab wound

Abbreviations: FAST focused assessment with sonography in trauma, *DPL* diagnostic peritoneal lavage

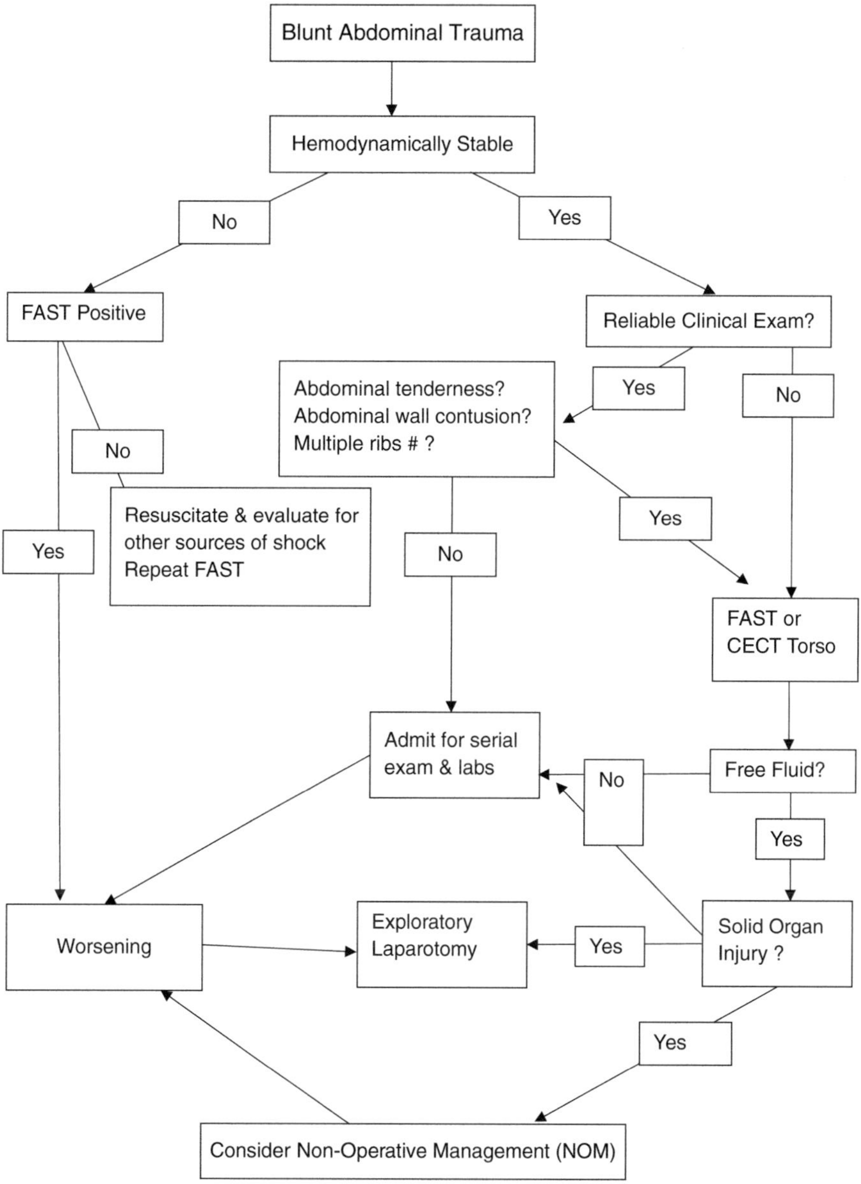

Fig. 11.3 Management algorithm for blunt abdominal trauma

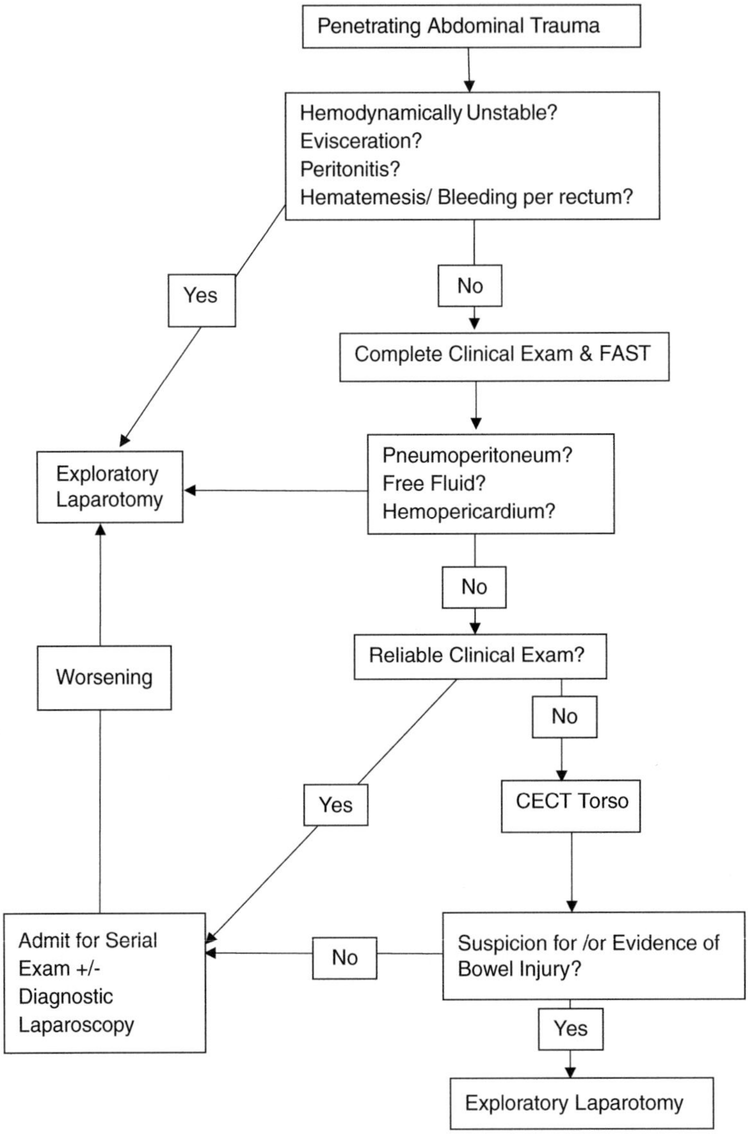

Fig. 11.4 Management algorithm for penetrating abdominal trauma

Pelvic Fractures and Tactical Management

Pelvic fractures in combat trauma are among the most lethal injury patterns due to their association with non-compressible hemorrhage, polyvisceral damage, and high-energy mechanisms. Accounting for up to 10% of all blunt trauma cases, pelvic injuries can result in up to 50% mortality when associated with hemorrhagic shock or open wounds. In battlefield settings, where imaging is not immediately available and surgical intervention may be delayed, the early recognition and stabilization of pelvic fractures are essential to prevent death from exsanguination.

Anatomical and Clinical Significance

The pelvis is a ringlike structure composed of the sacrum, ilium, ischium, and pubic bones. It contains major vascular structures (e.g., internal iliac arteries and venous plexuses), the lower urinary tract, rectum, and reproductive organs. Disruption of this ring—especially in open-book (AP compression) or vertical shear fractures—can lead to catastrophic hemorrhage from both venous and arterial sources.

Additionally, the retroperitoneal space, which cannot be compressed externally, can accommodate 3–4 L of blood before tamponade occurs. This makes pelvic bleeding both hidden and rapidly fatal if not controlled early.

Mechanism of Injury in Combat

Common mechanisms causing pelvic trauma in the field include:

- *Blast injuries (IEDs, landmines)*: Direct explosive force or body displacement leading to open-book or lateral compression fractures.
- *Falls from height*: Often lead to vertical shear injuries and sacroiliac joint disruption.
- *Motorcycle or vehicle collisions*: Rapid deceleration with anterior impact commonly causes open-book patterns.
- *Crush injuries*: Occur during structural collapse or armored vehicle rollovers.

In these settings, pelvic fractures often coexist with abdominal, thoracic, spinal, or extremity injuries.

Classification

While the Young-Burgess classification is used in trauma centers, for tactical care purposes, pelvic injuries can be grouped into:

- *Open-book (AP compression)*: Widened symphysis pubis; associated with venous hemorrhage.
- *Lateral compression*: Pelvic ring buckles inward; may injure internal structures like the bladder or urethra.
- *Vertical shear*: Hemipelvis displaced upward; disrupts major vessels and ligaments—most unstable type.

Understanding the mechanism helps anticipate bleeding source, associated injuries, and transport urgency.

Field Signs and Clinical Indicators

In the absence of imaging, providers must rely on physical signs and mechanism history. Key findings include:

- Unstable pelvic ring on gentle, single compression (*do not repeat if positive*).
- Shortened or externally rotated lower extremity.
- Perineal bruising or scrotal hematoma.
- Blood at the urethral meatus or high-riding prostate (suggests urethral injury).
- Hypotension unresponsive to fluids or external bleeding control.

FORCE Tactical Pearl
Remember, a normal exam does not rule out bleeding. Up to 25% of patients with severe pelvic hemorrhage may not show obvious external signs initially.

Tactical Field Management

1. *Pelvic Binder Application*

Pelvic binders or improvised pelvic wraps (e.g., cravat or bedsheet with windlass) must be applied over the greater trochanters, not the iliac crest. The binder stabilizes the pelvis, reduces pelvic volume, promotes clot formation, and improves hemodynamics. Application should occur immediately upon suspicion of pelvic fracture—ideally within the first 10 min of care.

Improvised binder method:
- Use a bedsheet or wide cloth (Fig. 11.5).
- Center it over the greater trochanters.
- Twist tightly, and then secure with knot, clamp, or windlass.

Caution Misplacement (too high) is ineffective and may worsen outcomes.

2. *Hemorrhage Control and Resuscitation*

   Pelvic fracture bleeding is often venous, though arterial hemorrhage may occur, especially in vertical shear injuries. The following steps are essential:
   - *TXA*: Administer 1 g IV within the first hour of injury; follow with a second dose if needed.
   - *Blood products*: Use whole blood or 1:1:1 component therapy if available. Avoid large volumes of crystalloids.

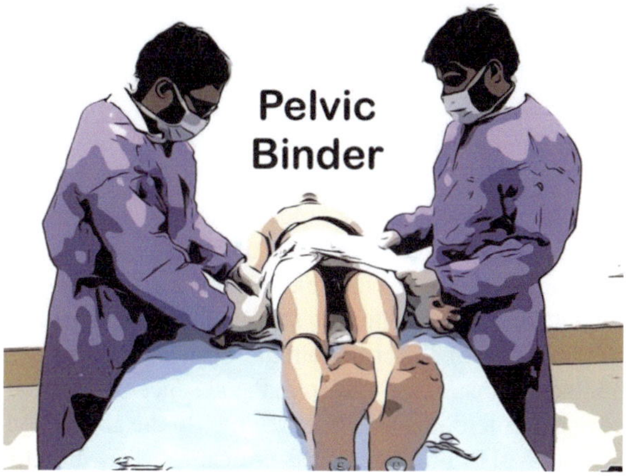

Fig. 11.5 Improvised pelvic binder using bedsheet

- *Permissive hypotension*: Target SBP 80–90 mmHg in the absence of TBI. This helps limit bleeding while maintaining perfusion.
- *Avoid catheterization*: If blood is present at the meatus or there is high suspicion of urethral injury, do not insert a Foley catheter in the field.
- *Antibiotics and tetanus*: In open fractures, begin broad-spectrum antibiotics and update tetanus prophylaxis when feasible.

3. *Prolonged Field Care and Evacuation*

   In prolonged care settings, continue to monitor for:
   - Increasing abdominal girth or worsening vitals (suggestive of ongoing hemorrhage).
   - Neurovascular status of the lower limbs.
   - Pelvic binder pressure points (to avoid ischemia).

Reassess every 15–30 min, document fluid balance, and ensure the patient is insulated against hypothermia. Pain management (e.g., ketamine and fentanyl lozenges) is essential to reduce movement and oxygen consumption.

Evacuation to surgical care is urgent if:

- The patient remains hypotensive after initial resuscitation.
- Associated injuries (e.g., open fracture and suspected bowel injury) are present.
- There is evidence of urethral disruption or perineal contamination.

Surgical Considerations in Higher Facilities

In settings with surgical capability, the following may be required:

- *Preperitoneal pelvic packing* for hemostasis in unstable patients.
- *Angiographic embolization* for arterial bleeding (if imaging available).
- *External fixation* of the pelvis to enhance stability.
- *Laparotomy* for associated abdominal injuries.

Surgical interventions should follow damage control principles, focusing on bleeding and contamination control before definitive repair.

Case Resolution

The 26-year-old infantry soldier, injured during a dismounted patrol by an IED blast, was stabilized in the field using structured MARCH assessment and damage control resuscitation principles. The immediate application of a high femoral tourniquet effectively controlled the massive hemorrhage from the right thigh. However, the presence of lower abdominal bruising, scrotal swelling, perineal ecchymosis, and pelvic instability—despite the absence of external abdominal wounds—raised strong suspicion for a pelvic fracture. In the absence of radiological tools, this constellation of clinical signs was critical for early identification and guided the timely application of a pelvic binder. Proper placement of the binder at the level of the greater trochanters helped tamponade venous bleeding and prevent further shearing injury to pelvic vessels. Delayed or misapplied pelvic stabilization in such settings could have resulted in ongoing hemorrhage, worsening shock, or further injury during transport.

The patient's abdominal distension and absent bowel sounds, coupled with a soft yet tender abdomen and signs of hypoperfusion, raised concern for internal hemorrhage rather than isolated gastric dilation. Although imaging was unavailable, the distension pattern, mechanism of injury, and associated pelvic trauma supported a presumptive diagnosis of solid organ or retroperitoneal bleeding. In this setting, bowel injury and gastric dilation—though possible—were less likely without vomiting, abdominal guarding, or high-pitched bowel sounds. Thus, abdominal hemorrhage was prioritized as the leading threat in the ongoing resuscitation plan.

The patient also presented with a GCS of 9, sluggish pupils, and an evolving head injury, necessitating a delicate balance during resuscitation. In such scenarios, field providers must maintain cerebral perfusion while avoiding over-resuscitation that could worsen abdominal or pelvic bleeding. The medic's goal was to sustain a systolic blood pressure between 100 and 110 mmHg, allowing enough perfusion for the brain while reducing further hemorrhagic loss. Whole blood transfusion was prioritized over crystalloid fluids to maintain oxygen delivery and clotting factors, while TXA was administered within the golden window to mitigate trauma-induced coagulopathy.

Repeat reassessments of respiratory status were crucial. The initial improvement after needle decompression suggested a partial pneumothorax relief. However, the provider remained vigilant for recurrence or signs of a missed hemothorax, particularly if respiratory status deteriorated again—an important consideration before deciding to reattempt decompression.

Throughout the prolonged care phase, the medic maintained reassessments every 15 min, closely monitoring mental status, abdominal girth, and hemodynamic trends. Thermal management prevented further coagulopathy and shock progression. Despite the high-risk polytrauma, structured field care, rapid interventions, and anticipation of complications likely improved this soldier's survival odds before definitive surgical care became available.

Key Messages

- Abdominal and pelvic trauma are leading causes of preventable death in combat settings due to occult hemorrhage and delayed diagnosis.
- Mechanism of injury, physical findings, and patient response are the foundation for triage in environments without imaging.
- Pelvic binders, TXA, and early fluid resuscitation are lifesaving in hemodynamically unstable pelvic injuries.
- Damage control resuscitation (DCR) principles—permissive hypotension, blood-first resuscitation, and minimal crystalloid—are vital.
- Prolonged field care protocols emphasize reassessment, warming, and packing for delayed evacuation.
- Evacuation should not be delayed when signs of intra-abdominal bleeding, altered mental status, or shock persist.
- Training and preparation—more than technology—determine survival in austere combat trauma care.

Conclusion

Combat trauma involving the abdomen and pelvis poses significant challenges due to its hidden nature and potential for rapid decompensation. In austere environments, the lack of imaging and surgical resources necessitates reliance on clinical signs, injury mechanism, and tactical decision-making. The MARCH framework and TCCC phases provide structure to initial assessment and intervention, emphasizing early hemorrhage control, airway stabilization, and damage control resuscitation. Pelvic fractures and intra-abdominal bleeding should be presumed when instability or shock coexist and managed accordingly with binders, TXA, and permissive hypotension. When imaging and surgery are delayed, prolonged field care and constant reassessment become critical bridges to definitive management. This chapter reinforces that with protocol-driven care, tactical awareness, and decisive action, medics and frontline providers can significantly reduce mortality and improve functional outcomes, even in the most extreme settings of combat trauma.

Bibliography

1. "Battlefield advanced trauma life support (BATLS)." *Journal of the Royal Army Medical Corps* vol. 146,3 (2000): 215–27. https://doi.org/10.1136/jramc-146-03-12
2. American College of Surgeons Committee on Trauma. ATLS: Advanced Trauma Life Support. 10th ed. Chicago: American College of Surgeons; 2018. ISBN: 978-0996826235

3. Auerbach PS, Cushing TA, Harris NS. Auerbach's Wilderness Medicine. 7th ed. 2 vols. Philadelphia: Elsevier; 2016. ISBN: 9780323359429
4. Butler, Frank K Jr et al. "Tactical combat casualty care 2007: evolving concepts and battlefield experience." *Military medicine* vol. 172,11 Suppl (2007): 1–19. https://doi.org/10.7205/milmed.172.supplement_1.1
5. Butler, Frank K Jr. "Tactical Combat Casualty Care: Beginnings." Wilderness & environmental medicine vol. 28,2S (2017): S12–S17. https://doi.org/10.1016/j.wem.2016.12.004
6. Feliciano DV, Mattox KL, Moore EE. *Trauma*. 9th ed. New York: McGraw Hill Medical; 2020. ISBN: 978-1260143355
7. Mabry, Robert L, and Robert DeLorenzo. "Challenges to improving combat casualty survival on the battlefield." *Military medicine* vol. 179,5 (2014): 477–82. https://doi.org/10.7205/MILMED-D-13-00417

Musculoskeletal Trauma: Sustaining Soldier Strength

12

Alli Sai Deepak and S. Shankarnath

Learning Objectives
Upon completion of this chapter, the reader will be able to:

- Classify musculoskeletal (MSK) injuries in the field into life-threatening, limb-threatening, and non-urgent categories.
- Perform rapid field assessment and triage of extremity injuries using the MARCH and FORCE principles.
- Apply hemorrhage control techniques, including direct pressure, hemostatic dressings, and tourniquet application.
- Execute field immobilization using both standard and improvised splinting materials for fractures and joint injuries.
- Identify signs of compartment syndrome and vascular compromise in limb-threatening injuries.
- Initiate antibiotic prophylaxis, pain management, and preservation of amputated parts for surgical reattachment.
- Differentiate and manage non-urgent injuries (e.g., contusions and sprains) to support early mobility and sustained combat readiness.
- Recognize crush injuries and crush syndrome in combat and disaster-related scenarios, especially following prolonged entrapment or structural collapse.
- Identify key clinical signs and early warning indicators of systemic deterioration, such as hyperkalemia, myoglobinuria, and acute kidney injury (AKI) and initiate appropriate management.

A. S. Deepak (✉)
Department of Emergency Medicine, Kasturba Medical College, Manipal, Karnataka, India

S. Shankarnath
Department of Trauma Surgery and Critical Care, JPN Apex Trauma Centre, AIIMS, New Delhi, India

N. T. Rai, S. Misra (eds.), *Frontline Operational Resuscitation and Combat Emergencies (FORCE) Manual*, https://doi.org/10.1007/978-981-92-1622-2_12

Introduction

Musculoskeletal injuries are the silent workhorses of battlefield trauma—*frequent, varied, and often underappreciated in their potential to disable*. In modern combat operations, MSK trauma accounts for a large proportion of non-fatal injuries, yet its consequences can be operationally catastrophic. Whether due to blunt trauma, penetrating wounds, blast exposure, or repetitive overuse, these injuries compromise both the fighting strength and the long-term health of deployed personnel.

Unlike other trauma categories, MSK injuries span a broad spectrum—from minor abrasions and sprains to traumatic amputations with crush injury and open fractures with vascular disruption. The initial response determines not only survival but also long-term limb function and rehabilitation outcomes.

Combat medics and responders must be equipped with a practical, tiered framework to rapidly assess, classify, and manage these injuries using the materials at hand. The FORCE model emphasizes decisive field intervention: bleeding control, fracture stabilization, neurovascular monitoring, and evacuation prioritization. Additionally, appropriate pain relief and antibiotic coverage can reduce secondary complications.

This chapter bridges core trauma principles with hands-on tactical strategies—enabling the provider to not just save lives, but to preserve the mobility and morale of the fighting force.

Case Scenario

During an early morning foot patrol in the dense, rain-soaked jungles of Assam, a 28-year-old rifleman from a counter-insurgency unit inadvertently triggers a concealed fragmentation device while inspecting a suspected tripwire along a narrow game trail. The explosion occurs at close range, violently propelling him backward onto the muddy forest floor. His teammates reach him within 2 min, finding him conscious but disoriented. His right arm has been traumatically amputated just below the shoulder, with bright red arterial spurting from the open stump. Multiple shrapnel wounds are also observed over the right thigh and chest wall, though his helmet and body armor have prevented more extensive thoracoabdominal injury (Fig. 12.1). Weather conditions and hostile surveillance delay planned evacuation by 45–60 min. A trained combat medic is the highest-level provider on site.

- *Care Under Fire (CUF)*
  Suppressive fire is maintained as the casualty is dragged to cover. A tourniquet is already in place above the amputation site but is visibly loose. The medic immediately repositions and tightens the combat application tourniquet (CAT) to high-humeral level, achieving full occlusion. Bleeding reduces significantly, though some deep tissue oozing persists. No further interventions are attempted until the threat subsides.

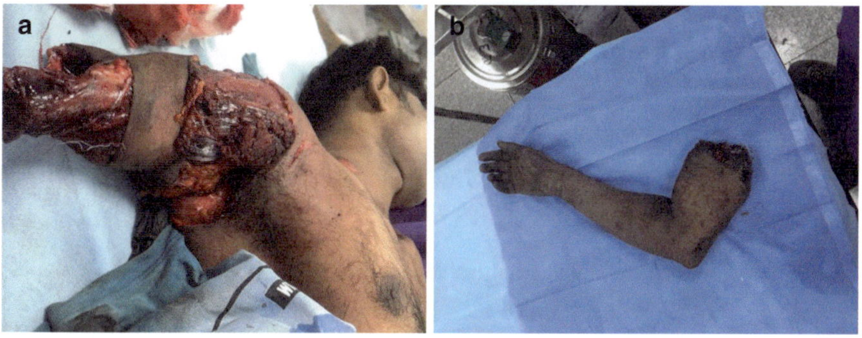

Fig. 12.1 (**a**) Soldier with traumatic amputation of the right upper limb secondary to IED blast. (**b**) Amputated upper limb

- *Tactical Field Care (TFC)*
  Following the MARCH sequence:
  M—Massive Hemorrhage: The traumatic amputation site continues to ooze blood. A hemostatic dressing is packed into the wound base and reinforced with pressure wrapping. Additional shrapnel wounds over the right thigh are addressed with compression bandages. Bleeding is controlled.
  A—Airway: The casualty is conscious and able to speak in short sentences. His airway remains patent. No signs of obstruction or facial trauma are noted.
  R—Respiration: Respiratory rate is elevated at 28/min. Breath sounds are equal bilaterally with no signs of chest wall instability or sucking chest wound. Oxygen is unavailable in the field, but no immediate respiratory compromise is observed.
  C—Circulation: The casualty is pale and diaphoretic. Radial pulse is thready on the left. Systolic blood pressure is estimated at 90 mmHg. An 18 G IV line is secured, and 500 mL of warmed Ringer's lactate is started slowly. Within 30 min, 1 g of tranexamic acid is administered IV. Pain is managed using titrated doses of IV ketamine to maintain consciousness while offering analgesia.
  H—Head Injury/Hypothermia: GCS is 15, but the soldier is mildly hypothermic (core temperature 35.5 °C). Rain and wet clothing increase the risk of further heat loss. Dry poncho liners and a Mylar blanket are used to insulate the casualty.
  Secondary Survey
  The amputated part is located, rinsed with sterile saline, wrapped in saline-moistened gauze, placed in a sealed waterproof bag, and stored in a second cool-water container for potential replantation. No other major trauma is found. Chest wall shrapnel wounds are superficial. The casualty continues to respond to verbal stimuli, with stable neurologic function.

- *Tactical Evacuation Care (TACEVAC)*
  Evacuation is delayed due to steep terrain and enemy presence. The casualty is monitored every 15 min for:
  - Changes in mental status or GCS.
  - Worsening pallor or hypotension.
  - Tourniquet effectiveness and wound saturation.
  - Risk of repeat hemorrhage or respiratory decompensation.

The field medic maintains permissive hypotension (SBP ~90 mmHg), avoids unnecessary crystalloid, and prioritizes blood products if available. IV cefazolin is administered. Analgesia and thermal insulation are continued. Evacuation is initiated as soon as tactical airspace is secured.

Reflective Questions

1. What are the step-by-step priorities in managing catastrophic hemorrhage and initiating circulatory resuscitation in the context of a traumatic amputation under combat conditions?
2. How should an amputated limb segment be preserved in the field to maximize chances for replantation at higher-level care?
3. What are the critical medications that should be administered within the first hour post-blast?
4. How does delayed evacuation in a tropical, wet environment alter your priorities for hypothermia prevention and wound infection control?
5. What are the early field indicators of evolving crush injury or compartment syndrome in blast casualties, and how can combat medics mitigate downstream renal complications?
6. How does the presence of traumatic amputation alter the likelihood or masking of concurrent crush syndrome in nearby soft tissues?

Classification of Musculoskeletal Injuries

Combat musculoskeletal (MSK) injuries span a broad spectrum of severity and demand a nuanced approach to triage. For tactical clarity and clinical relevance, these injuries are best classified into three categories:

Life-Threatening MSK Injuries

These injuries require immediate intervention as they pose a direct threat to life, usually due to massive hemorrhage. Delay in addressing these injuries can lead to rapid exsanguination and death in the field.

- *Examples*:
  - Traumatic amputation with arterial bleeding.
  - Open fractures with uncontrolled hemorrhage.

Junctional bleeding (groin, axilla) not amenable to standard tourniquet use.

- *Management priorities*:
  - *Hemorrhage control*: Apply tourniquets proximal to the injury (preferably CAT) or use junctional tourniquets/hemostatic gauze if in a non-tourniquet site.
  - *Direct pressure and packing*: Apply Axiostat®, Combat Gauze™, or equivalent into deep bleeding wounds (Fig. 12.2).
  - *IV/IO access and resuscitation*: Administer TXA (1 g IV), and start fluids (Ringer's lactate or NS) if there are signs of shock.
  - *Preserve amputated part: Wrap in moist sterile gauze, place in a sealed bag, and store in a cool environment (not direct ice contact).*

Limb-Threatening MSK Injuries

These injuries do not immediately threaten life but may result in permanent limb loss or dysfunction if not promptly managed. Timely intervention can prevent complications, such as compartment syndrome, vascular compromise, or infected open fractures.

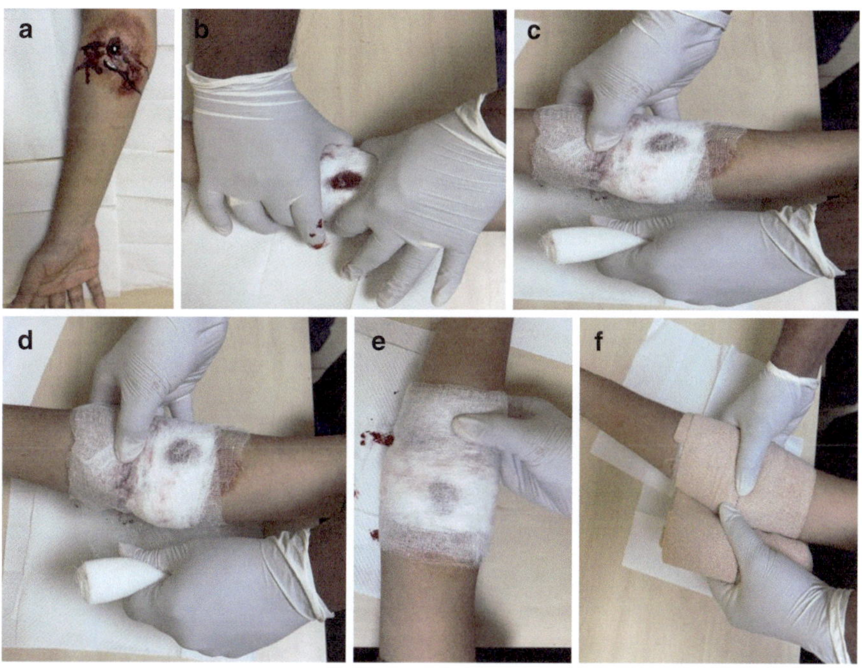

Fig. 12.2 Steps of direct pressure and packing. (**a**) Image showing arterial injury of the right upper limb around the elbow. (**b**) Application of gauze over the wound with pressure. (**c**–**e**) Application of roller gauze over the wound with firm pressure. (**f**) Application of crepe bandage/Israeli bandage over the wound

- *Examples*:
  - Open or unstable fractures with visible bone.
  - Crush injuries with prolonged entrapment.
  - Vascular injuries (absent distal pulse, cool pale limb).
  - Severe burns with circumferential involvement.
- *Management priorities*:
  - *Neurovascular assessment*: Check for pulses, capillary refill, and motor and sensory function.
  - *Limb splinting*: Immobilize the fracture using a SAM splint or improvised device.
  - *Realignment if necessary*: If distal pulses are absent, consider gentle manual traction to restore alignment.
  - *Early antibiotics*: Ceftriaxone 1–2 g IM/IV for open fractures.
  - *Analgesia: Administer ketamine (0.2–0.3 mg/kg IV) or fentanyl (IN/IV) for pain control.*

Non-urgent MSK Injuries

These injuries, while painful or functionally limiting, do not threaten life or limb and can often be managed conservatively in the field. The goal is to maintain mobility, reduce discomfort, and prevent secondary disability.

- *Examples*:
  - Simple sprains and strains.
  - Minor lacerations and contusions.
  - Closed fractures without deformity or neurovascular compromise. Superficial burns or abrasions.
- *Management Priorities*:
  - *RICE protocol*: Rest, Ice, Compression, Elevation when feasible.
  - *Splinting or elastic wraps*: To support joint or limb stability.
  - *Analgesia*: NSAIDs like ibuprofen (400–800 mg PO) and paracetamol (500–1000 mg PO).
  - *Wound care*: Clean, irrigate, and dress minor wounds. Monitor for signs of infection.
  - *Mobility assessment: Encourage early movement if safe to do so; provide* walking aids or load redistribution for field continuation.

FORCE Tactical Pearl
All musculoskeletal injuries must be monitored for progression. What starts as non-urgent may become limb- or life-threatening if bleeding resumes, swelling compromises perfusion, or sepsis sets in.

Assessment and Management of Life-Threatening Extremity Injuries

Life-threatening musculoskeletal injuries demand immediate control of hemorrhage and shock prevention, as delays can lead to rapid fatality. These injuries are most commonly associated with traumatic amputations, major vessel disruption, or junctional bleeding where standard tourniquets may not be effective.

Rapid Field Assessment

When approaching a casualty with suspected life-threatening extremity injury:

- Begin with the "M" in MARCH: Look for active, bright red arterial bleeding or amputated limbs.
- Expose the limb completely to visualize wound location, bleeding pattern, and injury extent.
- Assess distal pulses, skin color, and capillary refill—especially for partial amputations or deep lacerations.
- In junctional sites (groin, axilla), bleeding may be deep and non-visible—palpate and reassess frequently.

Hemorrhage Control: The First Priority-Tourniquet Application

Combat application tourniquet (CAT): Place 5–7 cm above the bleeding point, tighten until bleeding stops and distal pulse is absent:

Apply a second tourniquet if the first is insufficient.

Record the time of application on casualty's tourniquet or forehead using indelible marker (Fig. 12.3).

- *Junctional bleeding*:
  - Use Combat Gauze™, Axiostat®, or other hemostatic agents.
  - Pack the wound cavity firmly and apply sustained pressure for 3–5 min.
  - If available, use junctional tourniquets (e.g., SAM junctional tourniquet) over pressure points (femoral or axillary).

Field Resuscitation and Pharmacologic Support

- Establish IV or IO access (preferably 18G IV or tibial IO).
- *Administer 1 g TXA IV over 10 min (within the first hour of injury), followed by 1 g over 8 h if prolonged evacuation.*
- Begin fluid resuscitation with warmed Ringer's lactate or normal saline if SBP < 90 mmHg or mental status deteriorates.

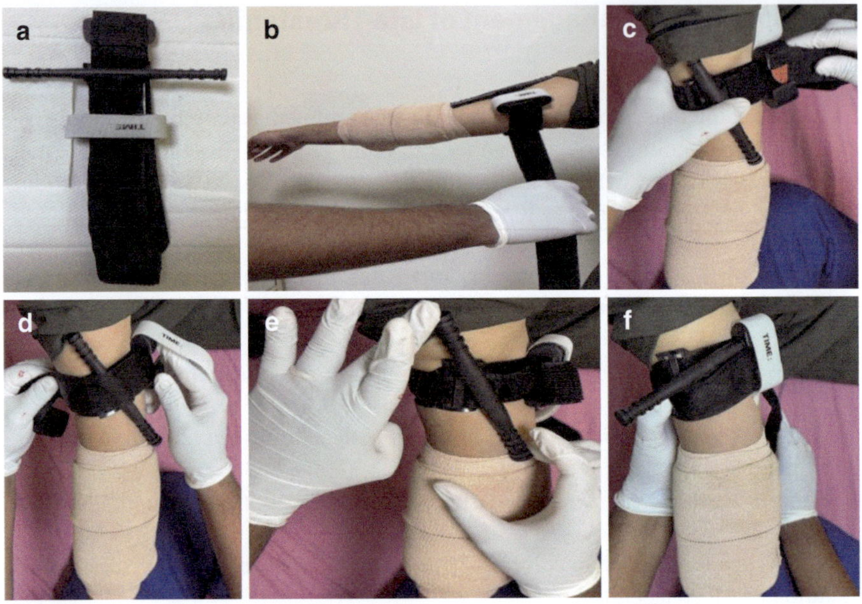

Fig. 12.3 Steps of CAT application. (**a**) Image showing CAT. (**b**) Pass the CAT around the arm 5–7 cm above the wound. (**c**) Pass the band through the buckle. (**d**) Fix the band tightly around the arm. (**e**) Rotate the windlass rod till the bleeding stops. (**f**) Fix the rod in the holder, attach the clip, and document the time of application

- Avoid fluid overload—*the goal is permissive hypotension in trauma (SBP 80–90 mmHg).*

Pain Management and Antibiotics

Pain control is essential for both physiological and psychological stabilization:

- *Ketamine IV*: 0.1–0.3 mg/kg (analgesic) or 0.5–1 mg/kg (sedation).
- *Fentanyl (IN)*: 800 mcg via mucosal atomizer device in divided doses if IV is not available.

- *NSAIDs/paracetamol* for non-severe cases.
- *Antibiotics*: For open fractures, crush injuries, and severe soft tissue wounds:
  - *Ceftriaxone +/− Metronidazole.*
  - *Ertapenem as a single agent in mixed injuries.*
- Monitor for respiratory depression, especially in closed environments.

Preservation of Amputated Parts

If the limb or part is salvageable:

- Rinse gently with sterile saline (avoid scrubbing).
- Wrap in sterile saline-soaked gauze, and place inside a clean, sealed plastic bag.
- Keep the bag in a cool container or ice chest—*do not allow direct contact with ice or water.*
- Label with casualty's name, time of amputation, and site of injury.
- Transport alongside the patient, ideally to a surgical-capable facility *within 6 h* (Fig. 12.4).

Evacuation Considerations

- Reassess tourniquet and hemostatic dressings during handoff.
- Monitor for signs of rebleeding, hypoperfusion, and shock deterioration.
- Document MIST (Mechanism, Injuries, Signs, Treatment) thoroughly.
- Prioritize rapid transport if amputation, uncontrolled hemorrhage, or deteriorating vitals are present.

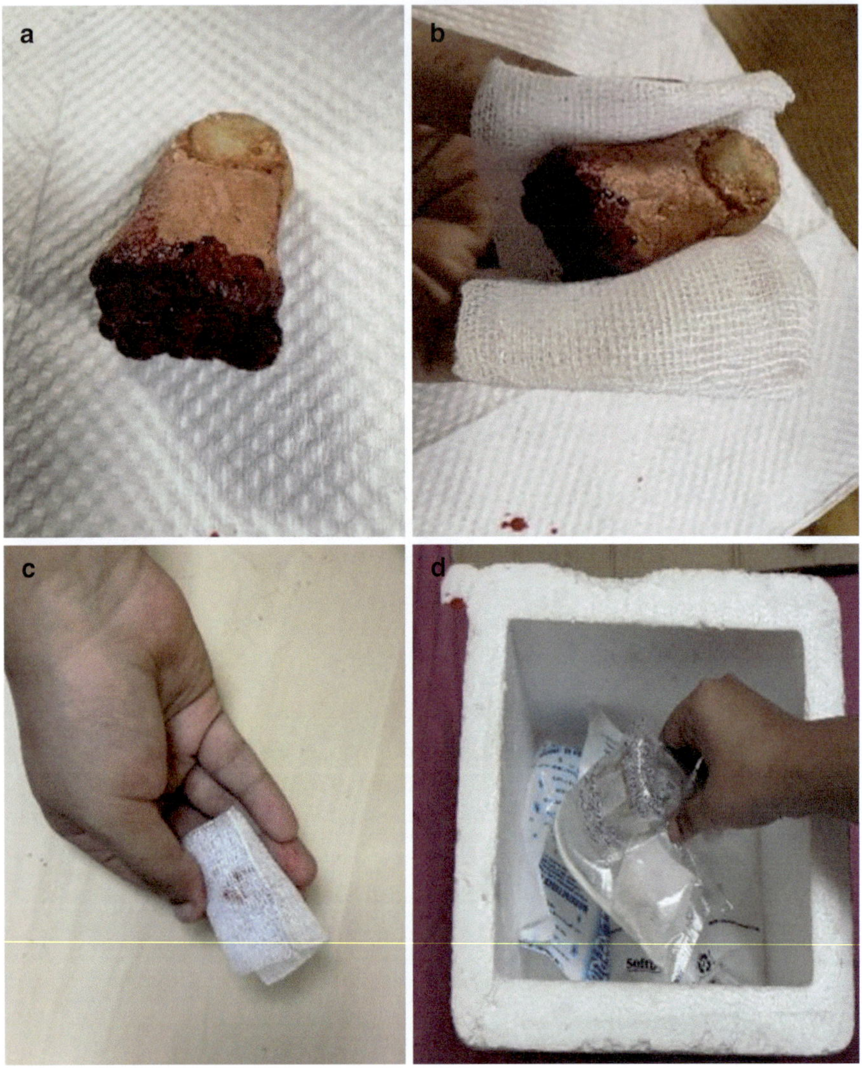

Fig. 12.4 Steps of preservation of amputated part. (**a**) Amputated digit. (**b**, **c**) Cover the amputated part with wet gauze. (**d**) Place the amputated part in a tightly sealed pack and place it in ice box

Assessment and Management of Limb-Threatening Extremity Injuries

Limb-threatening injuries are those that, if left unmanaged or improperly treated in the field, may result in loss of limb function, tissue necrosis, infection, or even amputation. While not as acutely fatal as uncontrolled hemorrhage, these injuries require rapid identification, neurovascular monitoring, and strategic stabilization.

Open Fractures and Grossly Unstable Injuries

Open fractures (bone visible through the skin or protruding) are common in blast and shrapnel injuries.

- *Assessment*:
  - Look for visible bone, deformity, severe swelling, bleeding, or exposed muscle/tendon.
  - Assess circulation (pulse, color, capillary refill) and neurological status (sensation, motor function) distal to the injury.
- *Management*:
  - Apply dry sterile gauze dressing over open wound—do not attempt to push bone back inside.
  - Irrigate gross contaminants if possible with clean water or saline.
  - Immobilize using SAM splints, rigid boards, or improvised devices (rifles, sticks).
  - Realign limb only if distal pulse is absent, applying gentle traction until circulation returns.
  - Administer antibiotics:
    - *Ceftriaxone 1–2 g IM/IV.*
    - Add *metronidazole* if large soft tissue wound or contamination.
  - Provide analgesia (e.g., ketamine or NSAIDs).
    Mark and monitor compromised limbs for signs of deterioration.

Vascular Compromise

Arterial damage may result from fractures, lacerations, or compartmental swelling (Fig. 12.5). Clinical signs of vascular injury are outlined in Table 12.1.

- *Red flags*:
  - Absent or weak distal pulses.
  - Cool, pale extremity.
  - Delayed capillary refill (>2 s).
    Cyanosis or mottling.

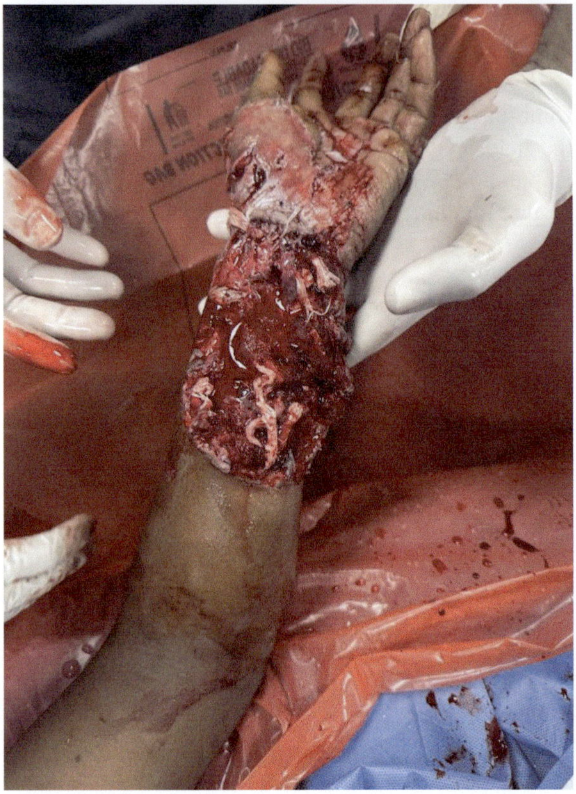

Fig. 12.5 Arterial injury to the left forearm with partial amputation and degloving

Table 12.1 Hard and soft signs of vascular injury

Hard signs	Soft signs
1. Absent or diminished distal pulses	1. Small, stable hematoma
2. Arterial bleeding	2. Injury to anatomically related nerve
3. Large expanding or pulsatile hematoma	3. Proximity of injury to vascular structure/fracture
4. Palpable thrill	
5. Distal ischemia (pain, pallor, paralysis, paresthesias, coolness)	

- *Management*:
  - If pulse is absent, attempt gentle realignment and splinting.
  - Apply loose dressing to prevent further tissue compression.
  - Initiate rapid CASEVAC.
    Continue pulse checks during transport and reassess every 15 min.

Compartment Syndrome

Compartment syndrome occurs when internal swelling increases pressure within a muscle compartment, cutting off blood supply and nerve function. It may develop over hours after a crush injury, tight splinting, or revascularization.

- *Five P's of compartment syndrome*:
  1. Pain out of proportion to injury.
  2. Paresthesia (tingling, numbness).
  3. Pallor (pale skin).
  4. Paralysis (weakness).
  5. Pulselessness (late sign).
- *Field clues*:
  - Severe pain unrelieved by immobilization.
  - Tense, swollen limb.
  - Inability to move fingers/toes.
    Loss of sensation.
- *Management*:
  - Loosen dressings or splints immediately.
  - Elevate limb to heart level (not above).
  - Avoid cold packs directly on the limb.
    Prioritize surgical evacuation—definitive treatment is fasciotomy, which is not a field procedure.
- *Evacuation priorities*
  Limb-threatening injuries should be escalated for early surgical intervention—ideally within 4–6 h if vascular compromise exists:
  - Reassess limb neurovascular status every 15–30 min.
    Monitor for evolving shock, rebleeding, or signs of sepsis.

Assessment and Management of Non-urgent Extremity Injuries

These injuries do not pose an immediate threat to life or limb and typically occur during routine operations, training exercises, or prolonged movement over challenging terrain. Proper field management prevents escalation and supports rapid return to duty or safe delayed evacuation.

Sprains and Strains

Sprains involve ligament injury around joints, while strains affect muscle or tendon fibers.

- *Presentation*:
  - Joint pain, swelling, and bruising.
  - Reduced range of motion.
  - Tenderness on movement or palpation.
    No bone deformity or loss of distal pulse.
- *Management*:
  - *RICE protocol* (Rest, Ice, Compression, Elevation), adapted for field settings:
    - *Rest:* Avoid weight-bearing.
    - *Ice:* Apply cold packs or cloth soaked in cold water (avoid direct skin contact).
    - *Compression:* Use elastic wraps, crepe bandage, or cloth strips.
      Elevation: Raise injured limb if feasible during rest.
  - *Splint or wrap* to support the joint.
  - *NSAIDs*: Ibuprofen 400–800 mg PO every 8 h as needed.
    Mobility: Encourage gentle use once acute swelling subsides.

Closed Fractures Without Deformity

Minor or stable fractures (e.g., hairline tibial fractures and metacarpal fractures) may present with localized swelling and pain but *no visible deformity* or neurovascular compromise.

- *Management*:
  - Immobilize with *SAM splint, cardboard, or improvised rigid material.*
  - Monitor for compartment syndrome signs.
  - Allow protected weight-bearing for upper limb fractures; restrict lower limb use.
    Analgesia and evacuation as needed depending on pain and operational role.

Minor Lacerations and Abrasions

Common during obstacle navigation, rope descents, or falls.

- *Management*:
  - Irrigate with clean water or saline to remove debris.
  - Apply antiseptic (e.g., povidone-iodine or chlorhexidine).
  - Dress with dry sterile gauze and secure with adhesive tape or elastic wrap.
  - Watch for signs of infection: redness, warmth, pus, and fever.

Contusions (Bruises)

Caused by blunt trauma to muscles or soft tissues.

- *Presentation*:
  - Tenderness, swelling, discoloration, and pain on movement. No open wound or significant deformity.
- *Management*:
  - Cold compress for first 24 h.
  - Elevation if limb involved.
  - Reassess for hematoma and compartment syndrome if swelling increases. Continue NSAIDs for 48–72 h.

Friction Blisters

Especially relevant in long-range foot marches or training deployments.

- *Management*:
  - Do not rupture unless painful or fluid-filled and interfering with function.
  - If ruptured:
    - Clean with antiseptic.
    - Apply non-adherent dressing and secure with tape.
  - Cover intact blisters with moleskin or hydrocolloid patch.

Field Recovery Considerations

- Allow self-ambulation where appropriate.
- Limit casualty load on CASEVAC unless escalation of symptoms.
- Educate on self-care: elevation, hydration, and dressing hygiene.
- Schedule reassessment if prolonged field care (>48–72 h).

Principles of Field Immobilization and Splinting

Immobilization is the tactical medic's primary tool for managing fractures, joint injuries, and unstable musculoskeletal trauma. It must be rapid, secure, and adaptable to the resources and terrain at hand. Whether using commercial splints or improvised materials, *the goals remain consistent: stabilize the injury, preserve neurovascular function, and prepare the casualty for movement.*

General Principles of Splinting

- Immobilize the joint above and below the injury site.
- Assess and document distal pulses, motor function, and sensation before and after splinting.
- Reassess frequently, especially if swelling or pain increases.
- Pad generously at pressure points to prevent soft tissue injury.
- Do not reduce dislocations or angulated fractures in the field unless there is a neurovascular compromise.
- Splint in the position found, unless distal circulation is compromised.

Materials for Field Splinting

- *Commercial tools*:
  - *SAM splints*: Moldable aluminum-core foam—lightweight and reusable.
  - *Vacuum splints*: Mold to limb when air is removed—excellent for air evac.
  - *Traction splints*: Primarily for femur fractures—require training and time.
- *Improvised materials*:
  - *Rigid materials*: Branches, metal rods, rifles (cleared), tent poles, and boards (Fig. 12.6).
  - *Padding*: Towels, uniforms, gauze rolls, and clothing.
  - *Securing tools*: Cravats, bandages, triangular slings, belts, and duct tape.

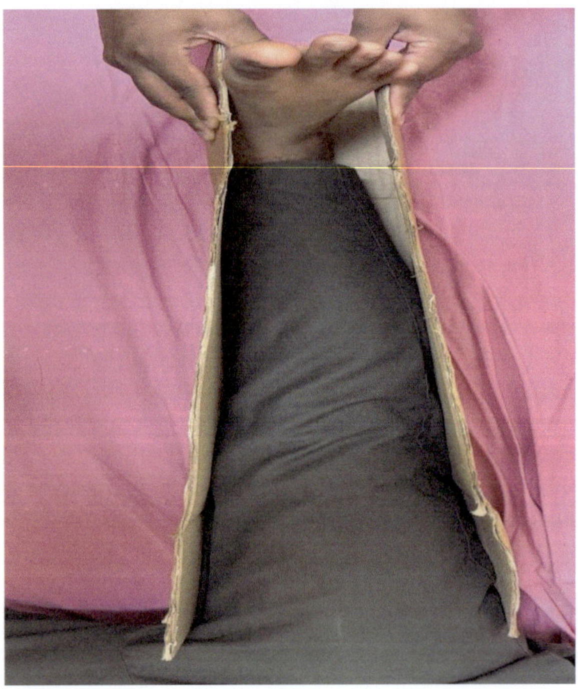

Fig. 12.6 Improvised splint for lower limb using cardboard

Stepwise Splinting Procedure

A. *Upper Limb (Forearm, Elbow, Shoulder):*
   Support arm in neutral or slight flexion.
   Use SAM splint or rigid board along posterior forearm and palm.
   Secure with elastic bandages or cloth ties—do not constrict.
   Sling and swathe to the chest for shoulder or upper arm injuries (Fig. 12.7).

B. *Lower Limb (Tibia, Fibula, Femur)*:
   - Do not attempt to walk or bear weight on injured leg.
   - For stable tibial fractures, apply SAM splint medially and laterally, padded well.
   - For femur fractures:
     – Use traction splint if trained and equipment is available.
     – If not, splint to the opposite leg with padding in between.
     – Secure with cravats or cloth strips at thighs, knees, and ankles (Fig. 12.8).

C. *Hand and Foot Injuries*:
   - *Hand*: Place in functional position (like holding a can), and splint dorsally.
   - *Foot*: Use boot as a natural splint or apply rigid sole and wrap.

D. *Pelvic Stabilization*:
   - Use *pelvic binders* or improvised belts over the greater trochanters.
   - Secure snugly but avoid compressing the abdomen.
   - Consider pelvic fractures in high-impact falls, blast injuries, or leg-length discrepancies.

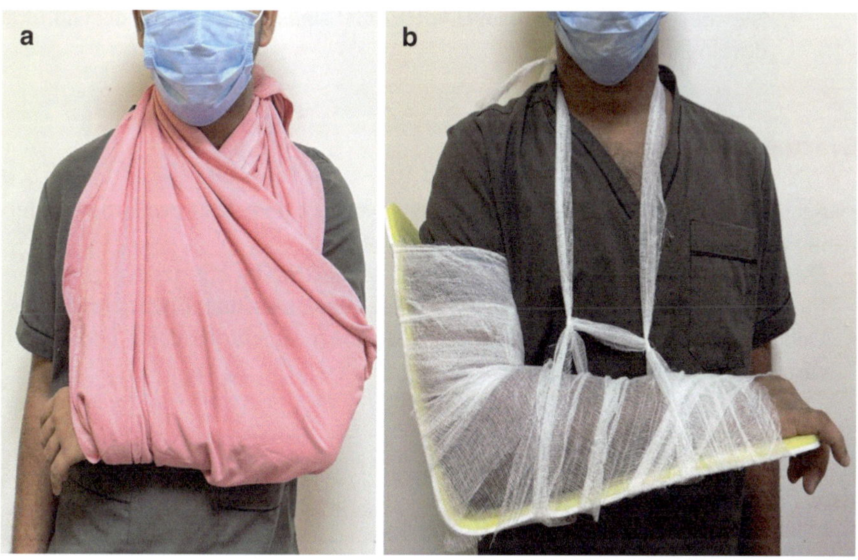

Fig. 12.7 Splinting technique for the upper limb. (**a**) Splinting of the left upper limb using a blanket. (**b**) Splinting of the right upper limb using a foldable splint

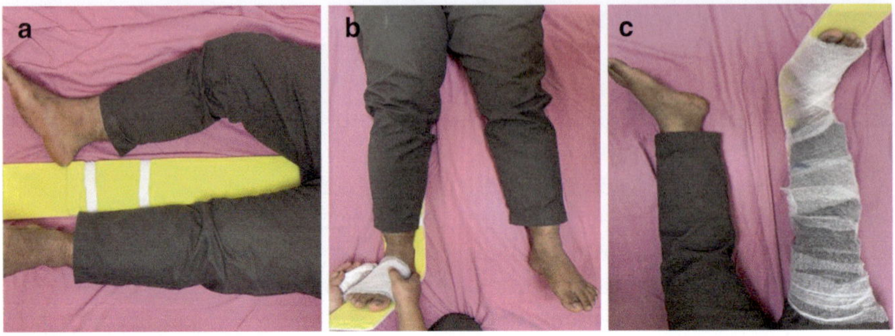

Fig. 12.8 Splinting technique for the lower limb. (**a**) Checking for the length of the splint for the limb. (**b**, **c**) Application of the splint and securing with roller gauze

Post-splinting Monitoring

- Recheck pulse, motor, and sensation every 15–30 min.
  - *Watch for:*
    - Numbness.
    - Color changes.
    - Increasing pain.
      Swelling or coldness distal to splint.
  - *If symptoms worsen:*
    - Loosen the splint slightly and reassess.
    - Elevate the limb and initiate CASEVAC if signs of compartment syndrome develop.

Evacuation Preparation

- Secure the splinted limb to a stretcher or casualty's body to prevent motion during transport.
- Elevate the limb if feasible, especially in lower extremity injuries.
- Protect splints from environmental exposure (mud, moisture, direct pressure).
- Document splint type, time applied, and pre–/postneurovascular findings on casualty card or handover sheet.

Crush Injuries in Tactical Settings: Management and Field Considerations

Crush injuries represent some of the most devastating injuries faced by soldiers and first responders operating in hostile, austere environments. They occur when a part of the body is subjected to prolonged compressive force, as seen during building collapses after blasts, vehicular rollovers, entrapments under debris, and structural failures in urban warfare.

In the Indian combat and internal security context — whether in jungles, mountains, urban counterinsurgency operations, or disaster relief missions — *the risk of crush injuries is ever present*. These injuries may initially appear deceptively stable but can evolve into life-threatening systemic collapse once the external compressive force is removed.

The critical danger lies not only in mechanical tissue damage but also in the systemic release of intracellular toxins that can trigger cardiac arrest, renal failure, metabolic derangement, and multi-organ dysfunction within minutes to hours. *Without aggressive, early field intervention — primarily in the form of fluid resuscitation and hyperkalemia management — even otherwise salvageable casualties can be lost.* Therefore, crush injury management in tactical settings demands rapid recognition, structured initial care, and seamless transition to evacuation while constantly anticipating deterioration even when external bleeding appears controlled. A combat provider's anticipation, preparation before extrication, and proactive resuscitation efforts often determine survival.

Pathophysiology

The underlying pathophysiology of crush injury involves a complex two-phase process:

1. Ischemic Phase (*Under Compression*)

   When muscles and soft tissues are compressed beyond critical pressure thresholds, perfusion ceases. This leads to:

   - Tissue hypoxia and anaerobic metabolism.
   - Accumulation of lactic acid, hydrogen ions, and reactive oxygen species.
   - Disruption of cellular membranes, resulting in leakage of intracellular contents, such as:
     - Potassium (K^+).
     - Phosphate.
     - Myoglobin.
     - Creatinine kinase (CK).

       Uric acid.

   Muscle ischemia typically begins within 1–2 h of compression but becomes irreversible after 4–6 h. The longer the entrapment, the greater the burden of toxic metabolites ready to flood the circulation once decompression occurs.
2. Reperfusion Phase (*After Release*)

   When the compressive force is removed, the previously ischemic tissue is rapidly reperfused. However, instead of restoring normal function, this can cause catastrophic systemic effects:

- *Massive release of accumulated potassium*, leading to fatal cardiac dysrhythmias.
- *Systemic inflammatory response syndrome (SIRS)* triggered by oxidative stress.
- *Myoglobin release* from muscle breakdown, filtered by kidneys, causing renal tubular obstruction and acute kidney injury (AKI).
- *Severe metabolic acidosis* from lactic acid and cell death products.
- *Capillary leak syndrome*, leading to hypovolemia, edema, and shock.
- *Key life-threatening outcomes*:
  - *Hyperkalemia* → cardiac arrest.
  - *AKI* → anuria, fluid overload, and uremic toxicity.
  - *Shock* → worsens tissue perfusion and perpetuates injury.
  - *Pulmonary edema* → due to fluid resuscitation complications, especially if blast lung coexists.

> **FORCE Tactical Pearl**
> *In crush injuries, the clock starts ticking long before the casualty is freed. Prepare early, resuscitate aggressively, and evacuate decisively.*

Mechanism and Risk Factors in Tactical Environments

Combat and operational contexts where crush injuries frequently occur include:

- Building collapses from IED blasts or shelling.
- Vehicle rollovers and crashes.
- Structural collapse during urban assaults.
- Cave-ins during tunnel operations.
- Earthquakes or landslides in mountain operations.

Contributing risk factors include delayed rescue, environmental extremes (heat, dehydration), and limited field resuscitation capability.

Clinical Recognition

Crush injuries should be suspected when there is:

- History of prolonged entrapment (>30–60 min).
- Visible limb deformities, swelling, and bruising.
- Tense, painful muscle compartments.
- Absent or weak distal pulses.
- *Systemic clues include:*

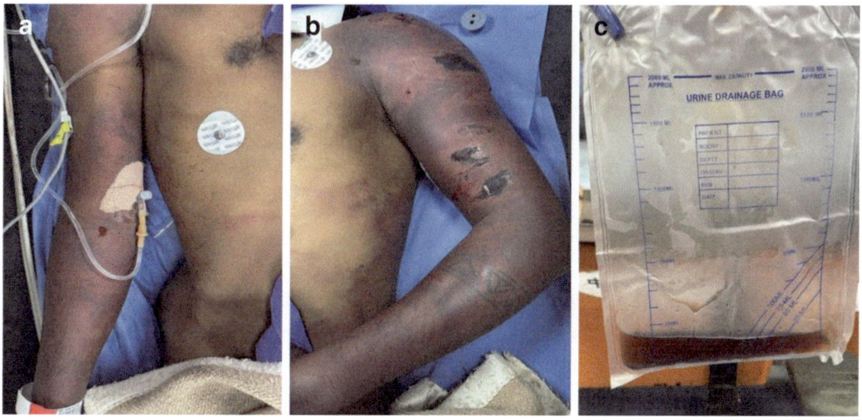

Fig. 12.9 (**a**, **b**) Soldier sustained crush injury to both upper limbs due to structure collapse and prolonged entrapment. (**c**) Tea-colored urine suggestive of rhabdomyolysis

- Hypotension and tachycardia (hypovolemia).
- Dark, tea-colored urine (myoglobinuria) (Fig. 12.9).
- Confusion or altered mental status.
- ECG changes: Peaked T-waves and widened QRS complexes (hyperkalemia).
- Reduced or absent urine output.

Field Management of Crush Injuries

1. *Initial Actions before Extrication*

   Start IV fluid resuscitation *before* or *during* extrication if feasible.

   Prepare airway adjuncts and monitor breathing.

   Anticipate sudden cardiovascular collapse at the moment of decompression.

   If the tactical situation demands urgent evacuation without full preparation, *prioritize bleeding control and fluid initiation at the earliest opportunity.*
2. *Bleeding Control*
   - Apply tourniquets high and tight for massive hemorrhage.
   - Pack open wounds with hemostatic gauze.
   - Control junctional bleeding if present (groin, axilla).
   - Record tourniquet time visibly.
3. *Aggressive Fluid Resuscitation*

FORCE Tactical Pearl

While hemorrhage remains the priority, awareness of hidden internal bleeding and crush-induced volume loss is essential.

- *Goal*: Prevent AKI, dilute toxic metabolites, and maintain renal perfusion.
  - *Preferred fluid*: Normal saline (0.9% NaCl).
    Avoid: *Lactated Ringer's (contains potassium) and colloids.*
- *Resuscitation strategy*:
  - Initial bolus: 1–2 L as rapidly as possible.
  - Maintenance: 500 mL/h, titrated to maintain urine output of at least 1 mL/kg/h.
  - Larger volumes (up to 6–12 L/day) may be needed in severe crush syndrome.
- *If prolonged field care (>4–6 h expected)*:
  - Continue high-volume fluids even without immediate signs of shock.
  - Use clinical parameters (urine output, mental status, capillary refill) for titration.

4. *Hyperkalemia Prevention and Management*

The sudden reperfusion of ischemic muscle releases potassium, causing life-threatening arrhythmias.

- *Field indicators of hyperkalemia*:
  - Weakness and paralysis.
    ECG: Peaked T-waves, bradycardia, and widened QRS.
- *Field management*:
  - Calcium gluconate IV: Stabilizes cardiac membranes.
  - Insulin (10 units IV) + 50% dextrose (50 ml IV): Drives potassium intracellularly.
  - Sodium bicarbonate IV (1 ampoule) if acidosis or ECG changes present.

These interventions should not delay evacuation if definitive care is within reach.

5. *Airway and Breathing Support*
   - Ensure airway is patent.
   - Administer oxygen if available.
   - Monitor respiratory effort closely: Pulmonary edema can develop from fluid overload or blast lung overlap.

Prepare for advanced airway management if GCS drops below 8 or respiratory status deteriorates.

6. *Circulatory Support and Urine Monitoring*
   - Monitor pulses and capillary refill.
   - Insert urinary catheter (if feasible) to assess output and detect myoglobinuria.
   - Cola-colored urine is an early sign of myoglobin-mediated renal injury.
     - *Urine output targets*:

- 1–2 mL/kg/h if myoglobinuria is present
- 100–300 mL/h ideal in moderate to severe crush cases.

> ***FORCE Tactical Pearl***
> *If urine output drops or becomes dark, escalate resuscitation and prioritize early dialysis at higher care levels.*

7. *Temperature Control*
   - Remove wet clothing.
   - Wrap casualty with thermal blankets or ponchos.
   - Preventing hypothermia is essential to maintain coagulation and reduce metabolic demands.
8. *Prolonged Field Care Adaptations*
   In delayed evacuation scenarios:

- Continue fluid administration aggressively.
- Reassess perfusion and neurologic status every 30–60 min.
- Manage wounds with sterile dressings and monitor for compartment syndrome development.
- Prepare for pain control (IV/IN ketamine preferred for hemodynamic stability).

> **FORCE Tactical Pearl**
> *If compartment syndrome is suspected (tense limb, worsening pain, loss of pulses) and evacuation is impossible, field fasciotomy may be lifesaving if performed by trained personnel.*

Definitive Care

Upon reaching higher facilities:

- Continue aggressive hydration.
- Serial monitoring of electrolytes and renal function.
- Dialysis initiation if anuria or refractory hyperkalemia develops.
- Early surgical debridement or fasciotomy if needed.
- Antibiotics and tetanus prophylaxis for open wounds.

Rehabilitation focuses on renal recovery, functional limb salvage, and management of psychological sequelae from prolonged entrapment and trauma.

Table 12.2 Operational scenarios, tactical considerations, and medical implications in crush injuries

Scenario	Tactical considerations	Medical implications
Mass casualty events	Prioritize casualties with signs of life (palpable pulse, spontaneous breathing)	Focus on triage and rapid extrication to prevent progression to crush syndrome
Urban collapses/ structural failure	Expect multiple entrapped victims with prolonged compression injuries	High risk of crush syndrome, compartment syndrome, and AKI
High-altitude/ jungle operations	Evacuation delays and dehydration accelerate rhabdomyolysis and systemic toxicity	Early IV fluid resuscitation essential; monitor for hyperkalemia and AKI
CBRN or terror-related blasts	Be alert for chemical contamination or radiologic exposure in addition to physical trauma	Decontamination may precede resuscitation; risk of multisystem involvement

Abbreviations: CBRN chemical, biological, radiological, and nuclear, *AKI* acute kidney injury

Special Tactical Considerations

In austere and combat environments, crush injuries often occur under unique and complex tactical scenarios that influence both the immediacy and approach to medical management. The risk of delayed extrication, prolonged compression, and systemic complications, such as rhabdomyolysis and acute kidney injury (AKI), is heightened in such contexts. Understanding the tactical landscape is essential to guide triage, anticipate complications, and tailor interventions accordingly. Table 12.2 outlines common operational scenarios associated with crush injuries, highlighting key tactical considerations and their corresponding medical implications to aid field medics and combat care providers in timely, effective decision-making.

Case Resolution

The 28-year-old rifleman injured during a jungle patrol in Assam presented with a traumatic arm amputation and multiple blast injuries to the chest and thigh. Rapid implementation of the MARCH algorithm under fire proved essential in prioritizing lifesaving interventions. The initial failure of the pre-applied tourniquet highlighted the critical need for reassessment of hemorrhage control devices. Once correctly placed and tightened to the high-arm level, the CAT effectively halted pulsatile bleeding. Persistent oozing from the stump warranted the use of a hemostatic dressing and pressure wrapping, reinforcing the step-by-step approach of hemorrhage control: direct pressure, wound packing with hemostatics, tourniquet optimization, and ongoing reassessment.

In managing circulatory resuscitation, the combat medic maintained permissive hypotension, targeting a systolic BP of ~90 mmHg to reduce the risk of dislodging clots while preserving end-organ perfusion. An 18 G IV line was placed, and warm

Ringer's lactate was infused slowly, with 1 g tranexamic acid (TXA) administered within the golden hour to reduce fibrinolysis and improve survival odds. This case highlights the importance of prioritizing TXA, analgesics (IV ketamine), and broad-spectrum antibiotics (IV cefazolin) within the first hour to stabilize casualties and prevent secondary complications, such as infection and shock.

The amputated arm was retrieved and preserved meticulously: rinsed with sterile saline, wrapped in saline-moistened gauze, sealed in a waterproof barrier, and stored in a cool water container—not directly on ice. This method optimizes tissue viability for potential replantation at a higher echelon of care. Early identification and preservation procedures are often overlooked but can critically influence functional outcomes post-evacuation.

Given the tropical and wet conditions, hypothermia prevention was aggressively pursued. Despite the ambient heat, rain-soaked clothing and immobilization placed the casualty at high risk. Insulating materials like Mylar blankets and poncho liners were used, a crucial intervention often neglected in tropical climates where paradoxical hypothermia due to evaporative heat loss can be fatal. Additionally, exposure to rain and organic debris heightened the risk of wound contamination. Prompt administration of IV antibiotics provided an essential prophylactic measure against early soft-tissue infection and sepsis.

Although the patient had no signs of entrapment, the blast force and delayed evacuation warranted vigilance for evolving crush syndrome or compartment syndrome. Early field indicators—such as tense, swollen muscle compartments, disproportionate pain, rising creatinine (if measurable), or dark-colored urine—were closely monitored. In this scenario, absence of visible entrapment did not eliminate the risk; instead, the mechanism of injury (close-range blast with limb trauma) mandated regular reassessment. While no immediate features of crush injury developed, the team prepared to initiate renal-protective measures (e.g., hydration protocols and urine alkalinization) if warranted.

This case illustrates how a traumatic amputation can mask adjacent soft-tissue injury. The amputation may shift attention away from more subtle indicators of compartment syndrome in proximal muscle groups, emphasizing the importance of full-body secondary survey—even under time and equipment constraints. Consistent reassessment during delayed evacuation, guided by tactical field care protocols, enabled the combat medic to stabilize the casualty, mitigate life-threatening complications, and preserve function and tissue viability for advanced surgical care.

Ultimately, through disciplined application of the MARCH sequence, early administration of key medications, wound preservation protocols, and proactive management of environmental risks, the casualty was delivered to a higher-level facility in stable condition, with a favorable trajectory for recovery and rehabilitation.

Key Messages

- Musculoskeletal injuries are highly prevalent in combat and require structured field triage into life-threatening, limb-threatening, and non-urgent categories.
- Life-threatening injuries, such as traumatic amputations and uncontrolled hemorrhage, demand immediate tourniquet use, hemostatic dressings, and resuscitation to prevent rapid fatality.
- Limb-threatening injuries, including open fractures and vascular compromise, must be identified early through neurovascular assessment and managed with splinting, antibiotics, and surgical referral.
- Non-urgent injuries, though not critical, can impact mobility and morale; prompt management with analgesia, support, and hygiene prevents long-term dysfunction.
- Field immobilization, using either commercial or improvised splints, is essential for fracture stability and safe transport. Always assess and reassess distal circulation and nerve function.
- Preservation of amputated parts using cool, sterile, sealed storage can support future reattachment or prosthetic planning—every minute matters.
- Ketamine is the preferred analgesic in field trauma for its safety, effectiveness, and minimal respiratory compromise.
- Prolonged field care protocols, including thermal protection, hydration, and infection prevention, are crucial when evacuation is delayed.
- Documentation (MIST) and communication ensure smooth transition to higher-level care and inform surgical decision-making.
- *Anticipate crush syndrome in any casualty entrapped for over 30 min*—initiate early saline resuscitation before extrication to prevent reperfusion injury.
- Recognize hyperkalemia as the most fatal complication; monitor for ECG changes, urine discoloration, and signs of renal compromise in the field.
- Prevent hypothermia, reassess regularly, and prioritize evacuation to facilities capable of managing electrolyte imbalance, renal failure, and systemic deterioration.
- Combat medics are force multipliers—when equipped with structured MSK injury protocols, they not only save lives but also preserve mobility, independence, and the operational strength of the unit.

Conclusion

Musculoskeletal injuries are among the most common and operationally significant wounds in the modern battlefield. While not always immediately life-threatening, they have the power to degrade combat effectiveness, compromise mission success, and permanently alter a soldier's life if improperly managed.

This chapter has outlined a tactical, tiered approach to extremity trauma—prioritizing hemorrhage control, fracture stabilization, neurovascular assessment, pain relief, and evacuation readiness. Whether dealing with an amputation, an open fracture, crush injury, or a minor sprain, the principles remain the same: *act early, stabilize smartly, and adapt to the environment with available resources.*

Combat medics are often the first and only responders at the point of injury. Their ability to differentiate between life-, limb-, and function-threatening injuries—combined with the skill to improvise splints, control bleeding, and preserve amputated parts—can mean the difference between recovery and permanent disability.

Through disciplined execution of FORCE-aligned protocols, we not only reduce mortality but also sustain the fighting strength, morale, and long-term resilience of our frontline troops. Mobility is mission critical—and every action taken in the first hour after injury shapes the outcome for the months ahead.

In musculoskeletal trauma, preserving soldier strength begins long before hospital care. It begins in the mud, the jungle, the desert, or the snow—*where precision under pressure becomes the true test of combat readiness.*

Bibliography

1. American College of Surgeons Committee on Trauma. ATLS: Advanced Trauma Life Support. 10th ed. Chicago: American College of Surgeons; 2018. ISBN: 978-0996826235
2. Army U.S. Tactical Combat Casualty Care Handbook. Version 5. Morrisville (NC): Lulu Press Inc.; 2017. 130 p. ISBN: 9781678198312.
3. Auerbach PS, Cushing TA, Harris NS. Auerbach's Wilderness Medicine. 7th ed. 2 vols. Philadelphia: Elsevier; 2016. ISBN: 9780323359429
4. Feliciano DV, Mattox KL, Moore EE. *Trauma*. 9th ed. New York: McGraw Hill Medical; 2020. ISBN: 978-1260143355
5. Long, Brit et al. "Crush injury and syndrome: A review for emergency clinicians." *The American journal of emergency medicine* vol. 69 (2023): 180–187. https://doi.org/10.1016/j.ajem.2023.04.029
6. Rajagopalan, S. "Crush Injuries and the Crush Syndrome." *Medical journal, Armed Forces India* vol. 66,4 (2010): 317–20. https://doi.org/10.1016/S0377-1237(10)80007-3
7. Sever, Mehmet Sukru, and Raymond Vanholder. "Management of crush victims in mass disasters: highlights from recently published recommendations." *Clinical journal of the American Society of Nephrology : CJASN* vol. 8,2 (2013): 328–35. https://doi.org/10.2215/CJN.07340712
8. St. John Ambulance Association (India), Indian Red Cross Society. First Aid Manual 7th Edition. Available from: https://www.indianredcross.org/publications/FA-manual.pdf
9. Tintinalli JE, Ma OJ, Yealy DM, et al. *Tintinalli's Emergency Medicine: A Comprehensive Study Guide*. 9th ed. New York: McGraw-Hill Education; 2019. ISBN: 978-1405296434.
10. Walters, Thomas J et al. "Management of Crush Syndrome Under Prolonged Field Care." *Journal of special operations medicine : a peer reviewed journal for SOF medical professionals* vol. 16,3 (2016): 79–85. https://doi.org/10.55460/AW4P-UO9F

Evacuation to Definitive Care and Airlift Operations

13

Romit Saxena, Manish Dhawan, Srikanth E R, and Sandeep Dhingra

Learning Objectives

At the end of this chapter, the reader should be able to:

- Understand the physiological changes and stressors associated with air medical transport.
- Identify key criteria for selecting air evacuation, including triage scoring and urgency stratification.
- Distinguish between elective, urgent, and emergent transport based on clinical scenarios.
- Describe the composition, capabilities, and limitations of Air Transport Teams (ATT) and Critical Care Air Transport Teams (CCATT).

(continued)

R. Saxena (✉)
Department of Paediatrics, Maulana Azad Medical College and Lok Nayak Hospital, New Delhi, India

M. Dhawan
Department of Anaesthesiology and Critical Care, Army Hospital (Research and Referral), New Delhi, India

Srikanth E R
Department of Critical Care Medicine, Christian Medical College, Vellore, Tamil Nadu, India

S. Dhingra
Department of Paediatrics, Army Hospital (Research and Referral), New Delhi, India

N. T. Rai, S. Misra (eds.), *Frontline Operational Resuscitation and Combat Emergencies (FORCE) Manual*, https://doi.org/10.1007/978-981-92-1622-2_13

- Recognize equipment, oxygen, and power requirements for prolonged in-flight critical care.
- Prepare patients effectively for transport, addressing airway, hemorrhage control, and stabilization.
- Apply principles of tactical aeromedical planning relevant to the combat forces and disaster situations.

Introduction

Aeromedical evacuation (AE) is a critical component of modern military and disaster response systems, enabling the rapid transfer of casualties from austere or high-threat environments to definitive care facilities. Unlike ground transport, air evacuation introduces a unique set of physiological, operational, and logistical challenges that demand meticulous preparation and trained personnel. The confined space within aircraft—be it rotary or fixed-wing—limits movement and access to the patient, while environmental stressors, such as vibration, noise, low humidity, and changes in barometric pressure, may exacerbate underlying injuries or destabilize already critical patients.

Acceleration and deceleration forces during takeoff and landing can influence cardiovascular function, particularly in hypovolemic or ventilated patients. Likewise, barometric pressure changes at altitude can lead to expansion of trapped gases, worsening conditions, such as pneumothorax, pneumocephalus, or bowel distension. Temperature regulation is often compromised in flight, increasing the risk of hypothermia—especially in trauma patients with hemorrhage.

Moreover, the lack of redundancy in power supply and oxygen sources during air transport necessitates careful calculation and backup planning to ensure continuous support for critically ill patients. As such, aeromedical evacuation is not merely a means of patient transfer—it is an extension of intensive care delivery in a dynamic, resource-limited setting.

This chapter explores the principles, protocols, and practical considerations of air medical transport in combat and disaster settings. It emphasizes physiological adaptation, equipment readiness, triage-based decision-making, and the critical role of trained teams in ensuring safe and effective casualty evacuation.

Case Scenario

During a dawn foot patrol in the remote, high-altitude valleys of North Sikkim, a 32-year-old para special forces operator triggers an improvised explosive device (IED) while stepping onto a suspected pressure plate embedded near a rock outcrop. The blast detonates directly underfoot, violently throwing him backward against a nearby tree and inflicting catastrophic injuries. His right lower limb sustains a

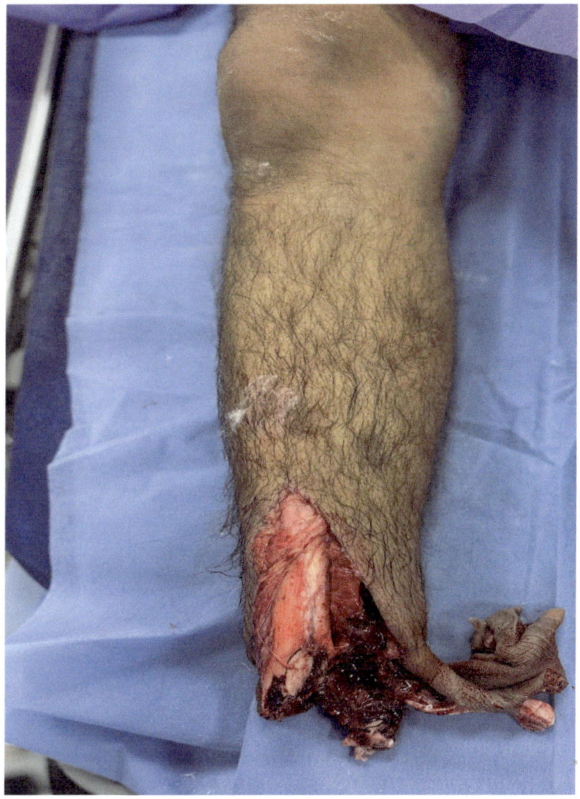

Fig. 13.1 Soldier with traumatic amputation of the right leg due to IED blast

traumatic amputation at the distal tibia, with visible arterial spurting, embedded shrapnel, and extensive open fractures (Fig. 13.1). Simultaneously, the force of the blast and secondary impact against the tree raise concern for thoracoabdominal trauma. Hostile threat remains active in the area, but his unit secures a safe perimeter, enabling the combat medic to begin immediate care under constrained field conditions.

- *Care Under Fire (CUF)*
  Initial suppression is maintained while the casualty is dragged to cover. A CAT tourniquet is applied above the knee. Combat gauze is packed into the proximal wound cavity, and a pressure bandage is applied, successfully arresting active hemorrhage. No further interventions are initiated until the threat is fully neutralized.
- *Tactical Field Care (TFC)*
  The medic proceeds with a structured MARCH assessment.
  Massive Hemorrhage (M): Bleeding from the traumatic leg amputation is reassessed. Despite the tourniquet, deep tissue oozing persists. The dressing is reinforced, and the tourniquet position is adjusted. Secondary bleeding sites from shrapnel wounds on the thigh are managed with pressure wraps.

Airway (A): The casualty is conscious and responsive to voice but groaning with visible blood at the lips. A jaw thrust confirms airway patency, though risk of compromise remains. A surgical cricothyrotomy kit is kept ready should deterioration occur during transit.

Respiration (R): Respiratory rate is elevated at 32/min with shallow effort. Breath sounds are asymmetrical—diminished on the right. A tension pneumothorax is suspected. Immediate needle decompression is performed in the right second intercostal space, followed by application of a chest seal. Oxygen saturation improves from 85 to 93%.

Circulation (C): Radial pulse is thready; systolic blood pressure is estimated at 90 mmHg. An 18 G IV is secured in the contralateral arm, and 1 g tranexamic acid (TXA) is administered over 10 min. A 500 mL bolus of warm lactated Ringer's is started and carefully titrated to maintain permissive hypotension.

Head Injury/Hypothermia (H): GCS is 14 (E4V4M6), with equal, reactive pupils. No scalp lacerations or visible skull trauma are identified. However, given the high-altitude environment, cold exposure, and blood loss, the casualty is already mildly hypothermic. He is wrapped in an insulated thermal kit with limb elevation and pelvic stabilization to mitigate retroperitoneal bleeding risk.

- *Tactical Evacuation Care (TACEVAC)*
  Rotary-wing evacuation is requested but delayed by 30–40 min due to overcast conditions and active surveillance near the landing zone. The casualty is transferred to a casualty collection point, where continuous monitoring is established with limited equipment. Oxygen delivery is not available, but ventilatory effort is reassessed every 10–15 min. Needle thoracostomy equipment is kept ready in anticipation of recurrence. Additional fluid resuscitation is withheld unless hypotension worsens. Communication is established with the rotary-wing team, and the receiving facility is pre-alerted for trauma bay readiness. En route preparations include packaging the patient for vibration, altitude, and cold tolerance during flight.

Reflective Questions

1. What clinical findings in this case justify urgent air evacuation over ground transport, and how does altitude influence this decision?
2. With a field-relieved tension pneumothorax, what precautions must be taken to prevent or manage recurrence during high-altitude air transport?
3. In the context of limited onboard oxygen and power availability in rotary-wing transport, what is the most feasible method of oxygen delivery?
4. How should the combat medic anticipate and manage altitude-related hypoxia or ventilation challenges during rotary-wing evacuation?
5. What are the implications of environmental exposure and barometric pressure changes on a patient with recent thoracic decompression and partial limb amputation?

Importance of Rapid Evacuation

For several decades, both trauma centers and military medical systems have emphasized the critical value of rapid evacuation and early intervention for patients with life-threatening injuries. Two foundational time-based concepts have emerged as cornerstones of trauma response planning: the *Platinum 10 Minutes* and the *Golden Hour*. The *Platinum 10 Minutes* refers to the ideal time window within which on-scene assessment, hemorrhage control, airway stabilization, and preparation for transport should be completed—minimizing delays and maximizing the effectiveness of early resuscitative efforts. Following this, the *Golden Hour* signifies the first 60 min after a traumatic injury during which definitive medical or surgical care must be initiated to significantly improve the chances of survival and functional recovery.

These time-sensitive frameworks have shaped the design of prehospital protocols, casualty evacuation chains, and triage algorithms in both civilian trauma systems and battlefield medicine. The overarching principle is clear: minimizing the interval between point of injury and access to definitive care—such as surgical control of hemorrhage, neurocritical intervention, or vascular repair—saves lives.

The mode and urgency of evacuation, however, must be tailored to each clinical scenario. Decisions are influenced by multiple operational and logistical factors, including the patient's hemodynamic stability and mobility, the presence of ongoing threats (e.g., hostile fire or environmental hazards), the availability and capability of the rescue team, the complexity of the terrain, prevailing weather conditions, and the distance to the nearest equipped medical facility. Efficient coordination among field responders, transport teams, and receiving centers is thus crucial for optimizing outcomes in critically injured patients.

FORCE Tactical Pearl

"Decide for Air Evac Early – Don't Wait for Deterioration"

Delayed decisions cost lives. If the casualty has active hemorrhage, thoracic injury, and altered mental status, or is at risk of deterioration due to remote terrain or tactical delays, prioritize air evacuation proactively.

Levels of Evacuation and Scoring Systems

In the FORCE model, *evacuation is not a single event but a staged, decision-driven process* that evolves with the casualty's condition, available resources, and tactical environment. The concept of *levels of evacuation* refers to the progressive transfer of a casualty from the point of injury (POI) to increasingly advanced medical care facilities, often across challenging terrain and under operational constraints.

At every stage of this continuum, triage plays a central role. It is not merely a classification tool but a dynamic decision-making process that balances clinical urgency against logistical and tactical realities. In resource-limited or mass-casualty settings, the goal of triage is clear:

optimize survival outcomes for the largest number of casualties, rather than attempting exhaustive care for every individual. This requires rapid prioritization, frequent reassessment, and the ability to adapt decisions as the situation evolves.

To support these decisions—especially in aeromedical settings—structured scoring systems are used to objectively assess patient severity and transport requirements. These tools integrate multiple parameters such as:

- Physiological status (vital signs, level of consciousness).
- Extent and pattern of injuries.
- Mechanism of injury (e.g., blast and high-velocity trauma).
- Anticipated risk of deterioration during transport.

Such scoring systems help determine not only whether evacuation is required but also the urgency, mode, and level of medical support needed during transit.

One commonly used framework (referenced in Table 13.1) stratifies patients based on cumulative scoring to guide air evacuation decisions:

- *Score ≥ 6 (high risk)*
  Indicates a critically ill casualty requiring *urgent or emergent aeromedical evacuation* with advanced in-flight care. These patients benefit from deployment of a *Critical Care Air Transport Team (CCATT)*, capable of providing intensive monitoring and interventions during transit.
- *Score 3–5 (moderate risk)*
  Represents patients who are relatively stable but carry a *significant risk of deterioration*. These casualties require *urgent evacuation with medical supervision*, typically managed by a trained Air Transport Team (ATT).
- *Score 0–2 (low risk)*
  Denotes clinically stable patients with *minimal likelihood of in-transit deterioration*. These cases can be planned for *elective evacuation*, without the need for specialized critical care teams.

While scoring systems provide valuable structure, *they are adjuncts—not substitutes—for clinical judgment*. In tactical settings, where environmental stressors (altitude, hypoxia, vibration, limited access) can exacerbate injury, even "stable" patients must be reassessed continuously.

Comparable tools, such as the *Modified Early Warning Score (MEWS)* used in critical care systems, similarly rely on physiological parameters to identify patients at risk of deterioration. These frameworks reinforce a common principle: *early recognition of instability allows timely escalation of care and safer transport planning.*

Table 13.1 Scoring system for ordering air evacuation/activation of AT/CCATT

S. no	Parameter	3	2	1	0	1	2	3
1.	HR		<40	40–50	51–100	101–110	111–129	>130
2.	Systolic BP	<70 or on inotropes	71–80	81–100	101–170	171–199	>200	
3.	Resp. rate	On mechanical ventilation	<7		9–18	19–22	23–29	>30
4.	Temp (°F)	≤94.8	95	95.2–96	96.2–101	101.2–102	102.2–103	>103
5.	CNS	Focal neurological deficits	Altered sensorium, agitation		Alert	Voice	Pain	Unresponsive
6.	O_2 requirement				Room air			Any O_2 requirement
7.	SpO_2	<91	92–93	94–95	≥96			

Scoring system for air evacuation:

Score 0–2: Elective evacuation with minimal manpower.

Score 3–5: Urgent evacuation with ATT.

Score ≥ 6: Urgent/emergent evacuation with CCATT.

Abbreviations: Resp. respiratory, *temp* temperature, *SpO_2* saturation of peripheral oxygen, *ATT* air transport team, *CCATT* critical care air transport team

[a]Adapted from Dhawan [9]

Another triaging tool includes *SALT* (Sort, Assess, Lifesaving Interventions, Treatment/Transport), which rapidly evaluates individuals based on their response to verbal commands, breathing status, and presence of severe bleeding. This early assessment allows for assigning color-coded tags to the injured, indicating the urgency and level of medical attention needed.

FORCE Tactical Pearls:

- Evacuation decisions are *dynamic and context dependent*, not score dependent alone.
- A "stable" casualty in the field may become unstable in-flight—anticipation is key.
- The *level of escort and monitoring during evacuation is as important as the destination.*
- Scoring systems guide decisions, but *experience and situational awareness define outcomes*

Modes of Transport

Medical evacuations can be performed by air or land and can involve a range of vehicles and equipment, including:

1. Ground ambulances.
2. Air ambulances: Fixed-wing or rotary-wing aircraft.
3. First-response vehicles: Fire engines, police cruisers, or sport utility vehicles.

The choice between ground and different air transport platforms depends on many factors, such as availability, staffing, infrastructure, costs, geography, distance, time, and weather conditions. Thus, the choice of transfer modality is a context-specific one. The most common vehicle used is the ground ambulance, which is categorized into three common varieties:

Type I: A standard truck (e.g., pick-up) chassis with a separate modular box to carry personnel, patients, and equipment.
Type II: An enlarged van-type vehicle.
Type III: A van chassis with an integrated modular box on the back for medical care and equipment.

Types and Indications

In general, air medical transport may be preferable if there are clinically essential savings in time to administering meaningful interventions. There are two significant types of aircraft for air medical transport.

1. Rotary-wing aircraft: Helicopters.
2. Fixed-wing aircraft: Airplanes.

Blumen et al. outlined a four-step guideline to determine the appropriateness of air medical transport:

1. *Assess the patient*: Evaluate the severity of the patient's injury or illness and consider the potential for rapid deterioration.
2. *Determine medical care needs*: Identify the medications the patient is currently taking and whether specialized equipment, such as mechanical ventilation or circulatory support, is necessary.
3. *Assess time sensitivity for transport*: Determine if reaching a definitive medical intervention is time critical.
4. *Consider logistics*: Evaluate factors, such as weather conditions, travel distance, and traffic. *Air medical transport is designed and best suited to clinical situations involving critically ill and complex patients with a high likelihood of deterioration, where there is a need to minimize time to a definitive intervention that will provide a clear benefit to the patient.*

Based on the patient's condition and severity of illness, the choice between rotary-wing aircraft (helicopters) or fixed-wing aircraft (aeroplanes) should be made following a risk and cost versus benefit analysis using criteria like travel distance, landing infrastructure, weather conditions, and clinical emergency.

Most guidelines recommend considering fixed-wing transport for longer distances, if airports and appropriate operation support services are available. In addition, there may be additional benefits of using fixed-wing aircraft under certain conditions, such as adverse weather. Fixed-wing aircraft can use instruments to fly in challenging weather that some rotor-wing aircraft cannot. Finally, in general, fixed-wing aircraft can lift more weight and carry additional specialized equipment and personnel, which may be a consideration.

Physiological Considerations during Air Transport

This is elucidated in Table 13.2 and Fig. 13.2.

FORCE Tactical Pearl
"Anticipate Altitude-Related Gas Expansion".

Pneumothorax, bowel gas, and pneumocephalus expand at altitude. Mitigate risk with preflight decompression, NG tube placement, or surgical preparation when feasible.

Table 13.2 Physiological stressors in air medical transport

Changes during air transport	System affected	Physiological stressor	Management considerations
Sustained acceleration or deceleration	Cardiovascular system	Upon exposure to positive G forces, blood will "pool" in the dependent areas resulting in decreased cardiac preload and decreased cardiac output and blood pressure Hypovolemia and positive pressure ventilation also reduce venous return and worsen hypotension	Optimizing preload prior to transfer; the use of pneumatic anti-shock suits; or by raising the patient's legs during the acceleration (thus limiting the vector acting in the z-axis). Well-filled patients tolerate transfer better than those who are hypovolemic
	Neurological system	During deceleration, the intracranial pressure increases due to action of cephalad forces; blood and CSF are pulled into the cranial cavity, leading to a rise in ICP and reduction in cerebral perfusion pressure, which may worsen secondary brain injury	Use appropriate ICP control measures especially during deceleration
	Respiratory system	During deceleration, there is an upward displacement of the abdominal organs, which leads to splinting of the diaphragm, decreased tidal volumes, increased airway pressures, and worsening gas exchange	Appropriate positioning of patient, and stabilization prior to transport, and empty stomach contents
	Equipment and medical personnel	Lines and tubes can become displaced	Transfer trolleys should be compliant with the appropriate regulatory requirements, and the patient should be secured appropriately (e.g., a five-point strap). Equipment should be securely stowed in lockers or on the floor against a bulkhead. During air transfers, staff should remain strapped during takeoff and landing, as well as during other periods of high risk (e.g., turbulence or low-level flying)

(continued)

Table 13.2 (continued)

Changes during air transport	System affected	Physiological stressor	Management considerations
Barometric pressure changes Gas expansion (gas contained in a fixed space will expand with increased altitude or decreased pressure, according to Boyles law ($P \propto 1/V$) and ideal gas equation $PV = nRT$	Lung	Pneumothoraces will expand as height increases, worsening gas exchange and potentially causing a tension pneumothorax	*ICD should not be clamped during a flight.* If the patient is at risk or has a proven pneumothorax, ICD should be inserted prior to flight, and skilled personnel, who can insert the ICD as necessary in-flight, should accompany the patient
	Bowel gas/ pneumoperitoneum	Patients with ileus, bowel obstruction, or following bowel surgery have increased bowel gas, and the expansion of this gas can distend the bowel, leading to perforation or anastomotic breakdown	Insertion of NG tube and keeping the same on free dependent drainage or flying with cabin pressurization
	Brain	Pneumocephalus and open head fractures can potentially expand, resulting in features of increased intracranial pressure	Watch for features of increased intracranial pressure
Noise and vibration from engine		Hearing loss and motion sickness *Ventilator auto-triggering*	Hearing protection for treating team and patients
Flicker vertigo	Affects crew more	Occurs in rotary-wing aircraft especially in transport crew. It can induce vertigo or motion sickness and even epilepsy in susceptible individuals. Nausea, vomiting, sweating, and light-headedness may be experienced	Patients' eyes should be protected from the flicker especially if they have a history of motion sickness or epilepsy
Extreme temperature	Risk of hypothermia	Air temperature decreases by roughly 2 °C per 1000 ft. Hypothermia can lead to worsening coagulopathy and cardiac arrhythmias	Monitor temperature Adequate heating equipment as blankets and heating devices should be present and flight tested
Humidity		Difficult to regulate humidity	Use of HME filters, routine eye care (with artificial tears) in prolonged air transfers

(continued)

Table 13.2 (continued)

Changes during air transport	System affected	Physiological stressor	Management considerations
Medical equipment		On ascent, the cuff pressure may increase, causing mucosal ischemia, and on descent, it decreases, leading to a cuff leak Other gas-filled equipment (e.g., pressure bags) should also be monitored as they are at risk of rupture	Cuff pressure should be measured regularly especially following changes in altitude or the cuff should be filled with saline All equipment used must be validated and approved for use in the air environment

PV = nRT, where P is pressure, V is volume, n is number of moles, T is temperature, and R is gas constant

Abbreviations: ICP intracranial pressure, *CSF* cerebrospinal fluid; *ICD* intercostal drainage; *NG* nasogastric; *HME* heat and moisture exchangers

[a]Adapted from Hale [12]

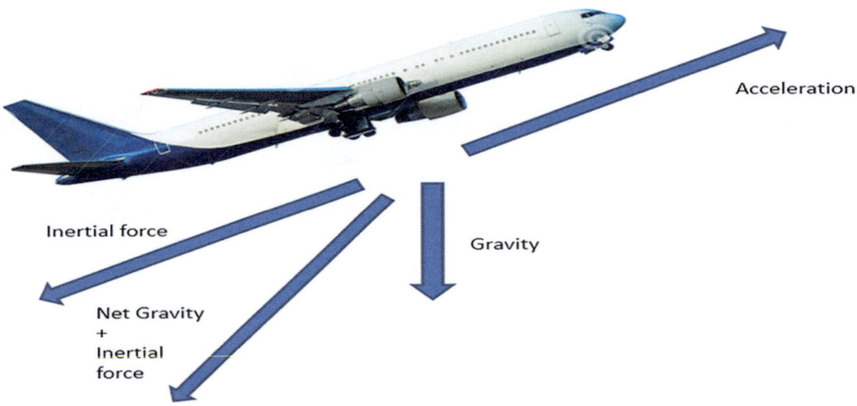

Fig. 13.2 Representation of various forces acting during aeromedical transfer in a fixed-wing aircraft like aeroplane

India's armed and paramilitary forces frequently operate in geographically challenging and logistically isolated environments, including high-altitude borders, dense forests, deserts, and insurgency-affected regions. In these settings, access to advanced medical care is often significantly delayed due to limited road infrastructure, difficult terrain, and long distances from secondary or tertiary care facilities.

While most casualties can be managed with initial stabilization and staged evacuation, a select group of critically ill or potentially unstable soldiers require rapid access to advanced diagnostics and definitive care. For such cases, time-sensitive aeromedical evacuation becomes a crucial link in the survival chain, enabling early transfer while maintaining continuity of care.

To address this need, specialized systems, such as the *Critical Care Air Transport Team (CCATT)*, have been developed. These teams represent a highly skilled but limited resource, designed to deliver intensive care capabilities within the constraints of an in-flight environment. Their role extends across a wide operational spectrum—from routine inter-facility transfers in remote areas to mass-casualty situations, disaster response, and active combat operations. In large-scale emergencies, multiple CCATT units can be mobilized simultaneously to facilitate the evacuation of several critically ill patients, ensuring scalable response capability.

The *Patient Transfer Unit (PTU)*, in conjunction with CCATT, is structured to safely transport stabilized yet high-risk patients from forward or remote locations to higher centers of care. Their primary objective is not merely transportation, but continuity of critical care during transit. This includes:

- Continuous physiological monitoring.
- Early identification of deterioration.
- Delivery of advanced interventions when required.
- Mitigation of physiological stressors associated with flight, such as hypobaric hypoxia, reduced humidity, and vibration.

The aeromedical environment itself poses unique challenges. Changes in cabin pressure, oxygen availability, and temperature can adversely impact patients with head injuries, thoracic trauma, or hemodynamic instability. Therefore, the role of PTU and CCATT extends beyond evacuation—*they function as mobile intensive care units, ensuring that patient stability is maintained from departure to handover.*

FORCE Tactical Pearls:

- In remote Indian settings, evacuation is often delayed—making in-transit care as critical as definitive care.
- CCATT is not just transport—*it is ICU-level care in motion.*
- *The decision to activate CCATT should be based on anticipated deterioration, not just current stability.*
- Flight physiology can worsen injuries—anticipation and preparation are key.

Aeromedical Evacuation (AE)

In combat and austere environments, timely aeromedical evacuation (AE) plays a critical role in improving survival and outcomes following traumatic injury. Choosing the appropriate mode of transport—rotary-wing (helicopter) or fixed-wing aircraft—depends on multiple operational and clinical factors, including distance, terrain, weather, patient condition, and available infrastructure. Each platform has distinct advantages and limitations that impact the speed, safety, and complexity

Table 13.3 Fixed-wing and rotary-wing/helicopter transport

Rotary-wing/helicopter	Fixed-wing aircraft
Advantages: Allows for rapid transfer for moderate distance. Accessible. Maneuverable.	Advantages: Speed. More cabin space. Maybe pressurized. Less noise and vibration. Can potentially avoid bad weather.
Disadvantages: Requires helipad. Not pressurized. Limited space. Noise and vibration. Unfavorable thermal environment.	Disadvantages: Expensive. Requires runway space. Needs road transport from airport to hospital.

of patient transfer. While helicopters are preferred for rapid point-to-point evacuation in difficult terrains if the distance is less than 250 km, fixed-wing aircraft offer advantages for long-distance transfers and are used if the distance is more than 250 km (Table 13.3).

Categories of Aeromedical Evacuation

In the tactical framework, aeromedical evacuation is categorized based on clinical urgency, patient stability, and resource requirements during transport. These categories help align evacuation decisions with both medical need and operational feasibility.

(a) *Medical Evacuation (MEDEVAC)*

MEDEVAC refers to the rapid evacuation of casualties from the point of injury to the nearest suitable medical facility, primarily aimed at enabling early resuscitation and stabilization. It is typically *time critical* and *most often conducted using rotary-wing aircraft (helicopters) to minimize delay.*

In operational settings, MEDEVAC is frequently initiated under uncertain or evolving clinical conditions, where *speed takes precedence over complete stabilization.*

(b) *Elective Aeromedical Evacuation (Elective AE)*

Elective AE involves the *planned transfer of clinically stable patients*, usually in the recovery or convalescent phase of illness or injury. These evacuations are undertaken when *specialized investigations, procedures, or expertise are not available locally*, rather than due to immediate life-threatening concerns.

Such transfers are *scheduled, resource optimized, and low risk*, with minimal likelihood of in-flight deterioration.

(c) *Urgent Aeromedical Evacuation (Urgent AE)*

Urgent AE applies to patients who are *stabilized but remain at risk of clinical deterioration.* These patients require *timely transfer to higher-level care*, even though immediate lifesaving intervention is not currently underway.

Typically, these casualties have:

- Secured airway (spontaneous or assisted).
- Controlled hemorrhage.
- Initial resuscitation completed.
- Stabilized fractures or injuries.

The emphasis in urgent AE is on *preventing secondary complications by avoiding delays*, ensuring that definitive care is accessed before deterioration occurs (Table 13.4).

(d) *Emergent Aeromedical Evacuation (Emergent AE)*

Emergent AE is reserved for *critically ill or potentially unstable patients*, where *delay in transfer may result in loss of life or limb*. These evacuations are initiated when *essential medical capabilities are unavailable at the current location*, necessitating immediate transport despite ongoing instability.

Typical scenarios include:

- Ongoing internal hemorrhage not amenable to immediate control.
- Vascular catastrophes (e.g., traumatic aortic injury) requiring specialized intervention.
- Conditions requiring advanced subspecialty care (e.g., interventional radiology and cardiothoracic or vascular surgery) not available in forward settings.

In such cases, evacuation occurs *in parallel with active resuscitation*, often requiring advanced in-flight monitoring and intervention by specialized teams.

Manpower Requirements

Patient transfer can be classified into Air Transport Team (ATT) and Critical Care Air Transport Team (CCATT), with different manpower requirements as outlined in Table 13.5.

Manpower, drugs, and equipment required in an emergent AE are the same as in urgent AE, depending on whether ATT or CCAT Team is to accompany the patient.

Table 13.4 Differences and considerations for elective and urgent aeromedical evacuation

	Elective AE	Urgent AE
Time of evacuation	Air transport is delayed sufficiently long after definitive therapy so that rigors of air travel are unlikely to result in medical decompensation of patients	Air transport as soon as possible within 24–48 h of requisition for AE
Availability of treatment	Some facilities may not be available at peripheral hospitals; such patients can be transferred to a tertiary care hospital where requisite facilities and expertise are available	The referring hospital is unable to keep the patient until full patient recovery or convalescence in the hospital due to: Nonavailability of specialized care like neurologist, neurosurgeon, cardiologist, nephrologist, or critical care specialist Limited resources of the hospital, i.e., hospital unable to sustain constant supplies of drugs or equipment for a longer duration of time, e.g., prolonged mechanical ventilation or requirement of long-term dialysis
Physical considerations	Elective AE may be undertaken when a difficult terrain separates the patient from a medical facility, e.g., 45-min flight over a mountain range may be safer than a 3-h ambulance ride over rough terrain	Recently treated, stabilized patient may decompensate due to disease condition, mode of injury, and even stress of AE
Examples	Stable dorsolumbar vertebral fracture without neurological deficit or open comminuted long bone fracture after initial stabilization for transfer to a trauma center	Severe head injury, postexternal ventricular drain (EVD) or decompressive craniectomy, polytrauma after initial damage control surgery, rhabdomyolysis with acute kidney injury requiring dialysis for transfer to a tertiary care hospital

Table 13.5 Differences between Air Transport Team (ATT) and Critical Care Air Transport Team (CCATT)

	Air Transport Team (ATT)	Critical Care Air Transport Team (CCATT)
Manpower	Doctor ±1 Critical care trained nurse 01 Operation room assistant 01 Medical assistants 02 Housekeeping staff 01	Critical care physician 01 Critical care trained nurse 01 Operation room assistant 01 Medical assistants 02 Housekeeping staff 01
Drugs and equipment	Resuscitation bag: Drugs, airways, Ambu bag/Bains circuit Oxygen bank with inverter/battery backup: 2–4 O_2 cylinders depending on en route O_2 requirement Multiparameter monitor with defibrillator IV fluids Routine drugs: Antibiotics, analgesics, etc.	Resuscitation bag: Drugs, airways, Ambu bag/Bains circuit Oxygen bank with inverter/battery backup: 2–4 O_2 cylinders Multiparameter monitor with defibrillator Transport ventilator Vasopressors, inotropes, anti-arrhythmic, antihypertensive injections, and anesthetic drugs Infusion pumps IV fluids and routine drugs: IV antibiotics, analgesics, etc. Drugs specific to the clinical condition
Role of each member		
Critical care physician	Have critical care knowledge and skills related to their primary medical specialty including anesthesiology, medicine, pulmonology, surgery, pediatrics, and emergency medicine Is the team leader. He is responsible for overall in-flight management of the patient, planning of the mission, and its execution	
Critical care nurse	Nurses preferably who are trained in basics of intensive care Assists the team leader in nursing care, administration of drugs, IV fluids, vasopressor/inotropic infusions, and other supportive care	

(continued)

Table 13.5 (continued)

	Air Transport Team (ATT)	Critical Care Air Transport Team (CCATT)
Operation room assistants (ORAs)	Assists the team leader and nurse in preparation of drugs, maintenance of airway, and handling of ventilator and other electro-medical equipment, drains, and catheters.	
Medical assistants	Assist the team in loading/unloading the patient and equipment in the ambulance or the aircraft and other supportive role like changing of oxygen cylinders, connecting the electro-medical equipment to the patient and to the inverter-battery (if required), operating the suction machine for clearing oropharyngeal secretions, maintaining the in-flight records of the patient, and preparing the handing-taking over summary to the receiving team at the airport	
Housekeeping staff	Handle biomedical waste, including cleaning of spills of blood, urine, vomitus, or drains as well as handling of sharps as per laid down policy. Responsible for handling luggage and ensuring the food and comfort of the patient and the team Assists the team in loading and unloading of the patient transfer unit (PTU)	
Important considerations: Management checklists of adverse events and complications is required to be in place. It is easy to categorize and take equipment as a part of specific pre-checked kits, for example, airway equipment, vascular access equipment, monitoring, medications, chest compressing devices if available, pneumothorax kit, and trauma kit.		

Unique Aspects of Air Transport

Specific considerations during air transfer besides having sufficient equipment include communication and radiofrequency interference. Sufficient oxygen should be calculated for the duration of the journey, with consideration given for any diversion or any eventuality. *It is advisable to always take three times the calculated volume of oxygen required and to have sufficient power supply, including battery source for the entire duration of the flight.* Patient, staff, and equipment safety remains most important, and all efforts should be made to secure all these three elements safely, and instructions of air crew should be always followed. All equipment must be secured for takeoff and landing and during flight when not in use. Each transport service providing aeromedical transfer should be compliant with standards, such as those set out by the European Aeromedical Institute or the Commission on Accreditation of Medical Transport Systems (CAMTS) Standards.

In a country like India, having a dedicated air ambulance can be challenging because of nonavailability of aircrafts specifically for air evacuation of critically ill patients, especially for long-distance missions. A dedicated air ambulance also turns out to be very expensive. Nowadays, Quick Conversion Kits (QCK) are available,

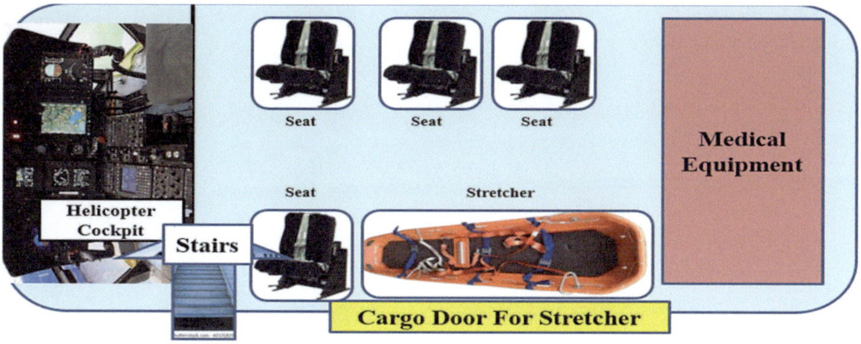

Fig. 13.3 Typical seating arrangement in six-seater aircraft

which can convert a fixed-wing aircraft or a helicopter into an air ambulance (Fig. 13.3). Broadly, the following are the details of equipment installed as part of QCK:

(i) *Platform*: In an aircraft whether fixed wing or rotary wing, platform forms the base on which one or two stretcher bases can be fitted on the two sides, respectively. This manufactured platform is aircraft specific and cannot be used in any other aircraft. For any modifications to the seating arrangements, manufacturers or agencies authorized by the OEM should be involved in creating a customized platform. The platform is used to fix the stretcher trolleys so that they do not move during takeoff, landing, or in-air turbulence (Fig. 13.4).
(ii) *Stretcher trolleys*: The stretchers are fitted with wheels and can be easily rolled in and rolled out with the stretcher bases. The stretchers are ergonomically designed with surfaces that can be cleaned easily. The head end of the stretcher can be elevated to any angle between 0 and 90°.
(iii) *Medical equipment carrier*: This is customized for the type of aircraft and is in the foremost part of the cargo compartment (Fig. 13.5) anchored to the internal airframe of the aircraft (Fig. 13.6).
(iv) *Cabinet for drugs and other consumable equipment*: This is provided to store expendable and nonexpendable medical items. In a rotary-wing aircraft, it is generally at the rear end of the cargo compartment between the two stretchers (Fig. 13.7).
(v) *Time for role conversion*: The configuration may take up to 4 h to convert the aircraft to an air ambulance.
(vi) *Power*: An adapter is connected to the aircraft power source. All the electromedical equipment on board derive power from this adapter. Once all the equipment is fully charged, the battery backup of each equipment can vary from 2 to 8 h. The charging of equipment can be done from the aircraft power source only when the aircraft engine is switched on. This power supply unit is specific to aircraft and requires modifications with addition of frequency converter to the aircraft. This feature may not be available on majority of aircraft.

Fig. 13.4 Platform for fixing stretcher trolley in a helicopter

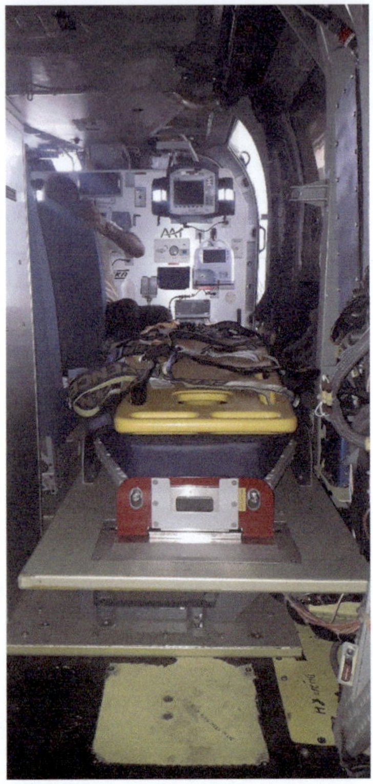

Fig. 13.5 Medical equipment carrier with ventilator, multiparameter monitor, and suction

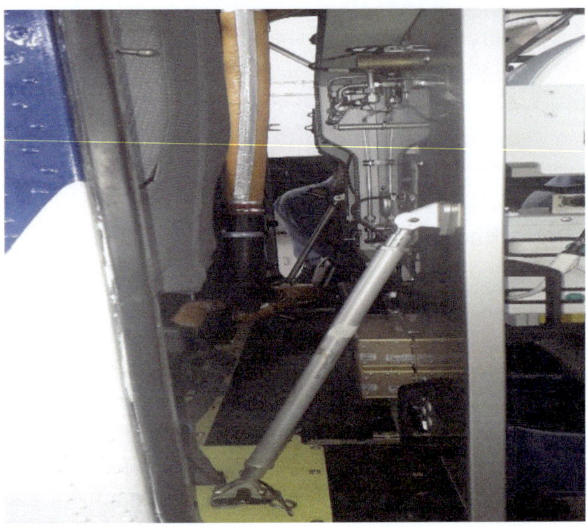

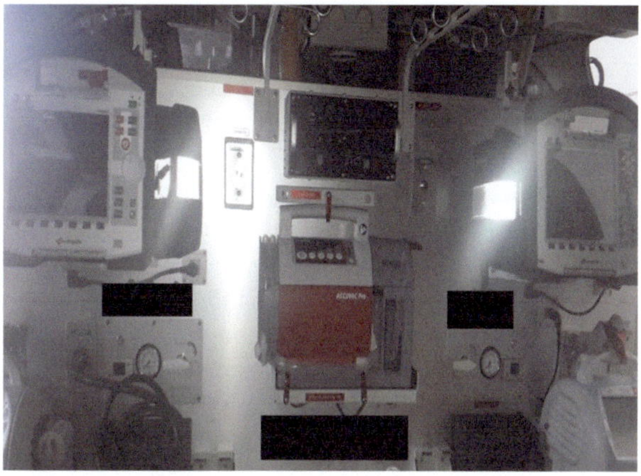

Fig. 13.6 Medical equipment carrier wall anchored to the internal airframe of the helicopter

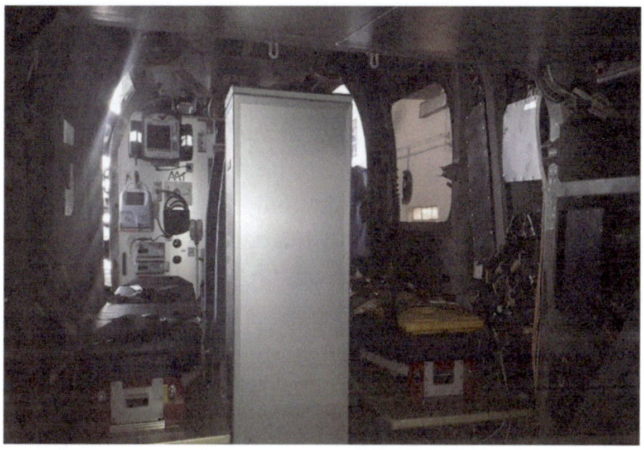

Fig. 13.7 Cabinet for drugs and other consumables at the rear end of helicopter

(vii) *Paucity of space*: Any CCATT consists of at least five to six personnel as described earlier. With the present QCK, there appears paucity of space to carry additional medical manpower, especially helicopters. Over and above, there may be paucity of space for aircraft tradesmen like a flight engineer who may be part of aircrew of most aircrafts.

(viii) *Use of automated CPR device*: Continuous high-quality CPR becomes extremely difficult during air evacuation as it involves space constraints and the healthcare workers being unbelted during flight making it unsafe for the crew especially in rotor wing transport. Therefore, some transfer teams now have an automated CPR device, device like a load-distribution band (e.g., *Autopulse®*) or a piston-based chest compression device (e.g., *LUCAS®* device), which takes care of the compressions while the medical team are safely secured to their seats during the critical phases of a flight as in takeoff, in-flight, and landing. Automated CPR devices have been tried by teams during transfer providing significant help by reducing hands-off time during resuscitation in addition to providing high-quality CPR during long flights or flight rescue maneuvers. Usually, the crew will decline transfer of such patients; however, if a high-acuity patient arrests during transport, then the need for mechanical CPR device may arise. The crew could decide on diverting to a landing facility or return to the primary hospital.

Oxygen Stations and Oxygen Cylinders

An average B type oxygen cylinder of 1320 L capacity gives a backup of approximately 2 h in a ventilated patient or up to 3.5 h if oxygen is given at a rate of 5 L/min through facemask. As a rule of thumb, *supplies up to three times the calculated requirements* should be carried along in any mission to cater for unforeseen problems like bad weather, technical snag in the aircraft, delay in receiving ambulance reaching the airport, or other administrative problems. So, if the estimated flying time of a mission is 2 h, at least three to four oxygen cylinders will provide a backup of approximately 6–8 h and should be carried for any safe transfer of a patient.

The CCATT should carry lightweight oxygen cylinders. Aluminum alloy oxygen cylinders are one such kind of lightweight cylinders. While these do reduce the weight as compared to conventional oxygen cylinders, they may not be airworthy certified. The weight of oxygen bank can be brought down further by using carbon composite oxygen cylinders, which weigh approximately 30% lighter than aluminum alloy cylinders and have higher holding capacity at a higher service pressure up to 300 bar. Using carbon composite cylinders may reduce the number of cylinders being carried to two instead of four, which can be fitted in the PTU by making minor alterations in the stretcher trolley of PTU.

The Mounted Medical Oxygen System (MMOS), which is used in certain types of aircraft, is now available (Fig. 13.8). It is a low-pressure portable liquid oxygen storage and gaseous delivery system that requires no external power. The MMOS has been successfully tested to work in tandem with commonly used ventilators. It requires no external power and uses just one 9 V battery for the quantity indicator.

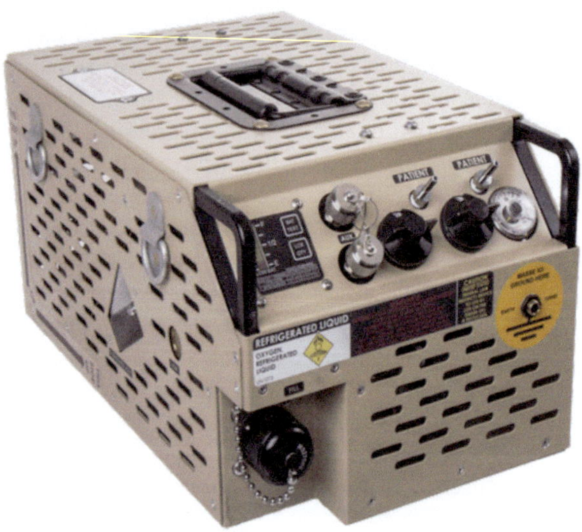

Fig. 13.8 Mounted Medical Oxygen Supply (MMOS)

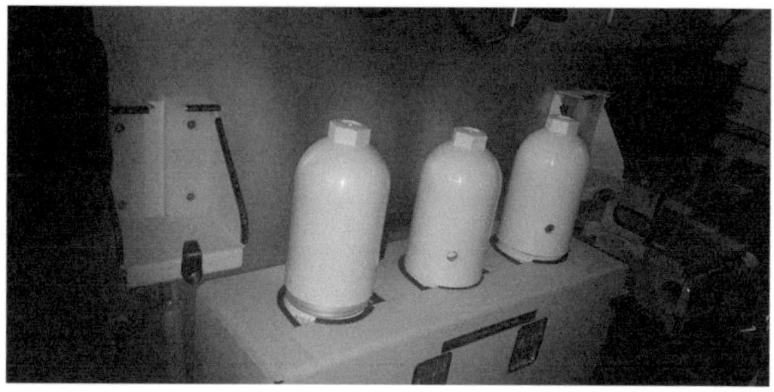

Fig. 13.9 Oxygen station in a helicopter

Oxygen Station Consists of 02–04 light weight oxygen cylinders, each with a varying capacity depending on the size and type of oxygen cylinder (Fig. 13.9). Outlet oxygen pressure for ventilator should be 4.5 bar, which is compatible with turbine-based transport ventilator. The cylinders are connected in series, with valve of only the first cylinder kept open. As the pressure of oxygen falls below a certain threshold level, a low-pressure indicator alarm gets activated, and the valve of the second cylinder needs to be opened to maintain steady flow of oxygen at the desired pressure. Once the second cylinder shows low pressure, the valve of third cylinder is opened. This would require frequent monitoring by the evacuation team. The cylinders should be certified for air worthiness and safety at high altitudes.

FORCE Tactical Pearl

"Three Times Oxygen Rule".

Estimate oxygen requirement for the full flight duration and carry at least 3× the calculated oxygen volume to compensate for weather delays, altitude, or technical issues.

Patient Transfer Units

Patient Transfer Units (PTUs) are used for casualty evacuation from remote locations/peripheral hospitals to tertiary care centers after initial management and stabilization in controlled conditions with availability of all critical care equipment for safe transportation of the patient. A PTU is a stretcher trolley-based self-sufficient unit, with a platform for monitors, ventilators, other equipment, and oxygen. The platform is referred to as *SMEAD* (Small Medical Emergency Aeromedical Device), which is mounted on top of the stretcher trolley (Fig. 13.10). It is used to mount the electro-medical equipment, including the multiparameter monitor with defibrillator, transport ventilator, suction machine, and infusion pumps.

Defibrillation during CPR is possible without interference to flight with modern navigation systems. This is done by usual standard safety procedures after informing the pilot.

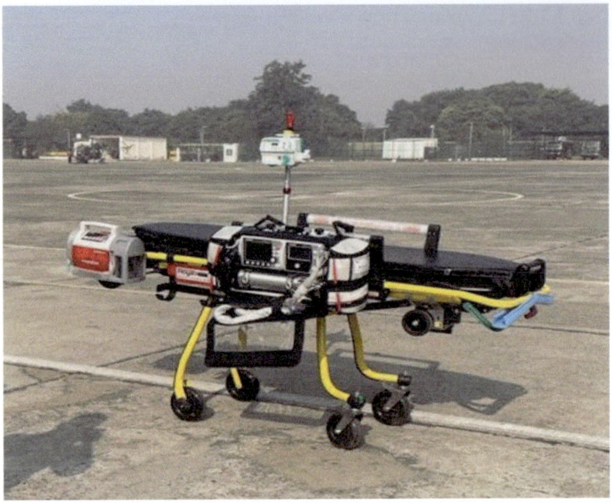

Fig. 13.10 Patient Transfer Unit (PTU): with light weight, airworthy electro-medical equipment mounted on a stretcher trolley. It includes Stretcher trolley, Defibrillator/AED with/without automated CPR device; Multi-parameter monitor, Transport ventilator, Oxygen source, Electric suction device with battery back-up and Infusion pumps

The Ventilator

The transport ventilators used in hospital settings are not compatible with altitude and thus will give increased tidal volumes with decreased barometric pressure, which occurs as the altitude increases. The cabin altitude of all transport aircrafts is maintained at 6000–8000 ft., which will result in a hypobaric environment, and will adversely impact the function of the ventilator, which could be an issue in patients with borderline respiratory function. An airworthy, lightweight ventilator, which compensates for decreased barometric pressure, is ideally suited for AEs.

Team Composition and Training Issues

Since air transport is a very specific kind of transport, it needs repeated training and updating. Providers, no matter how much skilled they are in resuscitation, need regular training, hands-on experience, and multiple graded simulations, before they can be certified for safe air transport. The experience gained over the years can be utilized to overcome the limitations and shortcomings encountered and enhance professional and administrative capabilities of the CCATT.

The CCATT needs to be well versed with critical care monitoring and procedures and at the same time possess sufficient knowledge of aviation medicine, particularly the effect of the flight environment on patient physiology and homeostasis, which is very often delicately balanced in the critically ill. The operations of CCATT using PTU are essential and vital steps forward in the safe and speedy evacuation of casualties from remote geographical areas. The capability of onboard monitoring, cardiorespiratory support, and intervention have permitted movement of casualties, which could not be transported in earlier years, resulting in saving more lives and limbs.

There are training courses that emphasize the above in the West, but commensurate training courses are the need of the hour in our country.

Case Resolution

Upon arrival at the designated landing zone (LZ), the casualty was immobilized using a vacuum mattress with full spinal precautions. A focused reassessment was performed—his airway remained patent, and the previously applied chest seal was intact with no signs of respiratory distress or new thoracic injury. Recognizing the risk of reaccumulation of air due to altitude-related gas expansion, the medical team ensured that a second needle decompression kit and chest drain setup were readily available during flight. His oxygen saturation was 92% on low-flow oxygen delivered through a nasal cannula connected to a portable field oxygen concentrator—an ideal choice in rotary-wing aircraft where electrical power is limited and oxygen resources must be conserved.

A second tourniquet was placed proximal to the initial one on the right thigh to ensure hemorrhage control redundancy. Vital signs showed a MAP of approximately 65 mmHg and thready peripheral pulses. To maintain organ perfusion without worsening bleeding, a second 500 mL bolus of warmed lactated Ringer's was administered during flight, adhering to principles of permissive hypotension.

Throughout the evacuation, the team closely monitored for signs of respiratory decline that could indicate recurrent pneumothorax—such as falling SpO_2, increasing respiratory rate, or tracheal deviation. Manual ventilation equipment and surgical airway kits were kept primed in anticipation of potential decompensation, especially given the patient's thoracoabdominal trauma. Effective communication was maintained with the receiving trauma center, which pre-alerted the vascular and orthopedic surgical teams for rapid intervention on arrival.

Upon landing, the casualty was transported directly to the operating theater. He underwent emergency fasciotomy, limb salvage procedures, and staged vascular repair. Imaging confirmed no expansion of the pneumothorax, and chest drainage was not required. Due to effective field hemorrhage control, airway management, TXA administration, and vigilant in-flight monitoring by the CCATT team, the casualty remained hemodynamically stable and neurologically intact.

Despite undergoing a below-knee amputation, the casualty survived with preserved cognitive function and no evidence of secondary brain injury or respiratory failure. This outcome was made possible by the early decision for air evacuation based on clinical indicators: traumatic amputation with active hemorrhage, thoracic injury with initial tension physiology, and limited tactical feasibility of prolonged ground transport. Oxygen delivery was optimized for the altitude, and equipment redundancy mitigated risk en route. This case exemplifies how decisive field interventions, supported by aeromedical planning and tactical foresight, can significantly reduce morbidity in hostile, high-altitude environments.

Key Messages

- Timely air evacuation saves lives, especially in remote, high-altitude, or tactically inaccessible terrain.
- MARCH protocol integration into preflight assessment is critical for determining readiness for transport.
- Chest injuries (e.g., tension pneumothorax) must be actively managed before and during flight due to air pressure variations.
- Airborne physiology affects gas exchange, perfusion, and wound dynamics—preparation and equipment must reflect these risks.
- Effective casualty monitoring and escalation planning during rotary−/fixed-wing transport are essential to sustain survival en route.

Conclusion

Air evacuation represents a vital bridge between field stabilization and definitive care. In combat settings, where terrain, weather, and threat delays complicate extraction, the ability to deliver continuous resuscitation during flight is mission critical. This chapter signifies the importance of preflight triage using MARCH and scoring systems, physiological anticipation, and redundancy in oxygen, power, and monitoring during aeromedical transport. *When seconds matter, it is not just the aircraft that moves the casualty—but the preparedness of the team inside it that truly determines survival.*

Bibliography

1. 2017_levels_of_evacuation.pdf [Internet]. [cited 2024 Nov 1]. Available from: https://www.wildmedcenter.com/uploads/5/9/8/2/5982510/2017_levels_of_evacuation.pdf
2. ATLS-10th-Edition.pdf [Internet]. [cited 2024 Nov 1]. Available from: https://saude.ufpr.br/labsim/wp-content/uploads/sites/23/2022/08/ATLS-10th-Edition.pdf
3. Aviation Medicine Course Manual. UCT/Stellenbosch university. 2006.
4. Blumen IJ, Lemkin DL, Association AMP. Principles and Direction of Air Medical Transport: Previously the Air Medical Physician Handbook [Internet]. Air Medical Physician Association; 2006. Available from: https://books.google.co.in/books?id=i9CoZwEACAAJ
5. Chapter 43. Aviation, High Altitude, and Space Physiology. In: Guyton and Hall Textbook of Medical Physiology. 12th ed.
6. Commission on Accreditation of Medical Transport Systems. Accreditation standards of The Commission On Accreditation of Medical Transport Systems. Eleventh edition [Internet]. 2018. Available from: https://www.camts.org/wp-content/uploads/2017/05/CAMTS-11th-Standards-DIGITAL-FREE.pdf
7. Critical Care Transfer Training Handbook [Internet]. Marylebone Road, London: Critical care network North west London; 2017. 1–42 p. Available from: https://www.londonccn.nhs.uk/media/1390/transfer-handbook-2017-nov.pdf
8. Custalow CB, Gravitz CS. Emergency medical vehicle collisions and potential for preventive intervention. Prehosp Emerg Care. 2004;8(2):175–84.

9. Dhawan M, Joshi MC, Dudeja P. Scoring system for activation of critical care air transport team for aeromedical evacuation. Med J Armed Forces India. 2021 Oct;77(4):397–402.
10. Gässler H, Kümmerle S, Ventzke MM, Lampl L, Helm M. Mechanical chest compression: an alternative in helicopter emergency medical services? Intern Emerg Med. 2015 Sep;10(6):715–20.
11. Goodman MD, Makley AT, Lentsch AB, Barnes SL, Dorlac GR, Dorlac WC, et al. Traumatic brain injury and aeromedical evacuation: when is the brain fit to fly? J Surg Res. 2010 Dec;164(2):286–93.
12. Hale JJ, Hall DP, Dunn MJG. Physiology of patient transfer by land and air. Anaesthesia & Intensive Care Medicine. 2019 Oct 1;20(10):595–9.
13. Hurd WW, Jernigan JG, editors. Aeromedical Evacuation: Management of Acute and Stabilized Patients [Internet]. New York, NY: Springer; 2003 [cited 2024 Nov 9]. Available from: http://link.springer.com/10.1007/b98827
14. Intensive Care Society. Guidelines for the transport of the critically ill adult. 3rd Edition. [Internet]. 2011. Available from: http://www.ics.ac.uk/ics-homepage/guidelines-and-standards
15. Jhamb , U, Saxena, R. Transport of sick kids :TaSK Module . IAP Presidential plan. Indian Academy of Pediatrics 2021. Ed. 1. 1–368.
16. Johnson D, Luscombe M. Aeromedical Transfer of the Critically Ill Patient. Journal of the Intensive Care Society. 2011 Oct 1;12(4):307–12.
17. Loyd JW, Larsen T, Swanson D. Aeromedical Transport. In: StatPearls [Internet]. Treasure Island (FL): StatPearls Publishing; 2020 [cited 2021 Jan 31]. Available from: http://www.ncbi.nlm.nih.gov/books/NBK518986/
18. Lutman C. CATS Aeromedical Transfer (Clinical): Clinical Guideline [Internet]. NHS Children's Acute Transport Service; 2018. Available from: https://cats.nhs.uk/wp-content/uploads/sog-aeromedicaltransfer.pdf
19. Lutman D. General Aeromedical Considerations : Standard Operational Guidance [Internet]. NHS Children's Acute Transport Service; 2018. Available from: https://cats.nhs.uk/wp-content/uploads/sog-generalaeromedical.pdf
20. Mattox KL, Moore EE, Feliciano DV. Trauma, Seventh Edition [Internet]. McGraw-Hill Education; 2013. Available from: https://books.google.co.in/books?id=nqYVYK1kohgC
21. Morris K, Wilson P, Fortune PM, Heward Y, Perrring J. Quality Standards for the Care of Critically Ill Children [Internet]. Paediatric Intensive Care Society and West Midlands Quality Review Service; 2015. Available from: https://pccsociety.uk/wp-content/uploads/2016/05/PICS_standards_2015.pdf
22. Nakajima M, Aso S, Yasunaga H, Shirokawa M, Nakano T, Miyakuni Y, et al. Body temperature change and outcomes in patients undergoing long-distance air medical transport. Am J Emerg Med. 2019 Jan;37(1):89–93.
23. National-Model-EMS-Clinical-Guidelines_2022.pdf [Internet]. [cited 2024 Nov 1]. Available from: https://nasemso.org/wp-content/uploads/National-Model-EMS-Clinical-Guidelines_2022.pdf
24. Paediatric and Neonatal Critical Care Transport Ed. Barry, P.; Leslie, A. Tavistock Square, London: BMJ Publishing Group;
25. Pietsch U, Lischke V, Pietsch C. Benefit of mechanical chest compression devices in mountain HEMS: lessons learned from 1 year of experience and evaluation. Air Med J. 2014 Dec;33(6):299–301.
26. Ramadas R, Hendel S, MacKillop A. Civilian aeromedical retrievals (the Australian experience). BJA Education. 2016 Jun 1;16(6):186–90.
27. Rash. Awareness of causes and symptoms of flicker vertigo can limit ill effects. Human factors and aviation medicine. 2004 Apr;6.
28. Ravi P, Joshi M, Dhawan M, Sud S, Vijai M. Critical care air transport team and patient transfer unit: A decade of experience of a zonal hospital. Journal of Marine Medical Society. 2019 Jan 1;21:121.
29. Rice DH, Kotti G, Beninati W. Clinical review: Critical care transport and austere critical care. Critical Care. 2008 Mar 5;12(2):207.

30. Riphagen S. PICU: Aeromedical Transfer : Clinical Guidance version 2.0 [Internet]. Available from: https://www.evelinalondon.nhs.uk/resources/our-services/hospital/south-thames-retrieval-service/Aeromedical-transfer-2017.pdf
31. Royal Flying Doctor Service. Clinical manual – Part 1 – clinical guidelines. January 2018 Version 8.0.
32. Royal Flying Doctors Service of Australia Western Operations: Medical Emergency Team (MET) Criteria. Pg. 40.
33. Schroeder PH, Napoli NJ, Barnhardt WF, Barnes LE, Young JS. Relative Mortality Analysis Of The "Golden Hour": A Comprehensive Acuity Stratification Approach To Address Disagreement In Current Literature. Prehospital Emergency Care. 2019 Mar 4;23(2):254–62.
34. Thomson DP, Thomas SH. G UIDELINES FOR A IR M EDICAL D ISPATCH. Prehospital Emergency Care. 2003 Jan;7(2):265–71.
35. Tintinalli JE, Stapczynski JS, Ma OJ, Cline DM, Meckler GD. Tintinalli's Emergency Medicine: A Comprehensive Study Guide, 8th edition [Internet]. McGraw Hill LLC; 2016. Available from: https://books.google.co.in/books?id=FNKLCgAAQBAJ
36. Transport of a critically ill patient [Internet]. Discipline of Anaesthesiology and Critical Care,School of Clinical Medicine , University of Kwazulu-Natal; 2017. Available from: https://anaesthetics.ukzn.ac.za/Libraries/ICU_1/FMM_No_2_-_03-02-2017_Transport_of_the_Critically_Ill_Patient_-_A_de_Castro.pdf
37. Transport of critically sick children to transplant centres Saxena R, Dhaliwal M, Ramnarayan P, Deep A - J Pediatr Crit Care [Internet]. [cited 2021 Feb 16]. Available from: http://www.jpcc.org.in/article.asp?issn=2349-6592;year=2018;volume=5;issue=3;spage=81;epage=90;aulast=Saxena

14 Tactical Care for Eye Injuries

Pradeeban S and Sreedevi Aravindan

Learning Objectives
By the end of this chapter, the reader will be able to:

- Conduct a focused tactical ocular examination in field conditions.
- Rapidly identify life- and vision-threatening eye injuries in combat.
- Classify ocular trauma and prioritize management based on injury severity.
- Implement protective strategies, such as eye shielding and prevention of intraocular pressure elevation.
- Initiate appropriate field-based treatments, including irrigation, infection prevention, and emergency decompression procedures.
- Recognize when to avoid further ocular manipulation and expedite specialist evacuation.
- Adapt tactical field care principles for ocular trauma in mass casualty and blast injury settings.

Introduction

In the unforgiving landscape of modern combat—be it dense urban alleyways, insurgency-prone jungles, or harsh mountainous borders—*traumatic ocular injuries have emerged as a critical yet often overlooked component of battlefield injuries*. Unlike other forms of trauma, where immediate life threats dominate the

Pradeeban S (✉) · S. Aravindan
Department of Emergency Medicine, AIIMS,
New Delhi, India

N. T. Rai, S. Misra (eds.), *Frontline Operational Resuscitation and Combat Emergencies (FORCE) Manual*, https://doi.org/10.1007/978-981-92-1622-2_14

provider's attention, eye injuries can silently cause permanent disability, degrade operational effectiveness, and compromise a soldier's future functional independence if not addressed swiftly.

The Frontline Operational Resuscitation and Combat Emergencies (FORCE) principles emphasize that *battlefield medicine must evolve beyond lifesaving interventions alone*. In the case of eye injuries, early recognition, minimal handling, immediate protective measures, and prompt evacuation are paramount—not only to preserve vision but also to maintain combat force integrity and long-term soldier rehabilitation.

In combat environments, such as the Indian subcontinent—where encounters can occur across varied terrains from snowy heights of the LOC to the labyrinthine slums of urban warfare—special considerations apply:

- Limited access to ophthalmologic care.
- Prolonged evacuation times due to terrain and threats.
- Resource constraints, where basic supplies must serve multiple critical needs.
- High risk of contamination, infection, and delayed secondary complications.

Tactical Combat Casualty Care (TCCC) protocols provide a structured, algorithm-driven foundation to manage such injuries. Integrating the MARCH sequence ensures that life threats are addressed first while still allowing for immediate sight-saving actions once stabilization permits. Special interventions, such as application of rigid eye shields, administration of systemic antibiotics, and recognition of evolving orbital compartment syndrome, must be embedded into the field responder's workflow alongside hemorrhage control, airway management, and hypothermia prevention.

This chapter delivers a combat-specific, field-adapted guide to managing ocular trauma—whether caused by blasts, gunfire, or blunt impact—within the operational realities faced by Indian forces. *Early, disciplined action can mean the difference between sight preserved and blindness, between return to duty and lifelong disability!*

Case Scenario

During a dawn counterinsurgency operation amidst the congested alleyways of Srinagar's old city, a 30-year-old special forces operator sustains a direct ocular injury following the detonation of an improvised explosive device (IED) concealed behind a roadside cart. The blast sends fragments of metal and glass into his face, embedding shrapnel deep into the left orbital region. The operator stumbles to the ground but remains conscious. His team neutralizes immediate threats and pulls him to cover.

- *Care Under Fire (CUF)*
  Suppressive fire is maintained as hostile engagement continues in the vicinity. A buddy operator manually drags the casualty behind a concrete barricade. Further intervention is deferred until the threat subsides.
- *Tactical Field Care (TFC)*
  As the situation stabilizes, the medic initiates a systematic MARCH assessment.
  Massive Hemorrhage (M): No active external bleeding is found. There is minor oozing from the periorbital laceration, but no arterial hemorrhage. Hemostatic dressing is not required.
  Airway (A): The casualty is able to speak and protect his airway. No facial fractures or signs of obstruction are noted.
  Respiration (R): Spontaneous breathing is present with a rate of 24/min. Bilateral chest rise is equal with no signs of pneumothorax or chest trauma.
  Circulation (C): Radial pulse is palpable but tachycardic at 120/min, likely due to pain and psychological stress. No other external bleeding or signs of hypovolemia are observed.
  Head Injury/Hypothermia (H): A focused neurologic assessment shows GCS 15. No loss of consciousness. The casualty is oriented and verbal but extremely anxious. Passive warming is initiated using a poncho liner to prevent hypothermia in the cold morning air.

Focused Ocular Assessment

The left eye reveals blood-stained sclera and distorted anatomy (Fig. 14.1). There is suspected globe rupture—evidenced by an irregular pupil, extrusion of uveal tissue, and rapid loss of vision. The casualty reports complete vision loss in the left eye. No damage is observed in the right eye, which is protected.

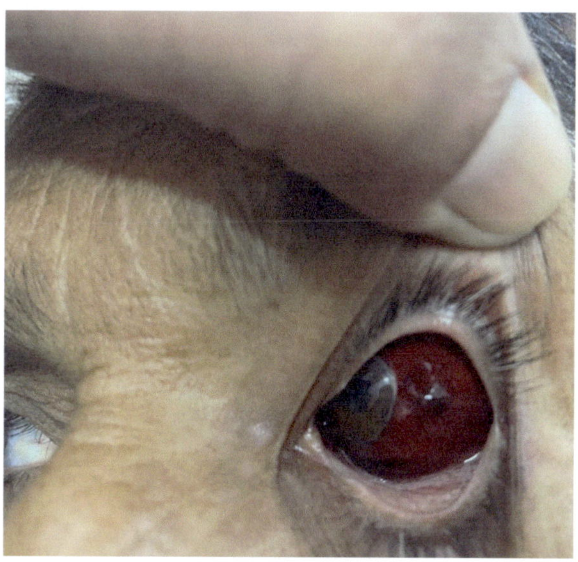

Fig. 14.1 Soldier with open globe injury to the left eye

A rigid eye shield is carefully placed over the left eye, ensuring no pressure is applied. The area is padded to avoid secondary trauma. No attempt is made to remove embedded foreign material.

- *Tactical Evacuation Care (TACEVAC)*
  A priority CASEVAC request is relayed for rotary-wing pickup from a rooftop LZ secured by an overwatch team. During the wait, the casualty is continuously monitored. Pain is managed using low-dose IV ketamine titrated to maintain consciousness without raising intraocular pressure. Broad-spectrum IV antibiotics are prepared and administered to reduce the risk of post-traumatic endophthalmitis. The eye remains shielded, and unnecessary handling is strictly avoided.
  A lateral canthotomy kit is kept on standby in case the operator develops signs of orbital compartment syndrome.

Reflective Questions
1. How do you distinguish between minor ocular trauma and a sight-threatening open globe injury when advanced diagnostics (e.g., slit lamp or ultrasound) are unavailable in the field?
2. What are the field management steps to protect a suspected open globe injury before evacuation to prevent irreversible damage?
3. In what clinical situations is a lateral canthotomy indicated, and what are the key steps for performing it safely under austere conditions when orbital compartment syndrome is suspected?

Basic Anatomy of the Eye

Understanding the basic anatomy of the eye helps in identifying the type and extent of an injury, making it easier to prioritize and treat effectively in tactical conditions.

The Globe The globe, also known as the eyeball, is spherical and encased within the bony orbit, with six extraocular muscles attached. The key anatomical structures are the following:

- *Cornea*: It is the clear and most anterior surface of the eye.
- *Iris*: It is a circular muscular structure present posterior to the cornea.
- *Pupil*: It is the central slit present in the iris through which light rays can pass.
- *Lens*: It is situated behind the iris used for the magnification of the image.
- *Retina*: It is the posterior-most structure from where the optic nerve arises.

There are two segments:

- *Anterior segment*: Present between the cornea and the lens. Consists of aqueous humor.
- *Posterior segment*: Present between the lens and the retina. Consists of vitreous humor.

Protective structures: Protect the eye from particles and trauma:

- Eyelids.
- Eyelashes.
- Bony orbit.

Blood Supply The eye receives blood from the ophthalmic artery, a branch of the internal carotid artery. Injuries compromising the blood supply are critical and require immediate attention.

Mechanisms and Types of Ocular Injuries in Combat

Ocular trauma on the battlefield arises from a spectrum of violent forces, each bringing distinct injury patterns and treatment challenges. Eye injuries can be further classified as described in Fig. 14.2. Understanding the underlying mechanism is crucial for anticipating complications, prioritizing interventions, and planning evacuation.

1. *Blast Injuries*
    - *Primary blast wave*: Overpressure from explosives can rupture the globe without external penetrating trauma.
    - *Secondary blast effects*: Shrapnel, dirt, glass, or metal fragments penetrate the eye, causing open-globe injuries.
    - *Tertiary blast injuries*: Blunt trauma from being thrown into hard surfaces can cause orbital fractures, retinal detachment, and optic nerve damage.
2. *Penetrating Trauma*
    - *Gunshot wounds*, shrapnel, and small high-velocity projectiles can perforate the cornea, sclera, or orbit.

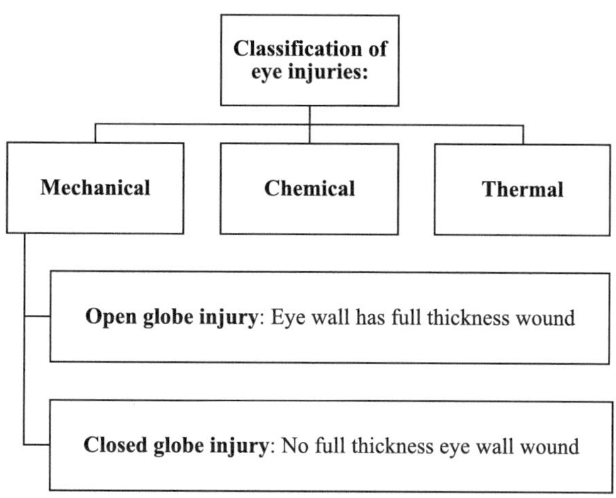

Fig. 14.2 Classification of eye injuries

- Such injuries often involve intraocular foreign bodies (IOFBs) and carry a high risk of infection (endophthalmitis).

3. *Blunt Trauma*
   - Impact from rifle butts, debris, or vehicular crashes can lead to:
     - Orbital fractures.
     - Hyphema (blood inside the front of the eye).
     - Lens dislocation.
     - Retinal detachment.
     - Traumatic optic neuropathy.
4. *Chemical and Thermal Injuries*
   - Caustic chemical sprays, fuel explosions, or incendiary devices can cause burns to the cornea and conjunctiva.
   - *Alkali burns* (e.g., *ammonia and lime) are particularly destructive and require immediate copious irrigation.*

FORCE Tactical Pearl

In combat settings, eye injuries are rarely isolated. Always integrate ocular assessment into the "H" phase (Hypothermia/Head injuries) of the MARCH sequence once life threats are controlled.

Assessment and Immediate Field Management of Ocular Injuries

MARCH Survey and Ocular Assessment

In tactical settings, the primary objective is to address life-threatening injuries first following the MARCH survey.

Ocular injuries are assessed once M, A, R, and C priorities are stabilized, during the H (Head and Hypothermia) phase.

Rapid Field Ocular Injury Assessment

- Is there visible eye trauma or swelling?
- Is the casualty complaining of vision loss, blurriness, double vision, or eye pain?
- Is there bleeding from the eye, eyelid, or periorbital structures?
- Are both pupils round, equal, and reactive to light?
- Is there obvious foreign material or protrusion from the globe?

Field Examination Techniques

Even without advanced tools, basic methods can yield critical information as described in Table 14.1.

Table 14.1 Field techniques for eye examination

Assessment	Field technique
Visual acuity	"Can you count fingers?" "how many fingers am I holding?"
Pupil shape and response	Shine a flashlight; check for unequal size (anisocoria), sluggish reaction
Eye movements	Ask casualty to follow your finger up, down, side-to-side.
External inspection	Look for lacerations, swelling, foreign bodies, protrusion (proptosis)
Globe integrity check	Avoid pressure on the eyeball. *If rupture suspected, DO NOT manipulate*

Key Warning Signs

- Irregular ("teardrop-shaped") pupil → likely globe rupture.
- Blood inside the front of the eye (hyphema).
- *Relative afferent pupillary defect (RAPD):* RAPD means optic nerve injury. Check by flashing light alternately directed into each eye, spending at least 2 s on each eye with a 1-s interval for transitioning—if the pupil dilates or does not constrict properly, RAPD is present in that eye. Notably, even in cases where the pupil in the injured eye is nonreactive, the presence or absence of RAPD can still be determined by observing the response of the unaffected pupil when the light is shone into the injured eye.
- Loss of light perception → severe optic nerve or globe injury.
- Severe eyelid swelling + inability to move eye → possible orbital fracture.

Immediate Field Management Principles

1. *Protect the Eye*
   - *DO NOT apply pressure if open globe injury is suspected.*
   - Shield the eye with:
     - Rigid eye shield (preferred; e.g., Fox eye shield).
     - If unavailable, *improvise using a cup or clean rigid object.*
   - Tape shield loosely around the orbit—not pressing on the eyeball (Fig. 14.3).
2. *Avoid Blind Bandaging*
   - *Never wrap both eyes unless absolutely necessary for bilateral injuries.*
   - Casualties must maintain situational awareness and balance (especially during evacuation).
3. *Pain Control*
   - Administer systemic analgesia (e.g., ketamine IV/IM if severe pain).
   - Avoid eye drops or ointments in the field without clear indications.
4. *Antibiotics (if Available)*
   - Broad-spectrum antibiotics should be started early if globe rupture is suspected.
   - Example: Moxifloxacin 400 mg orally once daily or IV equivalent.

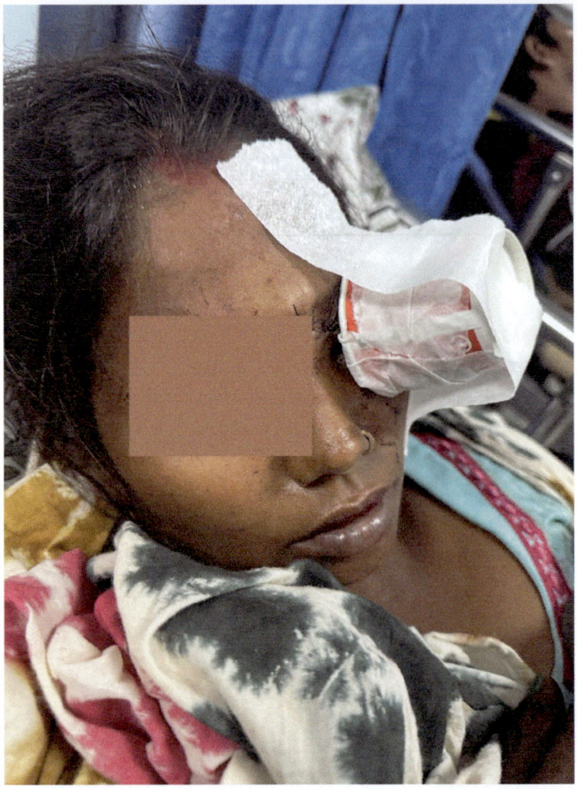

Fig. 14.3 Improvised eye shield applied on a civilian with globe injury

5. *Evacuation Planning*
   - *Priority I evacuation if:*
     – Globe rupture.
     – Visual loss.
     – Hyphema.
     – Orbital fracture with functional loss.
   - Maintain head elevation during transport (~30°) if feasible to reduce intraocular pressure.
   - Reassess vision and pupil response every 15 min during transport if possible.

Common Types of Ocular Injuries and Their Field Management

In combat and tactical environments, ocular injuries can be complex and devastating. Rapid identification and protective measures in the field can make the difference between preserved sight and permanent blindness.

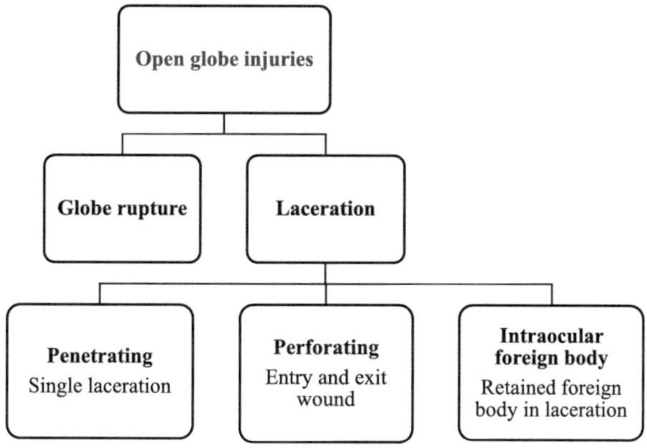

Fig. 14.4 Classification of open globe injuries

1. *Open Globe Injury (Globe Rupture)*

   Open globe injuries can be classified as outlined in Fig. 14.4.

   Field clues:

   - A visibly distorted shape of the eyeball, indicating structural disruption.
   - Obvious laceration of the eye or protruding contents (Figure 14.5a).
   - Irregular or "teardrop" shaped pupil.
   - *Iris prolapse*—where part of the iris protrudes through the wound (Figure 14.5b).
   - Marked decrease in vision.
   - Severe subconjunctival hemorrhage (blood under the white of the eye) encircling the entire globe.

   Immediate actions:

- *Protect*: Cover the eye with a rigid shield without applying pressure.
- *NPO*: Keep the patient nil per oral anticipating surgery.
- *Prevent IOP rise*: Avoid Valsalva, straining, and coughing.
- *Antibiotics*: Start systemic antibiotics (moxifloxacin/levofloxacin ± vancomycin).
- *Tetanus*: Administer prophylaxis for penetrating injuries.
- *Anti-Emetics*: Give ondansetron 4–8 mg to prevent vomiting-induced pressure spikes.
- *Analgesia*: Provide pain relief cautiously; avoid drugs raising BP/IOP.
- *Positioning*: Elevate head 30° to promote venous drainage.
- *Evacuate*: Urgent CASEVAC to an ophthalmic surgical center.

FORCE Tactical Pearl

If in doubt whether the globe is ruptured, assume it is and shield it.

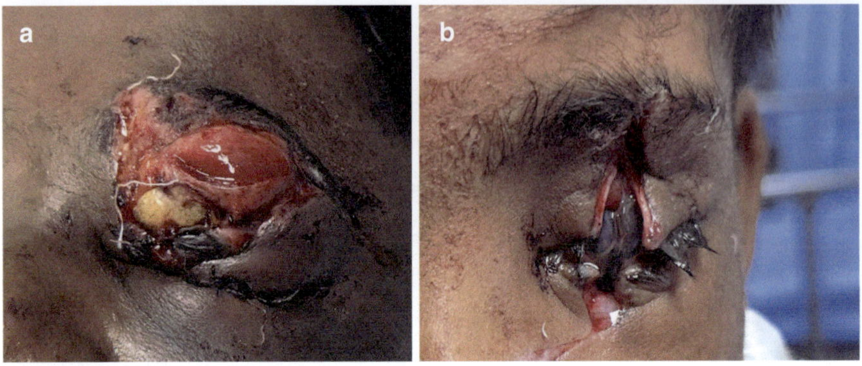

Fig. 14.5 (**a**) Eyelid laceration. (**b**) Iris prolapse

2. *Hyphema*—Bleeding into the Anterior Chamber
   Field clues:
   - Layer of blood visible in front of the iris.
   - Blurred or partial loss of vision.
   - Eye pain or photophobia (light sensitivity).

   Immediate actions:
   - Shield the eye gently.
   - Keep the casualty's head elevated (~30°) to allow blood to settle.
   - *Strictly no pressure or manipulation.*
   - Pain control with systemic analgesia.
   - *Evacuate urgently.*
3. *Orbital Fractures*
   Field clues:
   - Bruising/swelling around the eye.
   - Difficulty moving the eye (*especially upward gaze*).
   - Sunken or protruding eyeball (enophthalmos or proptosis).
   - Numbness over the cheek or upper lip (infraorbital nerve involvement).

   Immediate actions:
   - Protect the eye from further trauma.
   - If tension (swelling) threatens the optic nerve (orbital compartment syndrome suspected—decreasing vision, proptosis, hard globe), *lateral canthotomy may be life- and sight-saving if trained to perform.*
   - *Evacuate urgently.*
4. *Corneal Abrasion/Foreign Body*
   Field clues:
   - Sensation of "something in the eye".
   - Tearing, blinking, and eye tightly closed.
   - Visible foreign object on the cornea or conjunctiva (Fig. 14.6).

   Immediate actions:

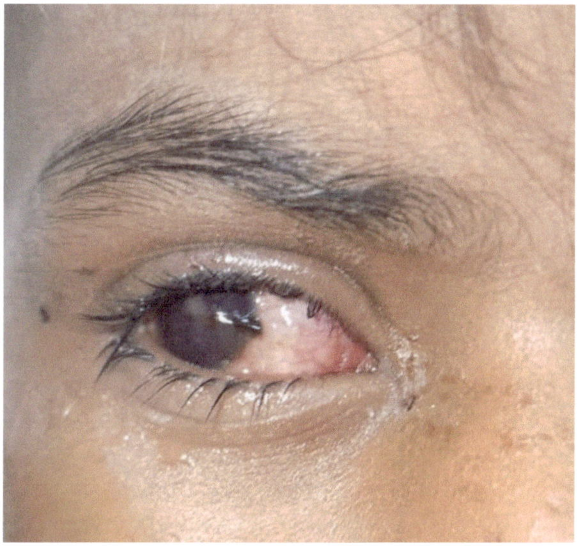

Fig. 14.6 Corneal foreign body

- Flush the eye gently with clean water or saline if available.
- If object remains embedded (especially metallic), *do not attempt forceful removal*.
- Protect the eye and evacuate if vision is compromised.

5. *Chemical Injuries*

   Field clues:

   - Exposure to irritants (e.g., riot control agents and explosions near chemicals).
   - Immediate severe burning, tearing, and redness.

   Immediate actions:

   - Immediate *copious irrigation* with any available clean water or saline.
   - Continue flushing for at least *15–20 min*.
   - Remove any contact lenses if easily removable.
   - Protect afterward and evacuate if severe damage suspected.

Evacuation Priorities for Ocular Trauma

In ocular trauma, time is critical—delays significantly increase the risk of permanent blindness. The evacuation priorities for ocular trauma in combat are as outlined in Table 14.2.

Table 14.2 Evacuation priorities for ocular trauma

Priority	Injury type	Evacuation notes
Priority I (urgent)	Open globe injury, suspected globe rupture, hyphema, orbital compartment syndrome	Immediate CASEVAC/MEDEVAC. *Early surgical intervention needed within 6 h for best outcomes*
Priority II (priority)	Corneal abrasion, minor foreign body, simple orbital fracture without vision threat	CASEVAC when feasible, ideally within 12–24 h. protect the eye during transport
Priority III (routine)	Mild conjunctival irritation, superficial injuries from dust/debris	Can delay evacuation if operational necessity dictates but monitor for infection signs

Case Resolution

The special forces operator was evacuated by rotary-wing aircraft to a forward surgical facility within 35 min of injury. During transit, his vitals remained stable, with heart rate gradually improving following IV ketamine administration for pain and anxiety. Neurologic status was intact (GCS 15), and the casualty remained oriented, cooperative, and shielded from external stimuli.

Field assessment clearly indicated a sight-threatening injury rather than a superficial ocular trauma. Key findings, such as loss of vision, blood-stained sclera, irregular pupil, eyelid laceration, and suspected extrusion, strongly suggested an open globe rupture, even in the absence of advanced diagnostic tools. In contrast, minor injuries typically present with foreign body sensation, conjunctival redness, or corneal abrasion but preserve visual acuity and lack full-thickness globe involvement.

A rigid eye shield was carefully applied to protect the injured eye, avoiding any pressure over the globe. This step was crucial to prevent extrusion of ocular contents. A pressure patch or manipulation in the field could have worsened the injury. The shield was stabilized with medical tape to the forehead and cheekbones, taking care not to disturb the wound.

Lateral canthotomy was considered but deferred, as the casualty showed no signs of orbital compartment syndrome. There was no proptosis, afferent pupillary defect, or rapidly worsening vision in the intact eye, and the eyelids were not tense. However, the medic was prepared to perform the procedure if any signs of increased intraorbital pressure emerged. If indicated, the canthotomy would have been performed by palpating the lateral orbital rim, clamping the lateral canthus, and cutting through the lateral canthal tendon using a #11 blade to relieve pressure.

Systemic antibiotics (IV ceftriaxone 1 g) were started en route to prevent endophthalmitis, a devastating complication of open globe injuries. Analgesia was continued using IV ketamine for its hemodynamic stability and minimal impact on intraocular pressure.

Upon hospital arrival, ophthalmologic assessment and CT orbit confirmed a globe rupture with partial uveal prolapse. The patient underwent surgical globe repair but ultimately lost vision in the affected eye. However, due to prompt field recognition, protective shielding, early antibiotic therapy, and controlled evacuation, the orbital structure was preserved, and cosmetic outcomes were optimized. The patient was later fitted with a prosthetic eye and returned to active duty in a noncombat role.

Key Messages

- *Eye injuries are medical emergencies, not secondary concerns*—Immediate shielding and stabilization are mandatory in tactical settings.
- *Rigid eye protection is critical*—Use a hard shield (improvised if necessary) to prevent further mechanical damage; never apply pressure.
- *Field visual assessment must be documented*—Even a crude acuity check (e.g., light perception and finger counting) guides triage and medicolegal documentation.
- *Globe rupture must be suspected in any penetrating periocular trauma*, blunt high-velocity trauma, or decreased vision post-explosion or gunfire.
- *Avoid irrigation if globe rupture is suspected*—Irrigation is reserved only for chemical burns or superficial foreign bodies without signs of open globe injury.
- *Avoid orally in penetrating eye trauma*—Anticipate possible surgical intervention under anesthesia.
- Combat providers and tactical physicians should be trained in emergency lateral canthotomy for orbital compartment syndrome to prevent irreversible blindness.
- *Triage priorities for eye injuries depend on severity*—Open globe injuries demand urgent CASEVAC, whereas minor abrasions may allow delayed evacuation.
- Hypothermia prevention, gentle handling, and minimal scene time are important even in ocular trauma—systemic instability can worsen ocular outcomes too.

Conclusion

Ocular injuries in tactical combat environments represent a unique and often underestimated threat to operational effectiveness and long-term quality of life. Vision loss can profoundly affect not only the combatant's future in service but also their overall rehabilitation potential. Swift, decisive action following the MARCH protocol, tactical casualty care phases, and basic ophthalmologic principles can dramatically alter outcomes—often preserving vision even under austere conditions.

Tactical responders must prioritize early recognition, immediate protection, avoidance of secondary injury, and timely evacuation to higher levels of care. Integrating simple field interventions like rigid eye shielding, basic visual assessments, and buddy-aid techniques into standard casualty management ensures that eye injuries are neither overlooked nor undertreated.

Bibliography

1. Eye Trauma: Initial Care (CPG ID:03), JOINT TRAUMA SYSTEM CLINICAL PRACTICE GUIDELINE (JTS CPG) https://jts.health.mil/index.cfm/PI_CPGs/cpgs
2. Feliciano DV, Mattox KL, Moore EE. Trauma. 9th ed. New York: McGraw Hill Medical; 2020. ISBN: 978-1260143355
3. Godbole, N. J., Seefeldt, E. S., Raymond, W. R., Karesh, J. W., Morgenstern, A., Egan, J. A., Colyer, M. H., & Mazzoli, R. A. (2018). Simplified Method for Rapid Field Assessment of Visual Acuity by First Responders after Ocular Injury. Military Medicine, 183, 219–223. https://doi.org/10.1093/milmed/usx175

Hand Injuries in Combat

15

Suvashis Dash

Learning Objectives

By the end of this chapter, the reader will be able to:

- Recognize common mechanisms of hand injuries in combat, including blast, crush, firearm, and avulsion injuries and understand their functional implications.
- Apply the MARCH protocol to assess, triage, and stabilize casualties with upper limb trauma in austere and high-threat environments.
- Demonstrate field management techniques for controlling hemorrhage, preserving amputated parts, and preventing contamination in open hand injuries.
- Perform and teach basic combat splinting techniques to immobilize hand and wrist injuries during prolonged field care and evacuation.
- Identify signs of tendon, nerve, and vascular compromise and understand documentation and referral priorities for surgical intervention.
- Understand the psychological impact of hand trauma in soldiers and recognize the importance of early psychological first aid and long-term rehabilitation.
- Integrate principles of functional preservation into field care, including proper positioning, early mobilization planning, and prosthetic considerations.

S. Dash (✉)
Department of Plastic, Reconstructive and Burn Surgery, JPN Apex Trauma Centre, AIIMS, New Delhi, India

N. T. Rai, S. Misra (eds.), *Frontline Operational Resuscitation and Combat Emergencies (FORCE) Manual*, https://doi.org/10.1007/978-981-92-1622-2_15

Introduction

Hand injuries are among the most common types of trauma in combat situations. Soldiers' hands are exposed to high-energy forces from explosions, ballistic impacts, and operational demands. Hands are critical for weapon handling, communication, and emergency care, making their protection essential. Impact of injuries, such as damage to bones, tendons, nerves, and blood vessels, can severely limit a soldier's functional capabilities. Such injuries can result in permanent disability or limb loss, affecting overall military effectiveness. Statistically upper extremity injuries, *particularly hand trauma, rank among the top three types of injuries on the battlefield.* Long-term implications of hand injuries can lead to prolonged recovery times, multiple surgeries, and extensive rehabilitation, influencing soldiers' quality of life and military operational readiness.

Combat environments pose a unique set of challenges when it comes to managing hand injuries. One of the most critical issues is the lack of adequate medical infrastructure in forward operating areas, which limits access to immediate surgical care and specialized intervention. The environment itself adds further complexity—battlefields are often filled with dust, debris, and unhygienic conditions that increase the risk of infection, especially in open or contaminated wounds. Many casualties also present with polytrauma, where hand injuries may be overshadowed by more visibly severe injuries, delaying definitive care.

Beyond the physical implications, hand injuries can have a profound psychological impact. The sudden loss of function—particularly in dominant hands—can lead to emotional distress, anxiety, and long-term adjustment issues, especially for combatants whose operational duties rely heavily on manual dexterity. These realities highlight the urgent need for focused training of both combat medics and frontline soldiers in basic field management techniques. Rapid stabilization, hemorrhage control, splinting, and sterile dressing application must become second nature to personnel operating in high-threat, resource-limited environments.

Tailoring hand injury management to combat settings requires not only clinical skill but also adaptability and foresight. Early intervention, infection control, and psychological reassurance, when delivered efficiently in the field, can significantly improve both survival and long-term functionality.

Case Scenario

During a close-quarters engagement in a high-threat insurgency zone, a 28-year-old para SF commando attempts to throw back a flash grenade that lands inside the perimeter compound. The flash grenade detonates prematurely as he attempts to throw it back, causing a near-complete traumatic amputation through the metacarpals (Fig. 15.1). The blast also results in shrapnel injuries to his upper chest and left thigh. The casualty is thrown backward, screaming in pain, with active bleeding from his mangled hand and disorientation from the blast concussion. The area remains partially hostile, requiring immediate extraction.

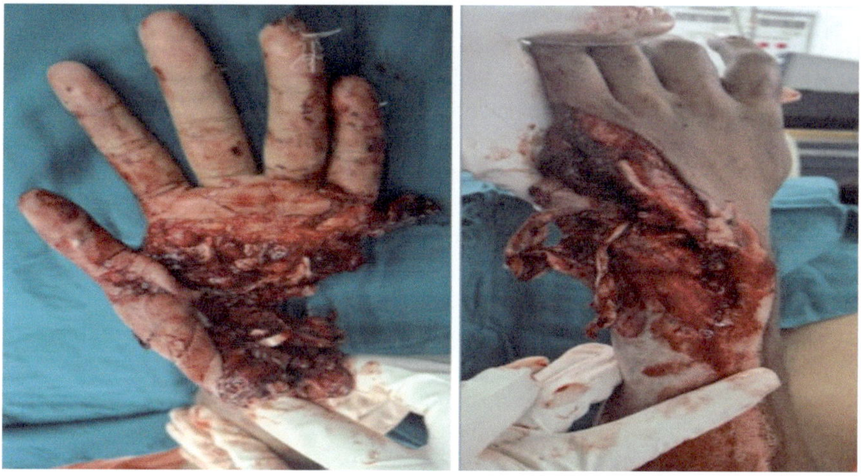

Fig. 15.1 Soldier with near-complete hand amputation due to premature grenade detonation

- *Care Under Fire (CUF)*
  Suppressive fire is laid down as two teammates manually drag the casualty to a covered position. A rapid blood sweep identifies severe hemorrhage from the left hand. A CAT tourniquet is applied mid-forearm. No other care is attempted until the firefight is controlled.
- *Tactical Field Care (TFC)*
  As the situation stabilizes, the medic initiates a systematic MARCH assessment.
  Massive Hemorrhage (M): The near-complete hand amputation continues to ooze despite the tourniquet. Hemostatic gauze is packed into the wound base, and a pressure dressing is secured over it. Additional shrapnel wounds in the left thigh are bandaged with compression dressings. Hemorrhage is controlled.
  Airway (A): The casualty is conscious, agitated, and shouting. No facial trauma is evident. Airway is patent and intact.
  Respiration (R): The respiratory rate is 30/min with shallow breaths. Equal chest rise is noted. A chest seal is applied to a small shrapnel wound over the left upper chest. There are no signs of tension pneumothorax.
  Circulation (C): The patient is pale and diaphoretic. Radial pulse is absent on the injured side but present on the right. SBP is estimated at 90/60 mmHg. A large-bore IV line is established. TXA (1 g IV) is administered within the first 15 min. A slow infusion of 500 mL Ringer's lactate is initiated.
  Head Injury/Hypothermia (H): GCS is 15. Pupils are equal and reactive. No signs of head injury. The casualty's rain-soaked uniform is removed and replaced with dry insulating layers and a Mylar blanket. A foil wrap is used to cover the injured extremity to reduce heat loss.
- *Tactical Evacuation Care (TACEVAC)*
  Evacuation is expected to take 40 min over uneven terrain. A splint is improvised using padded rigid material to immobilize the injured limb and prevent further

tissue damage. The casualty is secured in a lateral recovery position. Prophylactic antibiotics (e.g., IV cefazolin 1 g) are administered to prevent wound infection. Analgesia is initiated using titrated IV ketamine to control severe pain while maintaining consciousness. To address the casualty's visible psychological distress, the medic provides simple psychological first aid—offering reassurance, maintaining eye contact, and explaining the care process to regain a sense of control. The team continues regular monitoring of tourniquet effectiveness, perfusion, and mental status until handover at the LZ.

Reflective Questions

1. What are the correct field procedures to preserve an amputated hand segment for potential reimplantation during delayed evacuation?
2. Which clinical signs in the field should prompt the early administration of antibiotics, and what are the preferred choices?
3. What considerations guide the splinting and dressing of a traumatic hand amputation during prolonged casualty movement?
4. What psychological first aid techniques are most appropriate in managing acute emotional distress following traumatic limb loss?

Essential Anatomy for Managing Hand Injuries in Combat

- *Bone Structure Anatomy*
  1. *Phalanges*: Three segments in each finger, two in the thumb; allow dexterity for tasks like gripping. Combat fractures can cause misalignment, hindering fine motor skills.
  2. *Metacarpals*: Form the palm, anchor muscles, and provide grip. Commonly fractured in combat from blunt force, requiring stabilization.
  3. *Carpals*: Eight wrist bones providing flexibility and shock absorption; fractures limit wrist mobility, impairing weapon/tool use.
- *Soft Tissue Anatomy*
  1. *Muscle groups*: Forearm muscles for strength; intrinsic hand muscles for precision. Contusions/lacerations can weaken or cause spasm muscles, impacting essential movements.
  2. *Flexor and extensor tendons*: Flexors enable gripping; extensors allow opening. Shrapnel cuts can damage tendons, requiring suturing to avoid permanent motion loss.
  3. *Ligaments*: Stabilize joints and resist high impact; injuries (e.g., hyperextension) can weaken grip and control, impairing combat tasks.
- *Vascular and Nerve Supply*
  1. *Vascular supply (radial and ulnar arteries)*: The radial and ulnar arteries form the palmar arches to maintain blood flow; combat injuries can risk necrosis if blood supply is compromised.

Table 15.1 Ten-point quick assessment checklist for upper limb injury in combat settings

1. Initial observation: Look for visible signs of injury, bleeding, deformity, and abnormal positioning of the arm or hand.
2. Check for hemorrhage: Control severe bleeding immediately using direct pressure, bandages, or a tourniquet if necessary.
3. Pain-level assessment: Determine the level and type of pain to help identify underlying injuries, such as fractures or nerve damage.
4. Pulse check: Check distal pulses (e.g., radial and ulnar) to assess blood flow to the extremity. Absent pulses may indicate vascular injury.
5. Sensation test: Lightly touch fingers and forearm to test sensation. Loss of sensation can indicate nerve damage or severe trauma.
6. Motor function: Ask the soldier to wiggle fingers, bend the wrist, and move the arm if possible to evaluate muscle function and nerve integrity.
7. Skin temperature and color: Assess temperature and color to check for signs of compromised circulation. Pale or cold skin can indicate vascular compromise.
8. Capillary refill test: Press on the nail bed and observe how quickly color returns (should be <3 s). Delayed refill may suggest circulation issues.
9. Check for swelling and deformity: Observe for obvious swelling, deformity, or crepitus, which could indicate fractures or joint dislocations.
10. Immobilization decision: Based on the assessment, decide if the limb requires immediate immobilization to prevent further damage, especially before evacuation.

2. *Sensory-motor nerves*:
   - *Median nerve*: Controls thumb movement; damage impairs precision.
   - *Ulnar nerve*: Manages fine motor control in small/ring fingers; injury weakens grip.

     Radial nerve: Enables wrist/finger extension; injury causes wrist drop, reducing hand functionality.

Through quick assessment and intervention, field medical personnel can enhance outcomes and support the soldier's recovery. Table 15.1 provides a systematic approach to assess and stabilize upper limb injuries quickly in a combat environment in the Tactical Field Care phase.

Mechanisms of Hand Injuries in Combat

Hand injuries in combat often involve complex combinations of damage to bones, tissues, vessels, and nerves, which can lead to permanent functional loss.

1. *Blast and Ballistic Trauma*
   - *Sources*: Injuries primarily result from explosive devices (IEDs, grenades, landmines).
   - *Primary blast effects*:
     - Intense air pressure waves can damage soft tissues and bones without external penetration.

       May lead to complex fractures, dislocations, or traumatic amputations.

- *Secondary effects*:
  - Shrapnel and debris can cause deep lacerations and embed foreign objects.
  - Introduces contaminants, complicating wound management.
  - Challenges: Often involves open fractures with extensive soft tissue damage, necessitating immediate stabilization and specialized care.

    In ballistic hand trauma, begin with hemorrhage control using direct pressure or a tourniquet. Perform thorough wound irrigation to minimize contamination, followed by aggressive debridement to remove devitalized tissue. Stabilize fractures with splints and consider temporary fixation with K-wires if available. Administer broad-spectrum antibiotics and provide tetanus prophylaxis. Rapid imaging and early intervention prepare the patient for definitive surgical repair.

2. *Sharp and Penetrating Trauma*
   - *Causes*: Result from close-combat scenarios with knives, broken glass, or other sharp objects.
   - *Injury types*:
     - Tendon lacerations are common, especially in exposed areas like palms and fingers.
     - Nerve damage can cause sensory loss or paralysis.
     - Bone fractures may accompany soft tissue injuries, requiring precise alignment for healing.

       Treatment: Cleaning of the wound, stabilization with splint, and pain control. May involve microvascular repair and tendon grafting to restore function in later stage.
3. *Crush Injuries*
   - *Causes*: Commonly due to heavy machinery, vehicular accidents, or structural collapses.
   - Can severely damage tissues and compress muscles and nerves, potentially causing compartment syndrome.

4. *Fractures*: Can range from simple breaks to complex, comminuted fractures.

   Treatment: Requires immediate treatment to prevent tissue damage, including stabilization, decompression, and surgical alignment of bones (Fig. 15.2).
5. *Burns and Thermal Injuries*: Burns in combat can result from flame, chemical exposure, explosive blasts, and friction.
   - Flame and explosive thermal burns: Cause significant damage to skin and soft tissues. Lead to loss of skin and prone to infection.
   - Chemical burns: Occur due to exposure to hazardous substances. Can penetrate deeply and cause progressive tissue destruction.
   - Friction burns: Result in deep tissue injury from friction along with the body surface.

   Management of Burns
   - Immediate care:
     - Apply cooling techniques, such as running water at normal temperature to mitigate heat damage. Cover it with a clean cloth or dressing.

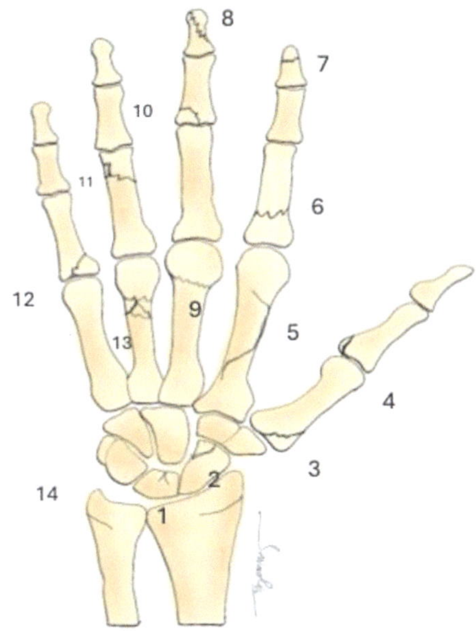

1. Distal End of Radius
2. Scaphoid
3. Base of the First Metacarpal (thumb)
4. Base of the Thumb Proximal Phalanx (Ppx)
5. Second Metacarpal (Index Finger) spiral
6. Proximal Phalanx of the Index Finger (IF Ppx)
7. Distal Phalanx of the Index Finger (IF Dpx)
8. Distal Phalanx of the Middle Finger (MF Dpx)
9. Neck of the Third Metacarpal (Middle Finger)
10. Middle Finger Proximal Phalanx (MF Mpx)
11. Ring Finger Proximal Phalanx (RF Ppx)
12. Little Finger Proximal Phalanx (LF Ppx)
13. Fourth Metacarpal (Ring Finger)
14. Ulna

Fig. 15.2 Annotated illustration of the skeletal structure of the hand, highlighting common fracture sites, including the distal radius, scaphoid, metacarpal bases, and proximal phalanges of the fingers. These markings serve as a reference for identifying specific fractures in hand trauma, aiding in precise diagnosis and targeted management

Perform decontamination when harmful chemicals come in contact with the skin.

- Long-term management:
  - Involves skin grafting to repair damaged areas
  - Requires strategies for scar management to minimize scarring
    Includes functional rehabilitation to restore mobility and dexterity

Special Considerations for Hand Burns

- Critical attention: Burn injuries to the hands necessitate specialized management due to their vital functional roles.
- Infection prevention:
  - Implement stringent hygiene practices to reduce infection risk in open burns.
    Closely monitor for signs of infection during the recovery process.

Initial Assessment and Triage for Hand Injuries in Combat

In combat zones, the initial assessment and triage are critical for managing hand injuries and stabilizing soldiers efficiently under challenging circumstances. Quick, systematic evaluations and prioritization allow medical personnel to address life-threatening conditions first, ensuring the best possible outcomes.

1. *Primary Survey*
   - *Goal*: The primary survey is aimed at immediate lifesaving interventions and stabilization.

     As per standard guidelines in previous chapters.
2. *Secondary Survey*—for the hand and upper limb
   - *Goal*: A focused, thorough evaluation of injuries beyond immediate life threats, with a specific emphasis on hand injuries.
   - *Inspection*: Visually examine the hand for signs of open fractures, lacerations, burns, or deformities. Look for discoloration or swelling, which may indicate underlying trauma or compartment syndrome.
   - *Palpation*: Carefully palpate the hand to identify areas of tenderness, instability, or crepitus that could signal fractures. Assess joint stability and alignment to help determine the extent of skeletal injuries.
   - *Range of motion testing*: Ask the patient to move their fingers if possible, or gently test passive movement. This allows for preliminary evaluation of tendon or nerve injuries and functional impairment.
   - *Vascular and nerve check*: Check distal pulses and capillary refill in the fingers to assess circulation. Perform a quick sensory and motor exam to evaluate for nerve damage; for example, assess thumb opposition for median nerve function, finger spread for ulnar nerve, and wrist extension for radial nerve integrity.
   - *Documentation*: Record findings clearly, as they will guide further management and are essential for continuity of care if the patient is evacuated.

3. *Triage Decision-Making*
   - *Goal*: Prioritize patients based on injury severity, potential for survival, and the resources available.
   - *Severity-based classification*: Assign categories such as *immediate* for life-threatening cases that require urgent intervention, *delayed* for injuries that can wait, and *minimal* for non-severe cases.
   - *Evacuation consideration*: Decide on evacuation necessity based on the hand injury's severity and potential for functional recovery. For instance, open fractures with vascular compromise may require immediate surgical intervention.
   - *Resource optimization*: In limited-resource settings, focus on the most salvageable injuries, applying basic splinting or dressing to stabilize noncritical wounds before transport. Complex injuries may be stabilized in the field with improvised splints, while efforts are concentrated on patients with a higher chance of recovery or preserving hand functionality (Table 15.2).
   - *Continual reassessment*: Conditions may change rapidly; reassess patients periodically, especially if evacuation delays occur or resources shift.

Table 15.2 Field dressing materials list

1. *Sterile gauze pads* (various sizes)—For wound coverage and absorption 2 × 2 in. small, large size
2. *Roll gauze bandages*—For securing dressings and providing compression: 4 and 6 in.
3. *Adhesive bandages*—For small cuts and abrasions
4. *Non-adherent gauze pads*—For covering open wounds without sticking to tissue paraffin gauze (10 × 10 cm)
5. *Elastic bandages* (ACE wraps)—For compression and immobilization
6. *Antiseptic wipes*—For initial wound cleaning and reducing infection risk
7. *Hemostatic gauze*—For rapid bleeding control
8. *Saline solution*—For irrigation and gentle wound cleaning
9. *Medical tape* (water-resistant)—For securing dressings
10. *Sterile gloves*—For maintaining hygiene during dressing changes
11. *Scissors* (blunt-tip)—For cutting gauze and bandages to size
12. *Tourniquet*—For hemorrhage control in severe cases

A structured approach to the primary and secondary surveys followed by strategic triage can help maximize outcomes in combat settings, ensuring that lifesaving interventions are prioritized and that resources are allocated effectively.

Immediate Management and Stabilization of Hand Injuries

In combat settings, effective immediate management and stabilization are crucial to preserving limb function and preventing complications. The following guidelines provide a step-by-step approach for controlling bleeding, ensuring wound cleanliness, immobilizing injuries, and managing pain, all tailored for field conditions.

1. *Hemorrhage Control*

   Goal: Quickly stop bleeding to prevent shock and maintain hand function.

   - *Direct pressure*: Press firmly on the wound with a sterile dressing or clean cloth. If bleeding continues, add more dressings without removing initial layers.
   - *Tourniquet*: For severe bleeding, place a tourniquet above the injury, typically on the upper forearm, avoiding joints. Tighten just enough to stop bleeding and note the application time.
   - *Hemostatic agents*: If needed, apply hemostatic gauze in the wound and press for a few minutes. Avoid repeated applications to prevent extra trauma.

2. *Wound Care and Debridement*

   Goal: Minimize infection risk and prepare the wound for eventual surgical intervention.

   Wound care and debridement

   - *Cleaning*: Rinse the wound with sterile saline or clean water. Avoid scrubbing, as it may spread contaminants.

- *Debridement*: Carefully remove visible debris and dead tissue with sterile tools. Limit debridement to avoid removing viable tissue.
- *Dressing*: Cover the wound with sterile or clean gauze, securing it loosely to accommodate swelling (Fig. 15.3).

3. *Immobilization Techniques*

   Goal: Stabilize fractures and prevent additional tissue damage during transport or while awaiting advanced care.

   - *Splinting*: Use rigid materials like sticks or cardboard for splints, positioning the hand with fingers slightly curled and the wrist slightly extended also called the *functional position of hand* (Figs. 15.4 and 15.5).
   - *Padding*: Place padding under the splint to prevent pressure sores, and wrap the hand gently.
   - *Securing the splint*: Use cloth strips or bandages to secure the splint, ensuring it is firm but does not restrict circulation. Check capillary refill or pulse.
   - *Hand elevation*

4. *Pain Management*

   Goal: Control pain to improve patient comfort and compliance without impairing their alertness.

   - *Oral pain relievers*: Administer ibuprofen or acetaminophen for mild to moderate pain. Avoid NSAIDs if bleeding is severe.
   - *Local anesthetics*: For severe pain requiring debridement, trained personnel can administer local anesthetics around the wound.
   - *Other techniques*: Encourage deep breathing and reassure the patient to reduce stress and discomfort.

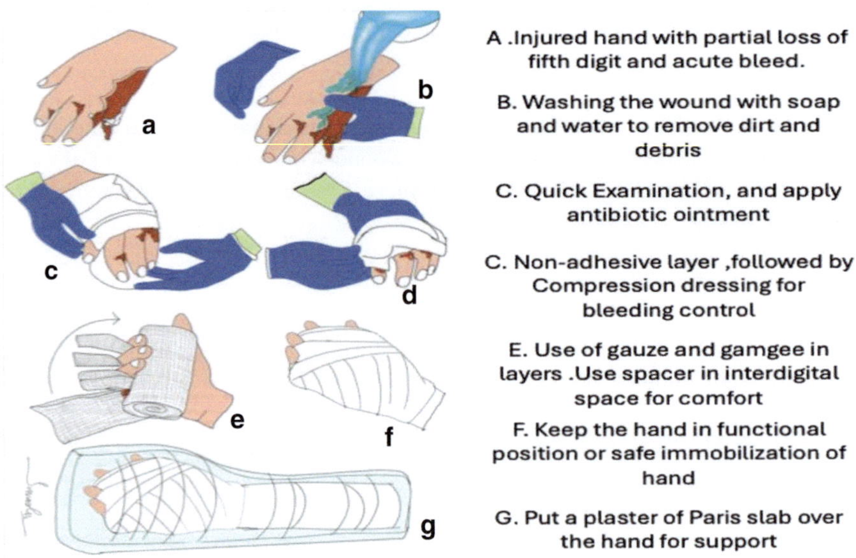

Fig. 15.3 Steps of wound care

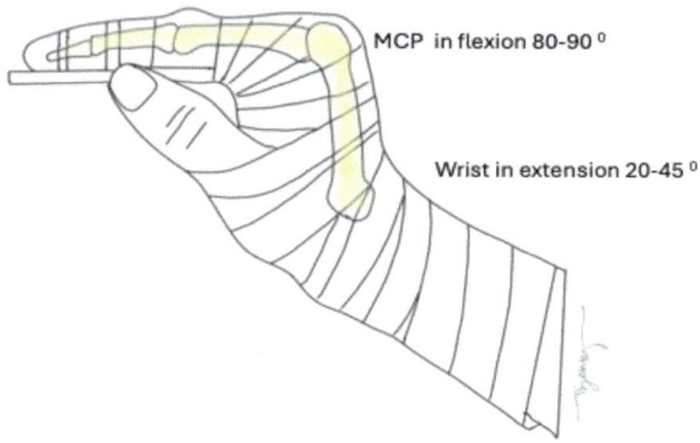

Fig. 15.4 Recommended hand positioning to minimize further deformity during splintage

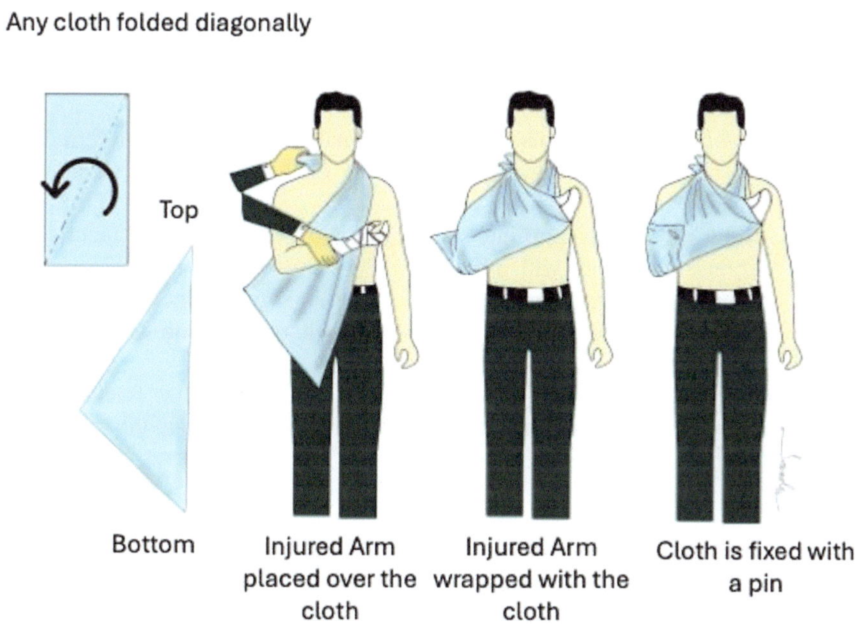

Fig. 15.5 Use of cloth to make sling for injured upper limb in combat scenario

Definitive Surgical Management

In combat zones, definitive surgical management of hand injuries requires a structured approach tailored to the unique challenges of the environment.

1. *Soft Tissue Repair and Reconstruction*
   - *Objective*: Restore function and appearance by repairing damaged muscles, tendons, and ligaments.

- *Primary repair*: If the injury is fresh and surgical resources are available, perform primary repair of soft tissues as soon as possible. This includes the following:
  - Muscle repair: Suture muscle edges using absorbable sutures, ensuring that the muscle fibers are aligned for optimal healing.
  - Tendon repair: Use tendon repair techniques, such as the Kessler or Krakow method, to approximate tendon ends. Reinforce repairs with nonabsorbable sutures for durability.

    Ligament repair: If ligaments are torn, use sutures or anchors to reattach ligaments to their insertion points. Consider using graft material if the ligament is extensively damaged.
- *Delayed repair*: In cases where initial repair is not feasible (e.g., due to contamination or delayed presentation), perform delayed repair after ensuring the wound is clean. Use flap techniques or grafts for reconstruction to provide coverage and restore function.

2. *Bone Fixation and Fracture Management*
   - *Objective*: Stabilize fractures to facilitate healing while considering the availability of surgical facilities (Fig. 15.6).
   - *External fixators*: In combat settings, external fixation is often preferred due to its minimal invasiveness and ease of application. Steps include the following:
     - *Application*: Insert pins into stable bone above and below the fracture site. Connect these pins with a rigid frame to stabilize the bone.

       Monitoring: Regularly assess the fixation for signs of infection or loosening. Adjustments may be necessary based on swelling or changes in alignment.
   - *Temporary stabilization*: Use splints or braces to immobilize fractures until definitive surgical intervention can be performed. Ensure that the splint does not compromise circulation.

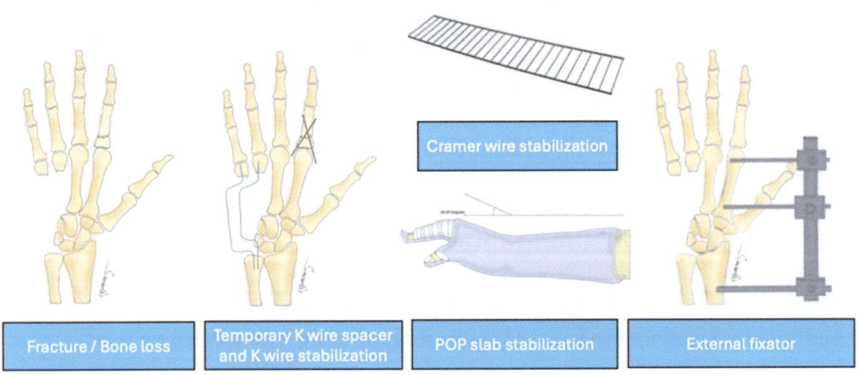

Fig. 15.6 Bony fixation methods for acute hand injuries, illustrating techniques like Cramer wire and pop slab for quick stabilization

- *Triage considerations*: Prioritize injuries based on the severity of fractures and potential for healing. In situations where advanced surgical care is unavailable, consider evacuation protocols for patients requiring complex interventions.

3. *Vascular and Nerve Repair*
   - *Objective*: Restore blood flow and nerve function to the injured hand.
   - *Vascular repair*: If blood vessels are damaged:
     - Surgical techniques: Use microsurgical techniques to perform end-to-end anastomosis for small vessel repairs. For larger vessels, consider using vein grafts or bypass techniques.

       Temporary measures: In urgent situations, apply vascular clamps to control bleeding while preparing for definitive repair.
   - *Nerve repair*: For nerve injuries, follow these steps:
     - Surgical intervention: Use epineurial or perineurial sutures to approximate the nerve ends. Ensure proper alignment to facilitate regeneration.

       Temporary solutions: If immediate repair is not feasible, consider placing a nerve conduit or using local muscle flaps to protect the nerve and maintain function until definitive repair can occur.
4. *Infection Control and Antibiotic Therapy*
   - *Objective*: Minimize infection risk, especially in wounds exposed to contaminants.

   Administer antibiotics as early as possible in cases of high-risk wounds. Guidelines include the following:
     - *Prophylactic use*: Initiate prophylactic antibiotics within 3 h of injury for high-risk wounds, particularly those contaminated with soil or fecal matter. Common choices include cefazolin or ampicillin-sulbactam.
     - *Tailored therapy*: Adjust antibiotic choice based on the patient's history and wound culture results. Consider the risk of resistant organisms based on local epidemiology.

       Wound management: Continuously monitor wounds for signs of infection, including redness, swelling, and discharge. Perform regular debridement as necessary to remove necrotic tissue and reduce bacterial load.

Definitive surgical management of hand injuries in combat zones requires a thorough understanding of the appropriate techniques for soft tissue repair, fracture management, vascular and nerve repair, and infection control. By following these structured approaches, medical personnel can effectively stabilize and treat injuries, maximizing the potential for recovery and function in challenging environments.

Rehabilitation and Functional Recovery

- *Early Mobilization and Physical Therapy*

  Early movement is key to preventing stiffness and promoting recovery. As soon as safe, encourage simple exercises like finger flexion and extension to improve circulation, reduce swelling, and maintain mobility. Use items like therapy putty or stress balls, if available, for gradual strengthening.

- *Splinting and Orthotics*
  Splints stabilize injuries, maintain alignment, and protect healing tissues. At combat situation, use any material available for the splintage. Use of custom or prefabricated splints based on the injury type, adjusting to allow safe movement as recovery progresses.
- *Psychosocial Support*
  Hand injuries impact mental well-being, especially for soldiers reliant on hand function. Offer access to counseling or peer support to help manage anxiety and restore confidence.
- *Return-to-Duty*
  Assess readiness for duty based on strength, dexterity, and pain levels. Functional benchmarks, such as task performance, should guide this process. A phased return with ongoing medical support ensures a smooth transition back to active roles.

Case Resolution

Upon arrival at the forward surgical post, the casualty was secured in a vacuum mattress, with spinal precautions in place. The avulsed hand segment, which had been gently rinsed with sterile saline, wrapped in moist sterile gauze, and sealed inside a double-layered waterproof bag placed in cool water (avoiding direct contact with ice), was transported alongside the patient and handed over clearly labeled for the surgical team. This meticulous field preservation maximized the viability of the part for replantation.

The casualty remained alert (GCS 15) but visibly distressed. In response to the psychological impact of sudden traumatic hand injury, the attending medic provided psychological first aid—maintaining calm, explaining each step of care clearly, ensuring effective pain control with IV ketamine, and reinforcing that efforts were ongoing to save his hand. This reassurance helped reduce panic and preserved the casualty's engagement with care.

On secondary reassessment, no additional life-threatening injuries were found. The injured hand and forearm had been stabilized in the field with a rigid padded splint, immobilizing it during transport to prevent neurovascular traction and further soft tissue injury.

In theatre, based on the short ischemia time, proper limb preservation, and the patient's hemodynamic stability, the surgical team proceeded with reconstruction. Debridement was performed to remove devitalized tissue and embedded shrapnel. Microsurgical neurovascular repair included arterial and venous anastomoses to restore circulation and nerve coaptation of the median and ulnar nerves. Fracture stabilization was achieved using a mini-external fixator spanning the metacarpal level (Fig. 15.7).

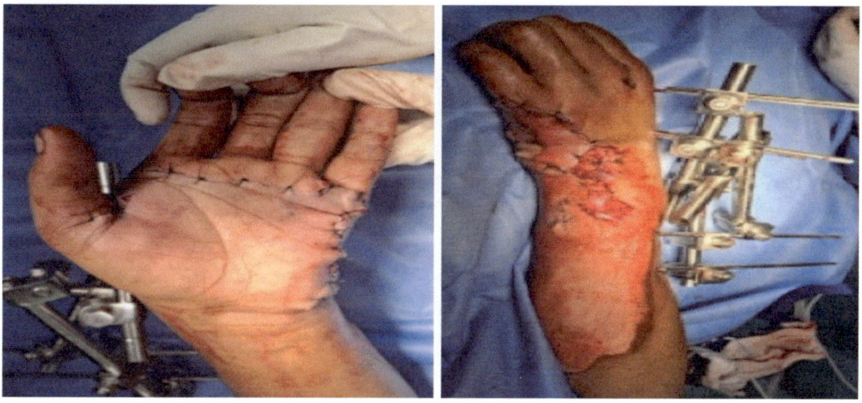

Fig. 15.7 Soldier's hand after debridement, reconstruction, and bony stabilization with an external fixator

During the immediate postoperative phase, the replanted limb demonstrated improved warmth, color, and capillary refill. The casualty remained stable and was transferred to a tertiary limb salvage center within 48 h for staged reconstruction and intensive rehabilitation.

Key Messages

- Hand injuries in combat are tactically disabling, with immediate and long-term impact on a soldier's operational capability, making early functional preservation a priority.
- Rapid hemorrhage control using tourniquets, hemostatic dressings, and pressure is vital in partial or complete hand amputations to prevent exsanguination.
- Amputated hand parts must be preserved properly—*rinsed, wrapped in moist gauze, sealed, and cooled without direct ice contact*—to optimize chances of reimplantation.
- Combat providers must be skilled in field assessment of tendon, nerve, and vascular damage and initiate splinting to prevent further functional loss.
- Timely administration of antibiotics and tetanus prophylaxis, along with sterile dressing of open wounds, reduces the risk of deep infections and septic complications.
- Pain management and limb positioning play a crucial role in minimizing secondary injury and improving patient comfort during prolonged evacuation.
- Psychological support at the point of injury is critical, as loss of hand function is associated with high emotional distress and identity disruption in combatants.
- Early surgical intervention, combined with rehabilitation and prosthetic integration, enables meaningful return to duty and long-term independence.

Conclusion

Combat-related hand injuries demand a *dual focus—saving life and preserving dexterity*. In the chaos of battle, a partially avulsed or amputated hand may appear secondary to other injuries, but its management determines not just survival, but how the soldier lives, fights, and functions after recovery. Combat providers must combine trauma triage principles with meticulous attention to tissue handling, splinting, and contamination control.

This chapter highlights that the *future usability of the hand is shaped in the first hour*—by the hands of a trained provider. From preserving the amputated part to offering psychological reassurance, every step in the field defines whether a soldier regains autonomy or adapts to loss. *The mission is not just to evacuate—but to restore capability, dignity, and purpose.*

Bibliography

1. Brown PW. War wounds of the hand revisited. The Journal of hand surgery. 1995 May 1;20(3):S61–S67.
2. Burkhalter WE. Care of war injuries of the hand and upper extremity: Report of the War Injury Committee. The Journal of Hand Surgery. 1983 Sep 1;8(5):810–3.
3. Dias JJ, Chung KC, Garcia-Elias M, Sabapathy SR, Tang JB. Recommendations for the improvement of hand injury care across the world. Injury. 2006 Nov 1;37(11):1078–82.
4. Eardley MW, Stewart CM. Early management of ballistic hand trauma. JAAOS-Journal of the American Academy of Orthopaedic Surgeons. 2010 Feb 1;18(2):118–26.
5. Mathieu L, Bertani A, Gaillard C, Chaudier P, Ollat D, Bauer B, Rigal S. Combat-related upper extremity injuries: surgical management specificities on the theatres of operations. Chirurgie de la Main. 2014 Jun 1;33(3):174–82.
6. Stahl S, Reis ND. Management of war wounds of the hand. Techniques in Orthopaedics. 1986 Jul 1;1(2):68–73.

Burns and Thermal Injuries in Combat 16

Midhun Mohan N and Aaditya Katyal

Learning Objectives

By the end of this chapter, the reader will be able to:

- Apply the integrated MARCH approach for rapid triage of burn casualties in combat environments.
- Recognize immediate life threats from burns, smoke inhalation, and coexisting traumatic injuries.
- Initiate effective prehospital interventions for thermal injuries, including airway protection, burn shock resuscitation, and hypothermia prevention.
- Distinguish between superficial, partial, and full-thickness burns using visual and sensory indicators under field conditions.
- Perform wound care, fluid management, and evacuation prioritization for burn victims during prolonged field care.
- Identify criteria for burn center referral and the role of tactical evacuation in severe burn cases.

Midhun Mohan N (✉)
Department of Emergency Medicine, Kozhikode District Cooperative Hospital, Kozhikode, Kerala, India

A. Katyal
Department of Emergency Medicine, Kasturba Medical College, Manipal, Karnataka, India

N. T. Rai, S. Misra (eds.), *Frontline Operational Resuscitation and Combat Emergencies (FORCE) Manual*, https://doi.org/10.1007/978-981-92-1622-2_16

Introduction

Burn injuries in combat zones present a unique blend of complexity and urgency. Unlike controlled civilian environments, combat burns often occur in conjunction with blast injuries, building collapses, vehicle fires, and chemical exposures, sometimes under active fire or delayed rescue conditions. The impact of burns on skin integrity, thermoregulation, immune function, and fluid dynamics makes them time-sensitive injuries with cascading complications.

In modern battlefield trauma care, the initial management of burns must align with MARCH (Massive hemorrhage, Airway, Respiration, Circulation, Hypothermia/Head injury) while remaining true to the ABCDE (Airway, Breathing, Circulation, Disability, Exposure) trauma protocol. This dual-lens assessment ensures that life-threatening injuries are addressed first while simultaneously accounting for progressive threats like airway swelling, burn shock, and toxic inhalation.

Crucially, burns are dynamic wounds–they evolve rapidly, may be deceptively deep, and often carry delayed systemic consequences. Early fluid resuscitation, thermoprotection, and airway management can drastically reduce mortality. Providers must also anticipate smoke inhalation, carbon monoxide (CO), and cyanide poisoning, especially in enclosed-space fires, and initiate supportive interventions despite resource constraints.

Case Scenario

During a joint counterinsurgency operation in the congested alleys of a semi-urban conflict zone, a fireteam breaches a reinforced building suspected to be an enemy stronghold. Shortly after entry, a secondary IED—rigged near the rear exit—detonates, triggering a structural collapse and fire. Amid the chaos, a soldier providing rear cover is struck by falling debris and trapped under a burning wooden beam. His uniform ignites, and he suffers extensive flame and contact burns before being extricated.

The environment is unstable, with thick smoke, compromised structures, and active small arms threat in the vicinity. The fireteam executes a tactical withdrawal to a covered courtyard, approximately 40 m away, to initiate medical care.

- *Care Under Fire (CUF)*
  Suppressive fire is maintained as teammates crawl into the collapsed room and drag the casualty out using a poncho and buddy drag. No immediate life-threatening bleeding is evident, but the soldier is groaning, with melted clothing and visible full-thickness burns to the lower limbs and back. No other interventions are performed until cover is achieved.
- *Tactical Field Care (TFC)*
  As the situation stabilizes, the medic initiates a systematic MARCH assessment.

Massive Hemorrhage (M): There is no external bleeding; however, significant skin sloughing is present over both legs and lower back, exposing underlying tissue. Deep burns are dry and leathery, raising concern for future compartment syndrome and delayed hemorrhage. The wounds are left uncovered for now, as priority shifts to airway and circulation.

Airway (A): The casualty is hoarse, with carbonaceous deposits around his nares and lips. He is able to speak but in short, strained sentences. The medic suspects evolving inhalational injury and airway edema. A nasopharyngeal airway (NPA) is inserted cautiously, and airway patency is monitored continuously. A surgical cricothyrotomy kit is kept ready in anticipation of worsening obstruction.

Respiration (R): The respiratory rate is 30/min, shallow, with intermittent wheezing and soot-tinged sputum. There are no signs of pneumothorax. Oxygen is not available in this field setting, so the casualty is positioned in a sitting posture to optimize ventilation.

Circulation (C): Radial pulse is weak; systolic blood pressure is estimated at 90 mmHg. Capillary refill is delayed. Signs point toward developing burn shock. The medic estimates total body surface area (TBSA) burned using the "Rule of Nines" and hand method: both legs posteriorly accounted for ~18%, posterior torso ~18% → approximately 36% TBSA. One large-bore IV is established. Fluid resuscitation is initiated with Ringer's lactate at a rate of 360 mL/h titrated based on urine output and clinical status.

Hypothermia/Head Injury (H): GCS is 13 (E4V4M5), and pupils are equal and reactive. There is no external head trauma, but the risk of smoke-induced hypoxia remains. The casualty is stripped of burned clothing, gently cleaned with saline, and wrapped in a clean poncho liner to reduce heat loss. Ambient rain and wind exacerbate hypothermia risk, so efforts are made to create a thermal barrier using plastic sheeting and body insulation from teammates.

- *Tactical Evacuation Care (TACEVAC)*

  Evacuation is delayed due to hostile activity near the extraction corridor. The medic prepares the casualty for movement over uneven terrain, reassessing airway status every 10 min. Burned areas are loosely covered with clean, nonadherent dressings and moist saline gauze, to prevent desiccation. The IV line is secured, and fluid volumes are carefully recorded. A running log of vital signs, fluid input, urine output, and GCS is maintained on waterproof notepaper.

  The casualty is reassured regularly to minimize anxiety, and preparations are made to escalate to airway intervention if his voice becomes progressively hoarse or mental status declines. CASEVAC is initiated once the corridor is deemed secure.

Reflective Questions

1. How do you estimate TBSA using field techniques like the Rule of Nines or hand method, and how does this guide your initial fluid replacement strategy?
2. What clinical signs would indicate a worsening inhalation injury requiring surgical airway intervention?

3. What field-appropriate analgesics are safe in suspected inhalation injury, and how do you titrate them while monitoring respiratory effort?
4. What are your immediate and ongoing priorities for monitoring and documentation when evacuation is delayed by over an hour in a severe burn casualty?

First Aid and Prehospital Care

In the combat setting, first aid for burn injuries must be rapid, prioritized, and resourceful. Burns rarely occur in isolation—they often accompany blunt trauma, blast injury, or smoke inhalation. As such, burn care begins not with the burn, but with a systematic trauma assessment using the MARCH approach, ensuring that life-threatening conditions are never missed in favor of visible wounds.

M—Massive Hemorrhage

Although burns may not bleed profusely, underlying blast or crush trauma may cause occult bleeding or expose vascular structures. Burned tissue may obscure deep lacerations or mask hemorrhage:

- Expose the casualty fully. Do not rely on visible bleeding—look under burned clothing.
- If bleeding is detected, apply:
  - Direct pressure with dry sterile gauze
  - Tourniquet if the limb is involved and bleeding is arterial
    Hemostatic agents if deep wounds are present

FORCE Tactical Pearl
Avoid moist dressings or creams in the field; they interfere with clot formation and may worsen hypothermia.

A—Airway with Cervical Spine Precautions

Airway compromise is the leading cause of death in burn victims—especially in enclosed fires where superheated air, chemicals, and particulates cause delayed swelling.

Red flags for airway burns:

- Soot around the mouth or nostrils
- Hoarseness or stridor
- Singed nasal hairs or eyebrows (Fig. 16.1)
- Carbonaceous sputum
- Burns on the face or neck
- Drooling or altered voice

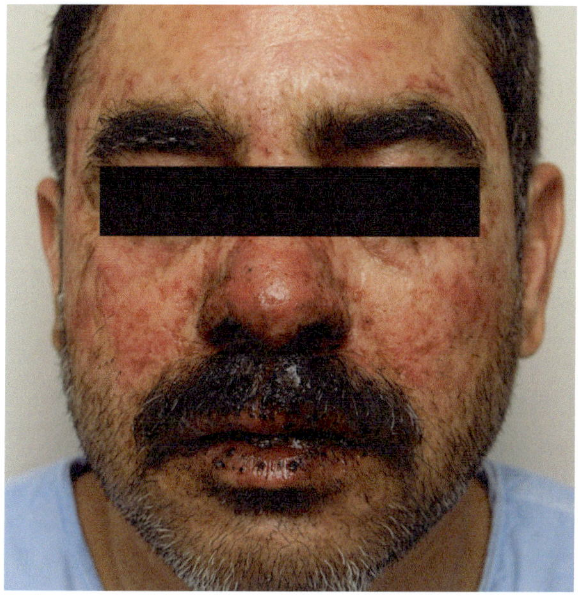

Fig. 16.1 Soldier with burns around the lips and singed facial hair

Field management:

- Perform jaw thrust with in-line spinal immobilization if airway needs to be opened.
- Administer high-flow oxygen if available—suspect CO or cyanide poisoning.
- If signs of airway edema are present and worsening:
  - Prepare for surgical cricothyrotomy—do not wait for full obstruction. Use bougie-assisted technique if trained and available.
- For conscious casualties with hoarseness but no severe distress, monitor closely. Swelling may develop over 30–60 min.

R—Respiration

Burns to the chest wall can restrict respiratory mechanics. Inhalation injury can also cause progressive respiratory failure, even if initial vitals are stable.

Field management:

- Assess the rate, rhythm, and depth of respiration.
- Observe for:
  - Burn eschars on the chest restricting expansion.
  - Wheezing, crackles, or decreasing breath sounds.
- If restrictive eschar compromises ventilation:
  - Be prepared to perform *escharotomy* in chest wall burns, using a scalpel along the mid-axillary line (only if trained).
- Oxygen is essential—but limited in field care.
  - Administer via non-rebreather mask or BVM.

FORCE Tactical Pearl
Suspect CO poisoning in enclosed space fires; consider hyperbaric oxygen post-evacuation.

C—Circulation

Burn shock is a combination of fluid loss, vasodilation, and third spacing. Unlike hemorrhagic shock, it evolves over hours—but early signs must not be missed.

Signs of early burn shock:

- Weak peripheral pulses
- Cool extremities
- Delayed capillary refill
- Altered mental status with preserved GCS

Field management:

- Secure large-bore IV or IO access (preferably in unburned limb).
- Initiate fluid resuscitation:
  - Use lactated Ringer's or normal saline (avoid D5W or hypotonic fluids).
  - In field: 500 mL bolus, repeat as needed based on perfusion and urine output.
  - Use *Rule of Tens* for adult burns >20% TBSA:
    - Start with 10× TBSA% in mL/h (for 70 kg adult).
      Adjust fluid based on mental status and radial pulse presence.
  - *TXA is not routinely needed unless associated trauma is present.*
    Keep track of urine output if catheterization is possible.

H—Head Injury/Hypothermia

Burn victims may have associated blast brain injury or carbon monoxide intoxication.

- Perform AVPU or GCS assessment.
- Watch for signs of neurological decline, which may indicate:
  - Hypoxia
  - Hypoperfusion
  - CO toxicity
  - Intracranial injury

Tactical considerations:

- Minimize morphine or fentanyl use unless airway is secured.
- Ketamine is preferred for burn pain—provides analgesia and amnesia and preserves respiration:
  - Dose: 0.2–0.5 mg/kg IV or IM

Once life threats are addressed, evaluate the extent and depth of burns.
Burn types:

- *Superficial (first degree)*: Red, painful, and dry
- *Partial thickness (second degree)*: blistered, wet, and painful
- *Full thickness (third degree)*: Charred, leathery, and painless

These are further elucidated in Figs. 16.2, 16.3, and Table 16.1.
Estimation:

- Use *Rule of Nines* (Fig. 16.4) or *Rule of Palms* (casualty's palm = 1% TBSA).

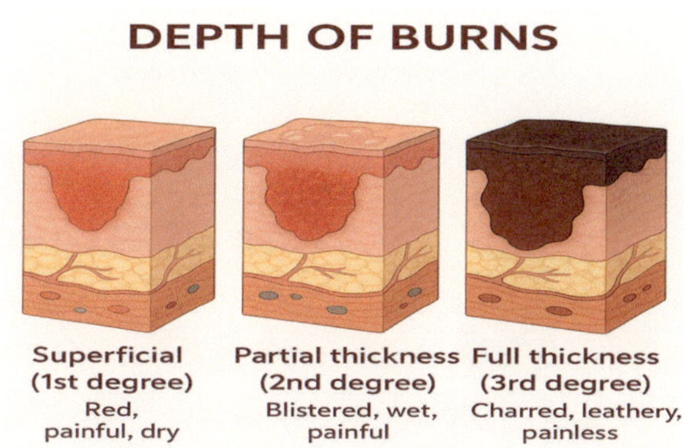

Fig. 16.2 Burn depth classification

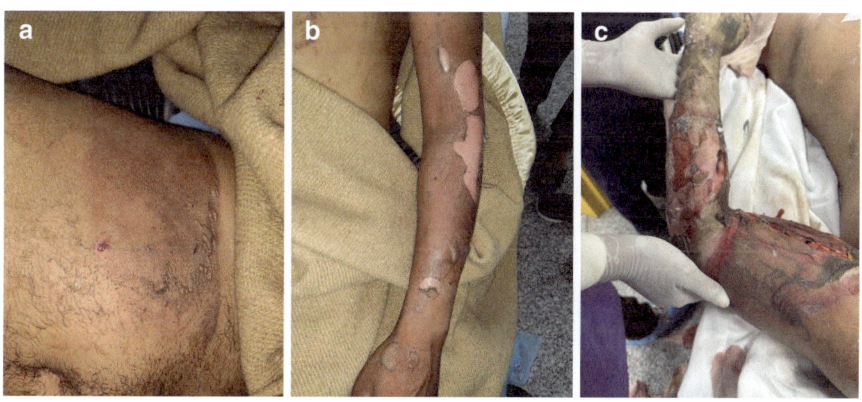

Fig. 16.3 (**a**) Superficial thickness burns to the flank. (**b**) Partial thickness burns to the upper limb. (**c**) Full-thickness degree burns to the upper limb

Table 16.1 Clinical features of each class of burns

Burn description	Appearance	Capillary refill	Pain/ sensation	Healing
Superficial thickness	Erythema For example, sunburns	Fast	+	7–14 days without scarring
Superficial partial thickness	Wet, pink with blisters	Fast *(Blanches with pressure)*	++	2–4 weeks without scarring or functional impairment
Deep partial thickness	Less wet, red +/– blisters	Sluggish or absent *(Does not blanch with pressure)*	+/–	3–8 weeks with severe scarring Needs grafting
Full thickness	Dry, white, or charred and black No vesicles or blisters	Absent *(Do not blanch with pressure)*	Absent	Severe scarring and contracture Needs grafting

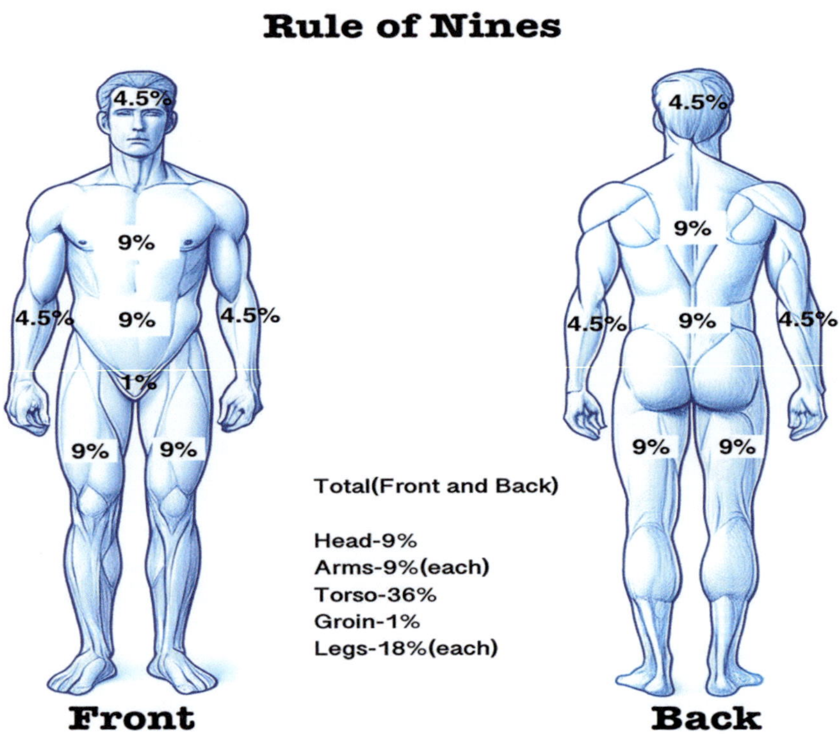

Fig. 16.4 "Rule of Nines" for burn estimation

Table 16.2 Emergency field care of casualty with major burns

Airway	Breathing	Circulation	Adjuncts
Early intubation if: Signs of airway obstruction (stridor, hoarseness of voice) Severe respiratory distress Oral cavity burns Severe facial burns Circumferential burns with edema in the neck Burns >40% TBSA Decreased level of consciousness Frequent reassessment is required as airway obstruction can evolve over time	Suspect smoke inhalation injury in enclosed space burns Continuous pulse oximetry with supplemental oxygen Mechanical ventilation as required Determine carboxyhemoglobin (COHb) level (if available)	Establishment of 2 large bore peripheral IV lines through unburned skin (if not possible burned area may be used) Cardiac monitoring Start IV Ringer's lactate (RL) solution as per Rule of Tens	Place a Foley catheter for monitoring urine output Insertion of nasogastric tube Administer tetanus booster Pain control Assess for other trauma

Initial Priorities in the Field Management of Major Burns

Major burn injuries represent a physiologically complex, multisystem emergency that requires rapid, structured, and disciplined resuscitation from the very first contact. The initial minutes are critical: airway edema can progress rapidly, respiratory compromise may be subtle yet life-threatening, and circulatory failure due to burn shock evolves over hours. A systematic approach—mirroring the principles of trauma care—ensures that life-threatening problems are addressed in the correct order of priority.

Table 16.2 summarizes the core actions and decision triggers in the early management of a casualty with major burns. Each domain—Airway, Breathing, Circulation, and Adjuncts—highlights essential interventions, indications for escalation, and the need for continuous reassessment.

Definitive Field Burn Management

Once the casualty is stabilized using the MARCH approach, the focus shifts to managing systemic effects of burns, preventing infection, and preparing for evacuation. In many combat scenarios, definitive care may be delayed due to hostile conditions, poor terrain, or evacuation logistics. *Therefore, burns must be managed as dynamic injuries, with close attention to evolving signs of deterioration.*

1. Fluid Resuscitation in the Field

In burns exceeding 20% total body surface area (TBSA), fluid loss from capillary leak becomes life-threatening. *The goal is to maintain perfusion without overloading volume*, especially when monitoring tools are minimal.

Field resuscitation principles:

- Start IV or IO fluids as early as possible—preferably Ringer's lactate.
- Use the *"Rule of Tens"*:
  - Estimate burn size to the nearest 10.
  - For adults >40 kg, give *10 mL × % TBSA burn per hour*, e.g., 30% TBSA = 300 mL/h.
  - *For every 10 kg above 80 kg, increase the rate by 100 mL/h.*
- Titrate based on:
  - Mental status (alert = adequate perfusion)
  - Radial pulse (present = acceptable SBP)
  - Urine output (if catheterized): aim for *0.5 mL/kg/h*

If available, the apps like Burn Navigator® can be used for patients weighing 40 kg or more to assist with fluid resuscitation. At the start of each hour, input the total fluid intake and urine output (UOP) values as prompted. The application will then calculate and recommend the appropriate isotonic fluid rate for the next hour.

FORCE Tactical Pearl

Burn shock may not peak until 8–12 h post-injury, so fluid needs may rise over time. Avoid under-resuscitation in the first 4 h—start early and adjust.

2. Burn Wound Care in Prolonged Field Settings

Burn wounds, especially full-thickness and partial-thickness injuries, are prone to infection, desiccation, and further tissue loss if not covered appropriately.

Wound handling protocol:

- Do not debride in the field—just remove loose debris and burned clothing.
- Irrigate gently with sterile saline only if significant contamination is visible.
- Apply dry, sterile dressings—ideally non-adherent (e.g., Adaptic™ and Telfa™).
- Use loose wrapping to allow for swelling and prevent compartment syndrome.
- If supplies are limited:
  - Use clean cloth or burn sheets as temporary dressing.
  - Separate digits with gauze in hand or foot burns to prevent webbing.
- *Do not apply creams, ice, or water—these worsen hypothermia and tissue damage.*

3. Pain Management

Burns are among the most painful injuries encountered in combat trauma. Adequate pain control improves physiological stability and reduces psychological distress.

Preferred field analgesia:

- *Ketamine (IV or IM)*: 0.2–0.5 mg/kg for analgesia; 1–2 mg/kg for sedation
- *Fentanyl (IN or IV)*: 800 mcg via intranasal atomizer or 25–50 mcg IV.
- *Paracetamol or NSAIDs* (if airway is secure and no renal compromise).

FORCE Tactical Pearl
Avoid morphine unless airway is secured, as it depresses respiration and worsens hypoxia.

4. Antibiotics and Infection Control
Routine antibiotics are not required for all burns, but are indicated if:

- Burns are >30% TBSA
- There is visible contamination or suspected infection
- There are associated trauma or field surgical interventions (e.g., cricothyrotomy and escharotomy)

Field choices:

- Ceftriaxone 1–2 g IV/IM daily.
- Add metronidazole 500 mg IV/IM if gastrointestinal or groin burns are present.
- In penicillin-allergic patients: Clindamycin + ciprofloxacin.

Sign of infection:

- Foul odor
- Increasing redness around edges
- Fever/chills
- Delayed healing or necrosis

5. Burn Complications
Even well-managed burns may develop complications. Watch for:

- *Airway obstruction* (progressive stridor, wheezing, cyanosis)
- *Burn shock* (despite fluid resuscitation)
- *Compartment syndrome* (circumferential burns of limbs or chest)
- *Sepsis* (tachycardia, hypotension, altered mental status)
- *Hypothermia* (burned patients lose heat quickly, even in warm climates)

Combat actions:

- Reassess every 15–30 min.
- Adjust fluid, oxygen, and pain meds as needed.
- Evacuate if airway status, perfusion, or neurological status deteriorates.

Table 16.3 Criteria for transfer to a burn center

Full-thickness burns
Partial-thickness burns >10% TBSA
Burns to the hands, face, genitalia, perinium, and major joints
Inhalation injury
Electrical and lightning burns
Chemical burns
Comorbidities complicating management

6. Evacuation Prioritization

Burn casualties should be prioritized for evacuation and transfer to a burn center if any of the following criteria are met (Table 16.3).

Evacuation guidelines:

- Cover with sterile dressings and insulate well against heat loss.
- Ensure fluids, analgesia, and airway tools accompany the patient.
- Document MIST and fluid balance.
- Preserve IV/IO lines and dressings during transport.

Case Resolution

Upon arrival at the designated extraction zone, the casualty is transferred onto a vacuum mattress with spinal precautions and elevated to a semi-Fowler's position to ease breathing effort. His clothing and dressings are gently assessed en route for saturation, displacement, or signs of secondary bleeding. The IV line remains patent, and the team closely tracks all inputs and vital signs during movement.

The total body surface area (TBSA) involved is reaffirmed using a combination of the Rule of Tens and the palmar method. In austere settings, each palm (including fingers) is approximately 1% TBSA. By approximating that both legs posteriorly contributed 18% and the posterior torso another 18%, the team estimated ~36% TBSA burns. Based on this, the Rule of Tens suggests initiating fluid resuscitation with 360 mL/h of Ringer's lactate (10× TBSA% = 360 mL/h for a 70 kg adult). This is titrated to maintain urine output of 0.5 mL/kg/h, monitored using visual estimation, as no Foley catheter is available in the field.

The casualty's respiratory effort remains labored, with increasing hoarseness and decreasing vocal clarity. The team notes progressive stridor, which—combined with soot in the nares and oropharynx and rising respiratory rate—suggests evolving airway edema and impending obstruction. While bag-valve-mask support is prepared, the surgical airway kit is kept ready. However, since the patient remains conscious and cooperative, no immediate intervention is made. Preparations are made to escalate to cricothyrotomy if respiratory fatigue, decreasing GCS, or inability to phonate is noted.

For analgesia, IV ketamine is chosen due to its minimal effect on respiratory drive and added dissociative benefits. It is given in titrated 20 mg boluses every 10–15 min, observing for signs of hypersalivation, dysphoria, or blood pressure lability. Opioids are avoided given the patient's borderline oxygenation and the risk of hypoventilation. The casualty is regularly reassured and oriented as part of psychological first aid, with team members communicating calmly and clearly to reduce anxiety and perceived isolation.

With evacuation delayed beyond an hour, documentation becomes critical. The medic maintains a field log noting:

- Time of injury and initial intervention
- Estimated TBSA and fluid volumes administered
- Hourly GCS, respiratory rate, pulse, and blood pressure
- Changes in airway signs or analgesia needs

The burn sites are covered with non-adherent saline-soaked gauze, replaced if contaminated. Hypothermia is prevented with a combination of Mylar blankets, a clean poncho liner, and body shielding from fellow soldiers. The burn shock progression is monitored via peripheral perfusion and serial GCS.

On arrival at the field surgical facility, the casualty is immediately intubated due to worsening airway edema and admitted to the burn ICU. Owing to early airway preparation, timely estimation of TBSA, fluid resuscitation, and vigilant monitoring in the field, the soldier survives the incident with stable hemodynamics and no airway-related complications.

Key Messages

- Burns in combat are dynamic injuries that often evolve in severity and frequently coexist with blast trauma and airway compromise.
- Apply the MARCH approach to prioritize life threats over visible burn injuries.
- Inhalation injury is a silent killer—look for early airway signs and be prepared for a surgical airway if obstruction is imminent.
- Begin fluid resuscitation early, using tactical adaptations of the Parkland formula such as the Rule of Tens.
- Use dry, sterile dressings and avoid creams, ointments, or wet wraps in the field.
- Burn casualties are extremely prone to hypothermia—even in warm climates. Preserve body heat.
- Ketamine is the analgesic of choice in the field, offering pain control without respiratory compromise.
- Evacuate early if burns involve critical areas and large surface area or are accompanied by airway or systemic signs.
- Combat providers must improvise—burn management is rarely about perfect tools but always about structured priorities.

Conclusion

Combat burns demand vigilance, decisiveness, and improvisation. While burns may not bleed, they threaten life through airway compromise, burn shock, and infection. They rob strength through pain and immobility and challenge providers to balance immediate needs with long-term survival.

This chapter has demonstrated how the MARCH-integrated ABCDE approach enables combat providers to identify and intervene on true life threats while managing evolving burn wounds under austere conditions. By focusing on airway protection, fluid resuscitation, thermal control, and wound coverage—while remaining tactically aware—combat providers can save lives, reduce suffering, and preserve the fighting strength of the unit.

Ultimately, the measure of success in burn care is not just survival, but functional recovery.

Bibliography

1. American Burn Association. National Burn Repository. [online]. Available from http://www.ameriburn.org/resources_publications.php.
2. American College of Surgeons Committee on Trauma. ATLS: Advanced Trauma Life Support. 10th ed. Chicago: American College of Surgeons; 2018. ISBN: 978-0996826235
3. Chung, Kevin K. MD; Wolf, Steven E. MD; Cancio, Leopoldo C. MD; Alvarado, Ricardo MD; Jones, John A. BS, BBA; McCorcle, Jeffery PA; King, Booker T. MD; Barillo, David J. MD; Renz, Evan M. MD; Blackbourne, Lorne H. MD. Resuscitation of Severely Burned Military Casualties: Fluid Begets More Fluid. The Journal of Trauma: Injury, Infection, and Critical Care 67(2):p 231–237, August 2009. https://doi.org/10.1097/TA.0b013e3181ac68cf
4. Thakur N, Misra S. *Pediatric Trauma Resuscitation Manual*. 1st ed. New Delhi: CBS Publishers & Distributors Pvt Ltd; 2023. 216 p. ISBN: 978-9356963979.

Managing Gunshot Wounds in Combat 17

Pancholy Kartik Nitin

Learning Objectives

By the end of this chapter, the reader will be able to:

- Identify key mechanisms and patterns of gunshot injuries in combat scenarios.
- Apply the MARCH protocol to assess and manage GSWs effectively in the field.
- Demonstrate appropriate use of tourniquets and hemostatic dressings for extremity and junctional bleeds.
- Recognize early signs of hypovolemic shock and initiate appropriate resuscitation, including TXA and fluid therapy.
- Manage pain safely and prevent hypothermia during prolonged field care.
- Prioritize patients for evacuation and adapt management based on environmental and tactical constraints.
- Understand when to convert or maintain a tourniquet during delayed transport.
- Reflect on common complications of GSWs and their prevention in field conditions.

P. K. Nitin (✉)
Department of Emergency Medicine, Max Super Speciality Hospital,
Dwarka, New Delhi, India

N. T. Rai, S. Misra (eds.), *Frontline Operational Resuscitation and Combat Emergencies (FORCE) Manual*, https://doi.org/10.1007/978-981-92-1622-2_17

Introduction

Managing gunshot wounds (GSWs) in combat is a true test of both medical expertise and tactical discipline. In the unforgiving reality of the battlefield—*where threats persist, evacuation may be delayed, and resources are limited—every second becomes a critical opportunity to impact survival.* Unlike controlled civilian environments, combat care must be delivered amidst chaos, uncertainty, and direct hostile engagement. It is under these extreme conditions that a provider's ability to assess, prioritize, and act systematically makes the defining difference.

The MARCH algorithm provides a structured, battle-proven framework to impose order in such moments of crisis. By following this sequence—Massive Hemorrhage, Airway, Respiration, Circulation, and Hypothermia/Head injury—combat providers can rapidly identify and treat life-threatening conditions in the correct order of urgency, ensuring that no critical intervention is missed even when working under extreme time pressure.

Gunshot wounds present varied and complex challenges: from catastrophic extremity bleeds to tension pneumothorax, to hidden internal injuries without obvious external signs. In each case, the tactical application of tourniquets, TXA administration, hypothermia prevention, and safe pain management must be immediate, methodical, and escalation ready. When performed correctly, these interventions do more than simply stabilize the casualty—they directly influence long-term outcomes, such as limb salvage, neurological preservation, and future operational capability.

This chapter reinforces that survival and functional recovery are achievable even in devastating gunshot injuries when care is timely, disciplined, and tactically sound. Field responders must internalize the principle that battlefield trauma care is not merely about managing injury—*it is about preserving the fighting strength, dignity, and independence of those who serve*. Every decision taken in the first 10 min of casualty care will shape not just the next hour—*but the next 10 years of that soldier's life!*

Case Scenario

During a coordinated clearing operation in a densely built urban zone of Kashmir, a 24-year-old infantryman manning a rooftop cover position is struck by unexpected small arms fire during movement between buildings. The soldier collapses on the narrow stairwell landing between floors, bleeding heavily from the upper left thigh. His teammates return suppressive fire and neutralize the remaining threat.

- *Care Under Fire (CUF)*
  Amidst intermittent hostile gunfire, the combat medic performs a manual drag to pull the casualty down the stairwell behind cover. A rapid MARCH sweep reveals no immediate threat to airway or respiration, but there is visible pulsatile bleeding from the proximal medial left thigh—suggestive of femoral artery injury. A

Combat Application Tourniquet (CAT) is applied "high and tight" on the affected thigh. No further interventions are performed until the area is secure.

- *Tactical Field Care (TFC)*

  Once the scene is stabilized and return fire has ceased, the medic initiates a structured MARCH assessment:

  Massive Hemorrhage (M): The gunshot wound lies near the groin crease—difficult for standard tourniquet efficacy. Though the CAT slowed bleeding, continued oozing persists, indicating a junctional location. The wound is packed with combat gauze and held under firm direct pressure for 3 min, followed by a pressure dressing. Bleeding is controlled with no further visible blood loss.

  Airway (A): The casualty is alert, speaking in short phrases, and follows commands. No facial trauma or airway compromise is noted. Jaw thrust confirms a patent airway. An NPA is prepared but not inserted as the casualty remains stable. The airway is monitored closely for deterioration.

  Respiration (R): The casualty's respiratory rate is 30/min but regular. Bilateral chest rise is symmetrical, with no crepitus, subcutaneous emphysema, or signs of tension pneumothorax. SpO_2 is 93% on room air. No chest wounds are visible. No intervention is needed.

  Circulation (C): The casualty is pale and diaphoretic, with a thready radial pulse and systolic BP estimated at 90 mmHg. A 16 G IV line is established, and 1 g tranexamic acid (TXA) is administered over 10 min. A 500 mL bolus of warmed Ringer's lactate is started slowly. A pelvic binder is also applied due to the proximity of the wound to the pelvic ring, to stabilize any occult pelvic fracture.

  Head Injury/Hypothermia (H): GCS is 15, with no visible head trauma or neurologic deficit. Wet and blood-soaked gear is removed. The casualty is dried, wrapped in a thermal casualty blanket, and shielded from wind exposure on the rooftop to prevent progressive hypothermia.

- *Tactical Evacuation Care (TACEVAC)*

  Evacuation is delayed by approximately 45 min due to narrow alleyways under threat and lack of rotor clearance. The casualty is positioned supine with the injured leg slightly elevated and immobilized using a rigid splint padded with a folded poncho and field dressing. The tourniquet site is left visible for continuous reassessment, and the medic documents time of application on both the dressing and the casualty's skin. Given the proximity of the wound to the femoral triangle, the team remains alert for signs of junctional bleeding recurrence, expanding hematoma, or compartment syndrome. The tourniquet is not converted in the field due to the continued risk of re-bleeding, limited resupply, and prolonged evacuation time. No attempt is made to extract the bullet. Pain is controlled with IV ketamine in titrated doses. The casualty remains conscious, reassured, and cooperative as the team prepares for rooftop sling extraction once aerial clearance is granted.

Reflective Questions

1. What considerations should guide the packaging and positioning of a casualty with a lower limb GSW during prolonged transport to prevent additional tissue damage or circulatory compromise?
2. When, if at all, should the tourniquet be converted to a pressure dressing in this casualty? What signs would support that decision?
3. Given the wound's proximity to the groin, how do you monitor for developing compartment syndrome or junctional bleeding despite initial control?
4. Should the bullet be removed in the field if it is palpable or visible within the wound, and what are the risks or consequences of attempting extraction before surgical care is available?

Mechanisms and Ballistics of Gunshot Wounds

Understanding the mechanics of ballistic trauma is critical in anticipating the extent and type of injury sustained. Gunshot wounds are not simply puncture injuries—*they represent a complex interaction of energy transfer, tissue density, and projectile dynamics*. In combat settings, the variability in weapons, engagement ranges, and ammunition types leads to a wide spectrum of injury patterns.

Key Ballistic Concepts

1. *Kinetic Energy Transfer*

   The damage caused by a bullet is proportional to its kinetic energy:

$$\text{K.E.} = 1/2mv^2$$

FORCE Tactical Pearl

Velocity plays a much greater role than mass. *A high-velocity rifle round causes exponentially more tissue destruction than a low-velocity pistol bullet.*

2. *Temporary Versus Permanent Cavitation*
   - *Temporary cavity*: A shockwave-created cavity where surrounding tissues are stretched or sheared, which can cause secondary damage to organs, vessels, or nerves
   - *Permanent cavity*: The actual wound channel where tissue has been destroyed
3. *Yaw, Tumble, and Fragmentation*

   Projectiles may *yaw* (turn sideways), *tumble* (rotate end over end), or *fragment upon impact—creating multiple wound tracks, unpredictable trajectories, and hidden internal injury.*

Common Combat Ballistic Sources

These are outlined in Table 17.1 and Fig. 17.1.

Tactical Relevance

- *Entry wounds* may appear clean and small, but internal damage could be extensive.
- *Exit wounds*, if present, often indicate a high-energy, through-and-through trajectory but do not always correlate with severity.
- *No-exit (retained bullet)* scenarios raise concerns for vascular proximity, organ injury, or fragment migration.
- *Junctional areas* (groin, axilla, neck) are especially vulnerable and difficult to compress manually.

Table 17.1 Common combat ballistic sources with typical injury patterns

Weapon type	Velocity	Typical injury pattern
Sniper rifle	Very high	Deep penetration, bone shattering, lethal torso hits
Assault rifle	High (700–1000 m/s)	Deep cavitation, long wound track, fragmentation
Handgun	Low (250–400 m/s)	Straight-line track, less cavitation
Shotgun (close range)	Low–medium	Devastating tissue destruction in wide pattern
Shrapnel (IEDs)	Variable	Multiple irregular wounds, embedded metal fragments

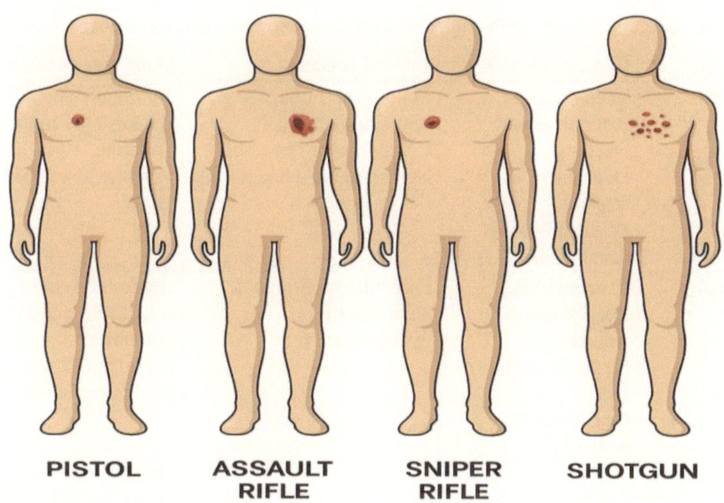

Fig. 17.1 Common combat ballistic sources with typical injury patterns

In combat, weapons vary from conventional firearms to improvised explosive devices (IEDs), often resulting in mixed-pattern injuries—combining blast, burn, and penetrating trauma. Accurate assessment and understanding of projectile dynamics help the provider anticipate complications and intervene early.

Types of Gunshot Injuries and Tactical Implications

Gunshot wounds (GSWs) can affect virtually any anatomical region, but their consequences vary widely depending on the site of impact, projectile energy, and trajectory (Table 17.2). In the combat setting, identifying the type of GSW helps guide field priorities—whether to stabilize and evacuate quickly or manage conservatively under fire.

Additional Considerations
In combat environments, ballistic injuries present with varied patterns and clinical complexities. Understanding the type of injury sustained is crucial in determining tactical priorities and potential field risks. Wounds may appear deceptively minor externally while concealing deeper, life-threatening damage. Through-and-through injuries, retained projectiles, and fragmentation patterns each carry distinct implications for bleeding, infection, and internal trauma. Moreover, bone involvement adds further urgency due to instability, hemorrhage, and risk of fat embolism. Accurate identification and classification of these injuries under battlefield conditions are essential for effective triage, timely evacuation, and lifesaving interventions. Table 17.3 outlines key features for operational decision-making.

Table 17.2 Gunshot injuries with clinical features, tactical concerns, and management priorities

Injury type	Clinical features	Tactical concerns	Management priorities
Extremity wounds	Visible wound Arterial/venous bleeding Deformity or fracture Possible loss of distal pulses	Major vessel injury (e.g., femoral/brachial) Compartment syndrome Nerve/tendon damage	Tourniquet application Hemorrhage control Splinting Vascular assessment
Junctional injuries	Massive bleeding Deep penetrating wounds Neck: air embolism risk Groin: possible pelvic injury	Difficult to tourniquet High risk of exsanguination	Hemostatic gauze Junctional tourniquet (if available) Pelvic binder Rapid evacuation

Table 17.2 (continued)

Injury type	Clinical features	Tactical concerns	Management priorities
Thoracic injuries	Chest entry wound Dyspnea Decreased breath sounds Late tracheal deviation Sucking/open chest wound	Tension pneumothorax Hemothorax Cardiac tamponade risk	Occlusive chest seal Needle decompression Prepare for respiratory failure
Abdominal injuries	Entry wound Abdominal tenderness/rigidity Hypotension Distension	Hollow viscus/solid organ injury Delayed shock Risk of sepsis	No oral intake IV fluids if hypotensive Early surgical evacuation
Head and neck injuries	Obvious trauma GCS decline Bleeding from nose/ears Airway obstruction	Airway compromise Cervical spine injury risk	Airway protection (NPA/cricothyrotomy) Cervical stabilization Early evacuation

Abbreviations: *GCS* Glasgow Coma Scale, *NPA* nasopharyngeal airway

Table 17.3 Tactical implications and field risks of ballistic injury types

Injury type	Tactical priority	Field risk
Through-and-through	May mask deeper tissue damage	Ongoing bleeding, infection risk
Retained bullet	Internal trajectory unknown	Hidden vascular or organ injury
Fragmentation wounds	Multiple wound paths	Embedded metal, infection, missed injuries
Bone involvement	Limb instability, bleeding	High pain, risk of fat embolism

Initial Approach and Field Management

The *MARCH algorithm* provides a structured, combat-tested framework for managing trauma in high-threat environments. When responding to gunshot wounds (GSWs), this sequence ensures that life-threatening conditions are prioritized and addressed systematically, even under pressure (Table 17.4).

M—Massive Hemorrhage

Uncontrolled bleeding is the leading preventable cause of death in combat. Extremity GSWs, junctional injuries, and femoral or brachial artery hits must be managed immediately.

Field actions:

- Apply a Combat Application Tourniquet (CAT) "high and tight" above bleeding sites.
- If bleeding persists or is junctional:

Table 17.4 MARCH survey considerations in a casualty with gunshot injury

Step	Focus	Considerations
M	Bleeding control	Arterial/venous hits, femoral/brachial bleeds
A	Airway protection	Neck/face/head trauma, unresponsive casualties
R	Lung integrity	Chest GSWs → pneumothorax/hemothorax risks
C	Perfusion/shock	Blood loss, TXA use, fluid restriction
H	Brain/temp protection	GCS changes, hypothermia post-hemorrhage

Abbreviations: *GSW* gunshot wound, *TXA* tranexamic acid, *GCS* Glasgow Coma Scale

  - Use hemostatic gauze (e.g., Combat gauze).
  - Apply direct pressure for 3 min.
  - Consider junctional tourniquets if available.
- Document time of tourniquet application visibly on the casualty.

A—Airway

Most GSWs do not compromise the airway unless the neck, face, or head is involved. However, unresponsiveness or trauma may necessitate early intervention.

Field actions:

- Assess airway patency—speak to the casualty.
- Use NPA (nasopharyngeal airway) if GCS > 8 and no facial trauma.
- Perform surgical cricothyrotomy if airway obstruction is suspected and cannot be relieved.
- Maintain cervical spine precautions in head/neck GSWs.

R—Respiration

Gunshot wounds to the chest can cause open pneumothorax, hemothorax, or tension pneumothorax—conditions that deteriorate rapidly without intervention.

Field actions:

- Expose and inspect the chest.
- Apply occlusive chest seals on all penetrating wounds.
- If tension pneumothorax is suspected (e.g., unilateral breath sounds, hypoxia, and hypotension):
  - *Use 14–16 G, 3.25″ needle and p*erform at:
    - Second ICS midclavicular (traditional)
      Fifth ICS anterior axillary line (preferred)
- Monitor for recurrence—*re-decompress if needed.*

C—Circulation

Shock from blood loss is common in GSWs. Providers must act quickly to maintain perfusion without over-resuscitating and diluting clotting factors.

Field actions:

- Check radial pulse, skin color, and capillary refill.
- Establish large-bore IV or IO access.

- Administer:
  - 1 g TXA (tranexamic acid) within 1 h of injury, IV over 10 min
    500 mL bolus of warm Ringer's lactate or Plasma-Lyte in shock
- *Avoid excessive fluids—the goal is to maintain mental status and radial pulse.*

H—Head Injury and Hypothermia

Head injuries from gunshots require rapid assessment of consciousness and pupil response. Simultaneously, hypothermia must be prevented, as it worsens coagulopathy and shock.

Field actions:

- Assess GCS and pupil reactivity.
- For altered mental status with penetrating trauma: Prioritize airway and early evacuation.
- Strip wet clothing, and apply Hypothermia Prevention Kit (HPK) or thermal blankets.
- Insulate from ground and wind—*maintain a core temperature of >36 °C.*

Hemorrhage Control and Tourniquet Strategy

Massive hemorrhage is the leading preventable cause of death in battlefield gunshot injuries. Timely intervention in the first few minutes can be lifesaving.

1. *Tourniquet Application*
   - *Indications*:
     - Arterial bleeding not controlled by pressure
     - Partial or complete traumatic amputations
       Bleeding in high-stress, high-threat situations
   - *Application*:
     - Apply *high and tight* on the limb—above the wound and over clothing if necessary.
     - Tighten until bleeding stops and distal pulse is absent.
       Mark time of application clearly (on forehead, tape, or casualty card).
   - *Conversion*:
     - Consider conversion to a pressure dressing *only* if:
       - Casualty is hemodynamically stable
       - No ongoing bleeding is seen after a 2-h window
         Conditions permit observation and reapplication if needed
2. *Junctional Wounds*
   - Sites: Neck, axilla, and groin
     - *Management*:
       - Apply direct pressure with hemostatic gauze.
       - Use junctional tourniquet if available (e.g., SAM Junctional Tourniquet).
         Consider pelvic binders for groin or pelvic hits.

3. *Bleeding from the Trunk or Non-compressible Zones*
   - Typically not managed definitively in the field.
   - Early TXA, rapid evacuation, and hypothermia prevention are key.

Antibiotic Management in Gunshot Wounds

Penetrating injuries, especially from gunshot wounds, pose a high risk of infection due to the introduction of bacteria, foreign material, and devitalized tissue into deep tissue planes. While definitive surgical debridement is the gold standard, early administration of field antibiotics significantly reduces the risk of wound infection and sepsis—especially in prolonged field care or delayed evacuation scenarios.

Indications for field antibiotics:

- Open fractures (e.g., femur and tibia)
- Wounds with visible contamination (e.g., soil, feces, and debris)
- Deep soft tissue GSWs, especially in the groin, axilla, or abdomen
- Junctional and perineal injuries
- Suspected bowel injury or peritonitis from abdominal entry wound
- Delayed evacuation >2 h

Preferred antibiotics and dosing:
This is as described in Table 17.5.

FORCE Tactical Pearl
Antibiotics are not a substitute for wound debridement. They are an adjunct to control bacterial proliferation until surgical care is available.

Administration tips:

Table 17.5 Empiric antibiotic recommendations for combat-related wounds and prolonged field care

Scenario	Antibiotic	Dose
Open wounds, soft tissue injury	Cefazolin or ceftriaxone	Cefazolin 2 g IV or IM Ceftriaxone 2 g IV/IM once daily
Suspected bowel involvement	Ceftriaxone + metronidazole	+ Metronidazole 500 mg IV/PO q8h
Penicillin allergy	Clindamycin or moxifloxacin	Clindamycin 600 mg IV/IM or moxifloxacin 400 mg PO/IV
Prolonged care >24 h in field	Continue above regimens q24h (max 48 h unless surgical care is reached)	

- Use IV or IM route depending on vascular access.
- In austere settings, reconstitute powdered formulations using sterile water or saline.
- If oral route is the only option, ensure casualty is conscious and tolerating fluids.
- Record dose, time, and route on casualty card for handover.

Management of an Embedded or Retained Bullet in the Field

In the field, providers may encounter gunshot wounds where the bullet is either embedded within soft tissue or suspected to be retained internally without an exit wound (Fig. 17.2). While the instinct may be to remove a visible or palpable projectile, current combat casualty care guidelines are clear: *Field removal of bullets is not recommended and should only be performed as part of definitive surgical care at an appropriate medical facility.*

Why Not in the Field?
Attempting to remove a bullet outside a sterile surgical setting can:

- Dislodge clots and restart bleeding, especially in vascular injuries

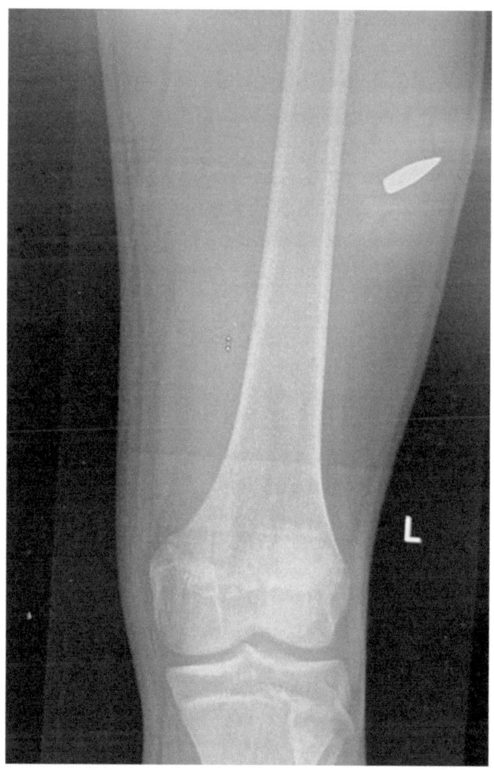

Fig. 17.2 Soldier with gunshot injury to the left thigh with embedded bullet as seen on X-ray

- Damage adjacent nerves, vessels, or bone
- Introduce infection into deep tissue planes
- Cause uncontrolled pain or unnecessary trauma
- Delay evacuation and divert attention from more urgent priorities

FORCE Tactical Pearl
Even if a bullet is visible or palpable, removal should not be attempted unless it directly impairs lifesaving interventions (e.g., *airway obstruction or interference with CPR).*

Recommended field actions:

- Do not probe the wound or explore to locate the projectile (Table 17.6).
- Control external bleeding with tourniquets, hemostatic dressings, and pressure.
- Stabilize the affected limb or area to prevent projectile migration.
- Document the presence of a suspected or known retained bullet.
- Communicate this information during evacuation using the MIST format.

Indications for Bullet Removal (Only at a Definitive Surgical Facility)

1. *Neurovascular compromise*
   Bullet is compressing or impinging on a major nerve or vessel, causing ischemia, neurologic deficit, or risk of limb loss.
2. *Intra-articular location (joint involvement)*
   Projectile is within a joint capsule, which may lead to chronic inflammation, arthritis, or functional impairment if not removed.
3. *Spinal canal involvement*
   Bullet or fragment located in the spinal canal or neural foramen, with potential or evident spinal cord compression.
4. *Ongoing infection or abscess formation*
   Retained bullet or fragment is acting as a nidus for sepsis, abscess, or chronic wound infection.

Table 17.6 Common myths and facts about bullet removal in the field

Myth	Fact
"If I can see or feel the bullet, I should remove it immediately"	*False*—Current guidelines advise against field removal. It should only be performed surgically
"Leaving a bullet inside is dangerous—It must come out right away"	*False*—Most retained bullets pose no immediate threat and are removed later during surgery
"Removing the bullet will reduce pain and speed up recovery"	*False*—Removal in the field may worsen bleeding, tissue injury, or infection risk
"I should probe the wound to locate the bullet"	*False*—Probing disrupts tissue planes, increases contamination, and delays evacuation

5. *Migration or embolization*
   Bullet has migrated (e.g., into the vascular system or vital organ), creating risk of embolism, infarction, or delayed organ injury.
6. *Chronic pain or functional impairment*
   Bullet is causing persistent pain, muscle spasm, or restricting motion—particularly in tendinous or muscular compartments.
7. *Toxicity from bullet composition (rare)*
   Bullets made of lead or containing other reactive materials may require removal if they pose systemic toxicity (e.g., in CSF or intraocular).
8. *Forensic or intelligence purposes (command directed)*
   Removal requested for identification, legal documentation, or operational intelligence, when tactically feasible and does not delay care.

FORCE Tactical Pearl
In tactical settings, the priority is not extraction of bullet but preservation of life, limb, and function. Bullet removal belongs in the operating room—not on the battlefield.

Hypothermia Prevention and Pain Management

Even in hot climates, blood loss leads to rapid heat loss and coagulopathy.

- Remove wet or bloody clothing.
- Use Hypothermia Prevention Kit (HPK) or thermal blankets.
- Insulate from ground.
- Maintain a core temperature of ≥36 °C.

Pain Management
Pain relief enhances casualty stability and facilitates further interventions.

Preferred Agent: Ketamine
- Dose: *0.2–0.5 mg/kg IV or 50 mg IM*
- Advantages:
  - Preserves airway reflexes
  - Maintains BP
    Provides dissociative analgesia

Alternatives (if stable)
- Paracetamol 1 g IV or PO
- Fentanyl 50–100 mcg IN or IV (caution in hypotensive cases)
- NSAIDs (e.g., ibuprofen) as adjuncts in non-bleeding wounds

Case Resolution

Upon stabilization under fire, the casualty was rapidly reassessed in a covered stairwell using the MARCH framework. The "high and tight" tourniquet over the proximal thigh successfully reduced arterial bleeding, though due to the junctional location near the groin, mild oozing persisted. Combat gauze was packed into the wound tract with sustained pressure, followed by a tight pressure bandage. Hemorrhage control was confirmed with no fresh soak-through at 10-min rechecks.

The casualty was positioned supine with the injured limb slightly flexed at the knee and hip to reduce tension across the groin and avoid exacerbating tissue damage. Foam padding was used under pressure points, and the limb was immobilized with a padded splint to reduce shear during CASEVAC. This careful packaging helped prevent additional disruption to clots or vascular compromise during movement.

Given the prolonged evacuation timeline of over 45 min, the provider considered—but deferred—tourniquet conversion. In this case, the wound was junctional, bleeding had initially been arterial, and the casualty remained borderline hypotensive. Conversion to a pressure dressing is typically considered only if all of the following are true: The casualty is stable, hemorrhage is fully controlled with secondary methods, and definitive care is imminent. None of these conditions were fully met.

The team continued frequent reassessments for compartment syndrome, watching for increasing pain out of proportion, progressive swelling, pallor, paresthesia, and loss of pulse in the distal limb. Although the initial control appeared successful, the wound's proximity to the femoral neurovascular bundle prompted high suspicion for delayed arterial spasm or clot displacement. The pelvic binder also served to stabilize the area in case of occult pelvic ring injury contributing to junctional bleeding.

The embedded bullet fragment was palpated near the wound tract, but was left undisturbed. Field extraction was deliberately avoided, as removal risks provoking uncontrolled bleeding, introducing infection, and disrupting tamponade.

The casualty was kept warm and calm and monitored for signs of deterioration. A mental status log, IV fluid input, pulse, capillary refill, and tourniquet checks were documented every 10 min. Evacuation was initiated once the area was cleared. On arrival to the forward surgical team, imaging confirmed a femoral vein laceration with tamponaded hematoma, and the embedded round was safely removed in the OR.

Key Messages

- Gunshot wounds require immediate, structured assessment using the MARCH protocol to address life-threatening priorities before definitive care is available.
- Early tourniquet application saves lives, particularly in extremity and junctional bleeds. Conversions should only be attempted under stable, monitored conditions.
- TXA administration within the first hour significantly improves outcomes in major bleeding and should be a standard part of initial field resuscitation.
- Fluid resuscitation must be goal directed—aimed at restoring perfusion (palpable radial pulse, intact mentation) without exacerbating coagulopathy.
- Hypothermia prevention is a critical adjunct, even in warm environments, as cold casualties bleed and clot poorly.
- Pain control enhances survivability and tactical cooperation; ketamine is the agent of choice for hemodynamically unstable casualties.
- Proper documentation and communication using MIST format ensures seamless handover and continuity of care during evacuation.
- Combat medics must balance lifesaving interventions with mission constraints, using available tools creatively to stabilize under fire.

Conclusion

Managing gunshot wounds in combat is a test of both medical skill and tactical discipline. In austere, high-threat settings, every second counts. The structured application of the MARCH algorithm allows medics to impose order on chaos—ensuring that bleeding is controlled, airways are secured, and circulation is preserved, even when resources are minimal.

This chapter reinforces that survival and limb salvage are possible even in complex GSWs when field interventions are timely, methodical, and appropriately escalated. From tourniquet use to TXA, hypothermia control to pain management, the principles outlined here form the backbone of battlefield trauma care.

When executed well, they not only save lives but also preserve function, independence, and combat readiness. *Every provider must remember: Your actions in the first 10 min determine the next 10 years of a soldier's life!*

Bibliography

1. Baker, S. P., O'Neill, B., Haddon, W., & Long, W. B. (1974). The injury severity score: A method for describing patients with multiple injuries and evaluating emergency care. *Journal of Trauma*, 14(3), 187–196. https://doi.org/10.1097/00005373-197403000-00001
2. Blackbourne, L. H., & Baer, D. G. (2008). Tactical combat casualty care in special operations. *Journal of Special Operations Medicine*, 8(3), 31–39.
3. Breen, R. A., & de Lemos, R. A. (2020). Hemorrhage control in combat: The role of pre-hospital hemostatic agents. *The Journal of Emergency Medicine*, 58(3), 420–428. https://doi.org/10.1016/j.jemermed.2019.12.037
4. Butcher, R. R., & Khan, N. (2016). Advances in the management of hemorrhagic shock and gunshot wounds in combat medicine. *Military Medicine*, 181(11), 1292–1302. https://doi.org/10.7205/MILMED-D-16-00132
5. Cotton, B. A., & Wade, C. E. (2011). Trauma-induced coagulopathy: A review. *Critical Care Clinics*, 27(3), 313–331. https://doi.org/10.1016/j.ccc.2011.04.005
6. Frykberg, E. R., & Plemmons, R. M. (2007). Battle injuries. *The Lancet*, 370(9585), 1–10. https://doi.org/10.1016/S0140-6736(07)61042-4
7. Gore, D. C., & Campbell, P. C. (2014). Tactical combat casualty care in Afghanistan: Insights from the battlefield. *Journal of Trauma and Acute Care Surgery*, 76(4), 1232–1238. https://doi.org/10.1097/TA.0000000000000191
8. Holcomb, J. B., & Hagmann, J. M. (2015). Damage control resuscitation: Current military perspectives. *Journal of Trauma and Acute Care Surgery*, 79(6), S-135–S-144. https://doi.org/10.1097/TA.0000000000000875
9. Kragh, J. F., & Wenke, J. C. (2009). Management of combat-related wounds: Current military perspectives. *Journal of Trauma and Acute Care Surgery*, 66(3), S-34–S-43. https://doi.org/10.1097/TA.0b013e31819856d9
10. Pruitt, B. A., & Barillo, D. J. (2015). Burn and trauma management in combat settings. *Burns*, 41(2), 295–303. https://doi.org/10.1016/j.burns.2014.09.006

Explosive and Blast Trauma Response 18

K. Rakesh Nayaka

Learning Objectives
By the end of this chapter, the reader will be able to:

- Understand the physics of explosive events and their physiological impact.
- Classify blast injuries based on mechanism and tissue involvement.
- Apply the MARCH algorithm in blast trauma care in tactical and resource-limited settings.
- Recognize critical life threats: hemorrhage, pneumothorax, blast lung, and airway compromise.
- Identify when and how to initiate damage control resuscitation, early evacuation, and definitive care.
- Execute triage and mass casualty management.

Introduction

In recent years, the Indian forces have faced increasing threats from explosive weapons—ranging from pressure-triggered IEDs in Naxal-affected regions, VBIEDs (vehicle-borne IEDs) in Kashmir, to cross-border artillery strikes in the north. The use of explosives has escalated both in frequency and lethality, often resulting in complex polytrauma and overwhelming casualty numbers.

K. Rakesh Nayaka (✉)
Department of Emergency Medicine, Amina Hospital, Ajman, United Arab Emirates

N. T. Rai, S. Misra (eds.), *Frontline Operational Resuscitation and Combat Emergencies (FORCE) Manual*, https://doi.org/10.1007/978-981-92-1622-2_18

Unlike gunshot wounds, blast injuries are unpredictable in nature and can affect multiple organ systems simultaneously. In such environments, structured protocols like the MARCH approach are crucial for systematic, efficient casualty management. *The goal is not just survival—but also preservation of combat function, minimization of preventable deaths, and rapid return to operational capability when feasible.*

The Indian context introduces additional layers of complexity: remote terrain, delayed MEDEVAC, minimal field resources, and variable levels of training among first responders. This makes it essential to adapt standard protocols to suit our realities while retaining core lifesaving principles.

This chapter combines the science of blast pathophysiology with combat-tested field medicine. It emphasizes a hands-on, priority-driven approach that can be executed by trained medics, first responders, or even trained buddies in combat situations. The integration of MARCH, TCCC phases (Care Under Fire, Tactical Field Care, Tactical Evacuation), and FORCE principles provides a coherent, Indianized framework for managing explosive trauma.

Case Scenario

During a routine counterinsurgency patrol in the dense jungles of Bastar, Chhattisgarh, a CRPF team is ambushed by a command-detonated improvised explosive device (IED) concealed beneath a forest path. The blast—believed to be a 15 kg ammonium nitrate device packed with metal fragments—is triggered by a pressure plate as the lead scout, a 28-year-old rifleman, advances. The explosion tears through the underbrush with devastating force. The casualty is thrown backward, landing supine amid broken foliage and soil debris. His right leg has been traumatically amputated below the knee, and he has sustained multiple penetrating fragment wounds across his left thigh and lower abdomen. The area remains unstable with hostile presence suspected nearby. A trained medic is first to reach the injured scout.

- *Care Under Fire (CUF)*
  Suppressive fire is returned by the patrol as the casualty is dragged to cover using a poncho. A rapid MARCH sweep is performed under fire. Bright red arterial bleeding is observed from the amputation site (Fig. 18.1), and hemostasis is initiated with a high-thigh Combat Application Tourniquet (CAT). Further interventions are deferred until the area is secured.
- *Tactical Field Care (TFC)*
  Once the situation is controlled, a detailed MARCH assessment is undertaken:
  Massive Hemorrhage (M): The right leg amputation site continues to ooze despite the tourniquet. Hemostatic gauze is packed into the stump, and a pressure dressing is applied. Concurrently, multiple shrapnel injuries to the left thigh are packed and dressed. Hemorrhage is successfully controlled.

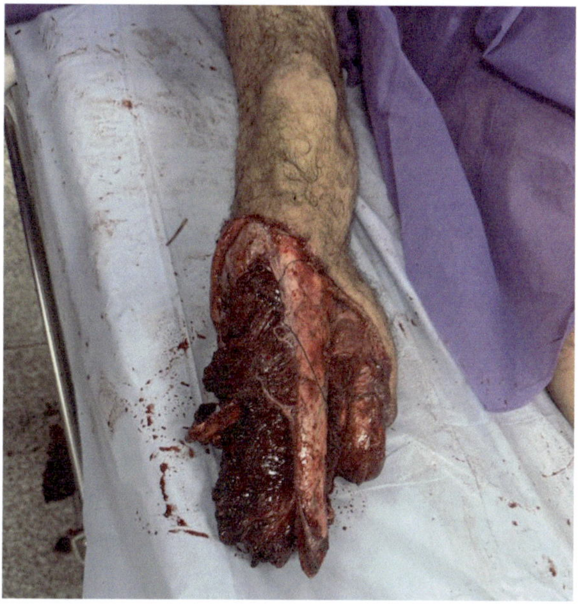

Fig. 18.1 A soldier with traumatic amputation of the right leg secondary to IED blast with active arterial bleeding

Airway (A): The casualty is semiconscious and speaking with a hoarse voice. Soot is present around his nostrils and lips, indicating likely airway burn. A nasopharyngeal airway is inserted to secure patency, while a surgical cricothyrotomy kit is prepared in anticipation of progressive airway edema and potential obstruction from inhalation injury.

Respiration (R): The respiratory rate is 32/min and shallow. Subcutaneous emphysema is palpable over the right chest wall. Suspecting blast lung with developing pneumothorax, the medic performs chest decompression at the fifth intercostal space (anterior axillary line). A marked improvement in oxygenation is noted post-procedure. Oxygen is unavailable in the field, but the casualty is placed in a sitting-angled posture to aid ventilation.

Circulation (C): The casualty's skin is pale and clammy. Radial pulse is weak, and systolic blood pressure is estimated at 80 mmHg. IV access is established, and 1 g of TXA is administered. A cautious 500 mL bolus of Ringer's lactate is given. A pelvic binder is applied due to the mechanism of injury and proximity of blast vector to the lower torso.

Head Injury/Hypothermia (H): GCS is 13 (E3V4M6). No external head injuries are visible. Wet, blood-soaked fatigues are removed. A foil thermal blanket is used for passive warming, and the casualty is insulated with dry jungle vegetation under the poncho to reduce heat loss in the damp environment.

- *Tactical Evacuation Care (TACEVAC)*

  Evacuation is delayed by 45–60 min due to difficult terrain and possible enemy presence along the extraction route. During this period, the medic:
  - Reassesses airway patency
  - Monitors respiratory efforts

– Maintains a fluid log and reassesses pulse pressure and mental status
Regularly inspects wound dressings and tourniquet site

The casualty is positioned laterally with the amputated stump elevated and secured to prevent further trauma during transport. CASEVAC is initiated once tactical corridor clearance is confirmed.

Reflective Questions

1. What indicators in this scenario suggest developing airway compromise, and when should a surgical cricothyrotomy be performed in such casualties?
2. Given the suspicion of blast lung and shallow breathing, how do you decide whether to administer fluids or withhold them to avoid worsening pulmonary injury?
3. What are the field strategies to manage and monitor a casualty with blast injury in a jungle setting with prolonged evacuation?

Explosion Mechanics

Understanding the mechanics of explosions is fundamental to managing blast trauma effectively. *Explosions are sudden, violent releases of energy that create a pressure wave, causing widespread damage across various organ systems.* In military and internal security operations, most blast injuries are caused by improvised explosive devices (IEDs), artillery, grenades, landmines, or vehicle-borne improvised explosive devices (VBIEDs)—common threats in Indian combat zones, such as Jammu and Kashmir, the Northeast, and Naxal belts.

Phases of a Blast Event

An explosion produces several distinct effects, each with specific injury patterns:

1. *Shockwave (Overpressure Wave)*
   - Travels faster than the speed of sound
   - Damages gas-filled organs: lungs, bowel, and middle ear
   - Can cause blast lung, tympanic membrane rupture, and air embolism
2. *Blast Wind (Dynamic Overpressure)*
   - Secondary to shockwave; causes displacement of bodies or debris
   - Responsible for tumbling injuries, fractures, and blunt trauma
3. *Thermal Effects*
   - Heat flash and flame injuries cause burns, inhalation injury, and combustion of clothing
4. *Fragmentation*
   - Generates shrapnel, bomb casing, or environmental debris (rocks, nails)
   - Responsible for penetrating injuries, amputations, and polytrauma
5. *Structural Collapse and Environmental Impact*
   - Triggers building debris, dust inhalation, or confined space effects
   - Can trap victims and delay rescue or airway management

Blast Pathophysiology

The human body is vulnerable to the pressure differentials caused by explosions. The pathophysiologic effects vary depending on the distance, medium (air, water, enclosed space), protective gear, and orientation of the casualty (Table 18.1).

Indian Context: Terrain and Tactical Considerations
In India, terrain-specific effects amplify the damage caused by blasts:

- *Jungle terrain (Chhattisgarh, Jharkhand)*: Claymore-style IEDs cause fragmentation injuries and delayed rescue.
- *Mountain environments (J&K, LAC)*: Pressure waves reflect off rocks, causing severe barotrauma and blunt injury.
- *Urban insurgency zones*: VBIEDs in enclosed spaces lead to mass casualties, airway burns, and blast lung.

Protective equipment (bulletproof vests, combat boots, and helmets) mitigates but does not eliminate injury. In most situations, first-line response is from fellow soldiers, not medic—highlighting the importance of basic combat lifesaver (CLS) training and structured casualty assessment using the MARCH algorithm.

Table 18.1 Organ-specific mechanisms and injuries associated with blast trauma

Organ system	Mechanism of injury	Common injuries
Ear (auditory)	Overpressure-induced barotrauma	Tympanic membrane (TM) perforation, ossicular chain disruption, cochlear injury, foreign body
Eye and orbit	Fragmentation, blast wave, or pressure differential	Globe rupture, orbital fractures, intraocular foreign bodies
Respiratory system	Primary blast wave, thermal inhalation, secondary penetration	Tension pneumothorax, hemothorax, pulmonary contusion, alveolar hemorrhage, smoke inhalation, sepsis
Gastrointestinal tract	Overpressure and blunt trauma to hollow and solid organs	Bowel rupture, mesenteric ischemia, liver and spleen lacerations, peritonitis
Cardiovascular system	Blast wave transmission through chest wall and pressure fluctuation	Septal rupture, myocardial contusion/ infarction, hypotension, commotio cordis
Renal system	Blast overpressure, crush injury, shock	Renal hematoma, laceration, acute kidney injury (AKI), rhabdomyolysis
Central nervous system	Acceleration-deceleration forces, pressure wave, embolism	Traumatic brain injury (TBI), concussion, stroke, spinal cord injury, air embolism
Musculoskeletal/ other	Penetrating shrapnel, blunt trauma, secondary blast effect	Amputations, long bone fractures, compartment syndrome, burns, degloving injuries

Classification of Blast Injuries

Blast injuries are classified based on the mechanism of tissue damage, not merely the external appearance. Recognizing the type of blast injury is essential for predicting complications and prioritizing interventions in the field (Table 18.2 and Fig. 18.2). In the combat setting—especially within Indian operations—*most casualties will exhibit multiple overlapping categories of injury.*

Table 18.2 Classification of blast injuries: mechanism, field clues, and management implications

Type of injury	Mechanism	Common organs affected/examples	Field clues/ tactical context	Management implications
Primary blast injury	Overpressure wave on gas-filled organs	Lungs: blast lung (alveolar rupture, hemorrhage) GI tract: bowel rupture, mesenteric tear Ear: tympanic rupture, vertigo CNS: TBI, air embolism	Sudden respiratory distress with no external wound Blood-tinged frothy sputum Ataxia/ confusion after blast Ear bleeding, deafness	Suspect blast lung and air embolism Administer oxygen if available Avoid aggressive fluid boluses Monitor neuro signs continuously
Secondary blast injury	Shrapnel or debris propelled by the explosion	Metal fragments, nails, stones Wooden stakes, wires Pipe bombs, embedded projectiles	Visible penetrating trauma Multiple foreign bodies Amputations or bleeding Most common in IEDs/VBIEDs	Control hemorrhage Apply tourniquets and hemostatic agents *Do not remove impaled objects* Prioritize for early evacuation
Tertiary blast injury	Physical displacement from blast wind into surfaces	Long bone fractures Spinal cord injury Blunt head trauma Crush injuries from debris	Fall downslope (mountain ops) Thrown into walls (urban) Found under rubble or debris	Spinal precautions Splint fractures Treat for crush syndrome Monitor for compartment syndrome if trapped or compressed
Quaternary blast injury	Nonmechanical effects of the explosion	Burns (thermal/ chemical) Smoke/toxin inhalation Dust contamination Acute stress reaction, PTSD	Soot in mouth/ nose Clothing melted to skin Respiratory distress post-enclosure Unexplained distress in non-wounded personnel	Prevent hypothermia Manage burns with dry dressings Treat airway early if inhalation injury is suspected Reassure and monitor for psychological impact

(continued)

Table 18.2 (continued)

Type of injury	Mechanism	Common organs affected/examples	Field clues/ tactical context	Management implications
Quinary blast injury	Biologic/chemical additives in explosive devices	Exposure to toxins, chemicals, or radioactive substances Systemic inflammation or unexplained organ failure	Seizures, multi-organ failure Unusual symptoms in multiple casualties Common in terror attacks with fertilizer or radiologic IEDs	Decontaminate if possible Supportive care Notify higher command for CBRN involvement Isolate affected individuals if contamination is suspected

Abbreviations: *GI* gastrointestinal, *TBI* traumatic brain injury, *VBIEDs* vehicle-borne IEDs, *PTSD* post-traumatic stress disorder, *CBRN* chemical, biological, radiological, and/or nuclear

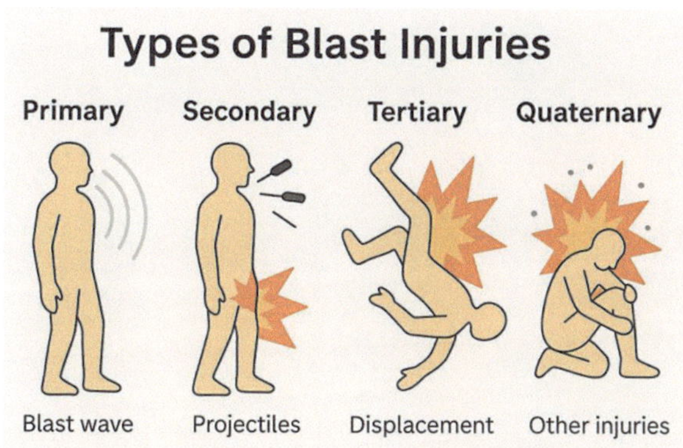

Fig. 18.2 Types of blast injuries

Factors Influencing Blast Outcomes

In Indian operational theatres—ranging from dense jungles and mountainous borders to urban conflict zones—blast injury outcomes are shaped not only by terrain and evacuation logistics but also by critical physical and tactical variables. Understanding these factors helps predict injury severity, allocate limited resources, and guide field interventions more effectively.

1. *Distance from the Explosion*
   - *Proximity is critical.* The overpressure generated by a blast diminishes rapidly with distance, following the *cube root law* (Fig. 18.3).
   - Even a few meters farther from the detonation point can make the difference between survivable tympanic rupture and fatal injury (Fig. 18.4).
   - Casualties closest to the epicenter are most likely to suffer primary blast injuries, including barotrauma, pulmonary rupture, and internal hemorrhage.

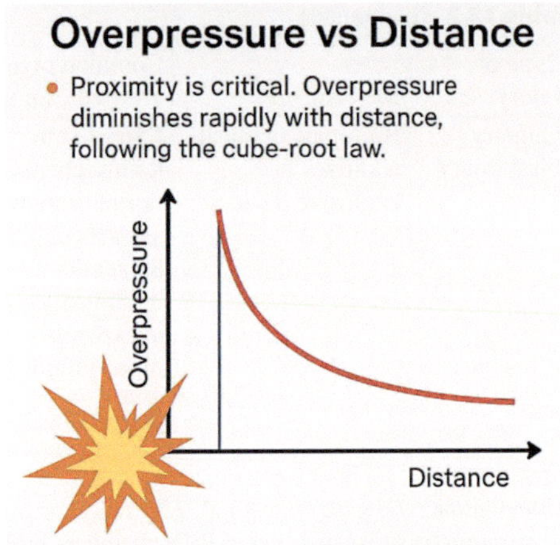

Fig. 18.3 The cube root law

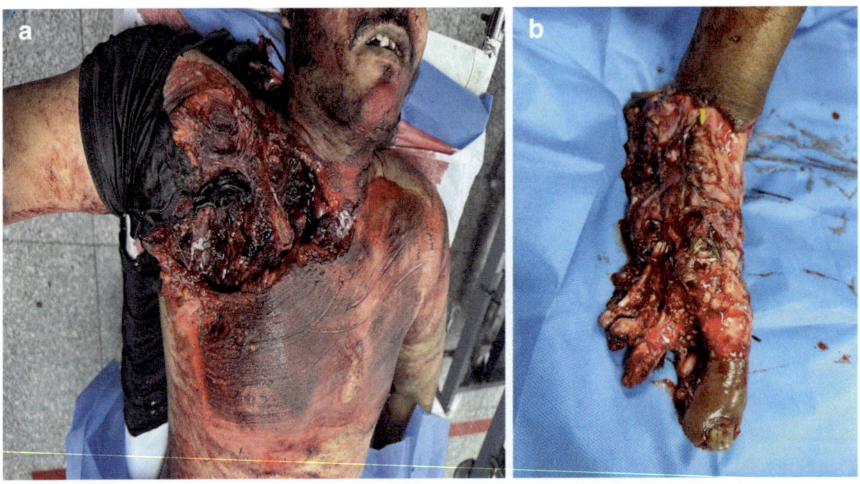

Fig. 18.4. (**a**) A soldier with chest injury from grenade blast. (**b**) Another soldier with lower limb injury following IED explosion

FORCE Tactical Pearl

In an ambush with multiple casualties, prioritizing those closest to the blast site for early airway and respiratory assessment is critical—blast lung may be present even without external trauma.

2. *Enclosed Versus Open Spaces*
   - *Confined explosions (inside rooms, vehicles, bunkers, buses) dramatically amplify the intensity of the blast wave, increasing mortality and severity of injuries.*

- Overpressure waves reflect and converge, causing multiple rebounds inside the body—especially the lungs, ears, and gut.

FORCE Tactical Pearl
In enclosed settings, even without external wounds, always suspect internal blast injury. Proceed with high suspicion of respiratory or GI tract compromise.

3. *Reflection of Blast Waves from Surroundings*
   - Solid surfaces like rock faces, concrete walls, or armored vehicles can reflect and concentrate the blast wave.
   - *This leads to localized pressure doubling, increasing the risk of severe internal injury in those adjacent to walls or barriers.*

FORCE Tactical Pearl
A soldier thrown against a bunker wall may suffer more internal trauma than a peer in open terrain. These cases demand early respiratory support, chest decompression kits, and conservative IV resuscitation.

4. *Quantity and Type of Explosive*
   - *Explosive load*
     - The larger the explosive charge, the greater the overpressure radius and injury distribution.
       In IED-laden ambushes in Naxal areas, explosive weight may range from 5 to 50 kg, creating catastrophic structural and personnel damage.
   - *Type of explosive*
     Explosives may be further subclassified as outlined in Table 18.3.

FORCE Tactical Pearl
When Intel suggests military-grade explosives or RDX, prepare for multi-casualty triage, high incidence of blast lung, amputations, and need for multiple tourniquets and airway interventions.

5. *Embedded Shrapnel and Intentional Fragmentation*
   - *Most insurgent and terrorist explosive devices are designed with embedded shrapnel*—metal ball bearings, nails, wires, or plastic shards.
   - These are responsible for secondary blast injuries: penetrating trauma, embedded foreign bodies, and high-risk infections.

Table 18.3 Type of explosives

Explosive type	Velocity of detonation	Examples	Injury severity
Low-order explosives (LE)	<1000 m/s	Gunpowder, petroleum-based IEDs	Moderate
High-order explosives (HE)	>4500 m/s	TNT, RDX, military-grade VBIEDs	Severe

6. *Environmental and Operational Overlays*
   - *Heat + blast*: Increased risk of burn shock and fluid loss.
   - *Rain/mud + blast*: Higher incidence of contaminated open wounds and risk of sepsis.
   - *High altitude + blast*: Rapid decompensation due to already compromised oxygenation—*blast lung at 10,000+ ft is often fatal without oxygen support.*

FORCE Tactical Pearl

In Indian combat zones, the outcome of a blast is shaped as much by environmental physics as by clinical decision-making. Recognizing the blast dynamics, terrain interactions, and explosive type can allow the provider to predict life threats and apply the MARCH algorithm with precision.

Tactical Field Management

In high-threat environments, such as counterinsurgency zones, LoC engagements, or jungle ambushes, prehospital blast trauma care is often performed with limited equipment, personnel, and time. Structured, algorithm-based field management using the MARCH protocol allows providers to address the most preventable causes of death in a prioritized sequence in TFC phase.

M—Massive Hemorrhage

Goal: Immediate control of life-threatening bleeding:

- Tourniquets (e.g., CAT) should be applied "high and tight" to limbs with heavy bleeding or amputations.
- In cases of junctional hemorrhage (groin, axilla), use:
  - Hemostatic gauze (QuikClot Combat Gauze®, ChitoGauze®) + 3 min of firm pressure
    Improvised junctional tourniquets or pelvic binders, if available
- Reassess for tourniquet effectiveness and note the time of application visibly.
- Avoid tourniquet removal in the field—maintain until surgical facility is reached.

A—Airway

Goal: Ensure airway is open and protected:

- If the casualty can speak, the airway is open—monitor only.
- In semiconscious casualties:
  Use jaw thrust and insert nasopharyngeal airway (NPA) if no contraindications (e.g., facial trauma).
- For casualties with facial burns, smoke inhalation, or maxillofacial disruption, prepare for surgical cricothyrotomy if airway compromise is imminent.

R—Respiration

Goal: Identify and treat life-threatening thoracic injuries:

- Expose and inspect the chest for:
  - Entry/exit wounds → apply occlusive chest seals.
    Asymmetrical rise → suspect tension pneumothorax.
- If tension pneumothorax is suspected:
  Perform needle decompression at the fifth ICS AAL or second ICS MCL using a 14–16 G needle (≥3.25″).
- *Suspect blast lung in patients with:*
  - Frothy blood from the mouth
  - Hypoxia
    No visible trauma

C—Circulation

Goal: Support perfusion and prevent shock.

- Establish IV/IO access (18 G cannula or field IO device).
- Administer:
  - 1 g TXA IV over 10 min, ideally within 1 h
    500 mL warmed crystalloid (RL or Plasma-Lyte) only if radial pulse is absent or GCS is declining
- Apply pelvic binder if:
  - Blast involved lower torso
  - Pelvic instability is suspected
    No obvious external bleeding but signs of shock persist

H—Head Injury/Hypothermia

Goal: Prevent secondary brain injury and coagulopathy:

- Evaluate GCS and check pupils regularly.
- Do not delay evacuation for suspected TBI—surgery is definitive.

- Remove wet/bloody clothing and wrap the casualty in:
  - Poncho liner
  - Foil or space blanket
    Body heat from another responder, if hypothermia is advanced

Secondary Assessment and Extended Field Considerations

Once initial MARCH-based assessment is complete, perform a rapid secondary head-to-toe survey:

1. *Neurologic Check*
   - Reassess GCS every 15–30 min.
   - Monitor for new deficits: Unequal pupils, worsening confusion, and limb weakness.
2. *Fractures and Immobilization*
   - Splint long bone fractures with SAM splints or improvised materials (rifles, sticks, rolled ponchos).
   - Elevate and pad the injured limb if possible.
   - Avoid tight bandaging that may cause compartment syndrome.
3. *Burn Management*
   - Cover with dry, clean dressings—avoid creams or ointments.
   - Administer pain relief (e.g., ketamine 30 mg IV or IN).
   - Monitor for signs of airway burns or fluid loss in TBSA >10%.
4. *Impaled Objects/Shrapnel*
   - *Do not remove any embedded fragments in the field.*
   - Stabilize with dressings and document for surgical team.
5. *Bladder/Bowel Monitoring (Prolonged Care)*
   - For prolonged field care:
     - Monitor for urinary retention or gross hematuria (pelvic trauma).
       Shield the perineum from debris and contaminants.

Definitive Care

Following evacuation, focus shifts from resuscitation to definitive surgical care, organ support, and recovery planning.

1. *Surgical Prioritization*
   - Reassess tourniquets and bleeding sites.
   - Perform vascular repair or amputation based on viability.
   - Conduct exploratory laparotomy for suspected internal hemorrhage.
   - Remove shrapnel only if:
     - Causing neurovascular compromise
     - Located in joints or vital cavities

Required for forensic/operational reasons

2. *Chest and Airway Management*
   - Insert chest tubes for pneumothorax/hemothorax.
   - Initiate lung-protective ventilation for blast lung.
   - Consider tracheostomy for prolonged ventilator support or airway burns.
3. *Burn and Wound Care*
   - Calculate %TBSA and guide fluids using Parkland formula.
   - Administer broad-spectrum antibiotics for deep/contaminated burns.
   - Perform early escharotomy/fasciotomy if circulation is threatened.
   - Ensure adequate analgesia and caloric intake.
4. *Neurological and Spinal Injury Care*
   - Obtain CT/MRI for GCS < 15 or focal deficits.
   - Monitor for raised ICP, seizures, and cerebral edema.
   - Immobilize spine and involve neuro/ortho specialists early.
5. *Crush Syndrome Management*
   - Maintain IV hydration and urine output.
   - Alkalinize urine (sodium bicarbonate).
   - Monitor for hyperkalemia and AKI, and consider dialysis if needed.
6. *Psychological and Functional Recovery*
   - Screen for acute stress/PTSD.
   - Begin counseling, debriefing, and psychiatric referral.
   - Start physiotherapy, prosthetics, and occupational rehab early.
   - Decide return-to-duty based on physical and mental recovery.

Triage and Mass Casualty Management of Blast Injury

Blast incidents frequently result in multiple casualties with varied injury patterns—ranging from minor shrapnel wounds to life-threatening hemorrhage and blast lung. In such scenarios, effective triage is critical to ensure optimal use of limited resources and to prevent loss of life due to under-prioritized injuries.

Key Principles of Triage in Blast Events

I. *Sort casualties rapidly based on severity*, not arrival time.
II. *Prioritize interventions for those with life-threatening but treatable conditions* (e.g., airway burns and junctional hemorrhage).
III. *Use MARCH during triage to identify and intervene in immediately reversible causes of death.*

Triage Categories

These are described in Table 18.4.

Tactical Considerations

- *Triage tags or field markings* (e.g., *color-coded cloth strips) help maintain clarity in low-light/jungle settings.*

Table 18.4 Triage categories in blast injuries: characteristics and field examples

Category	Characteristics	Examples in blast injury
Immediate (red)	Life-threatening injuries requiring urgent intervention	Airway compromise, active arterial bleeding, tension pneumothorax
Delayed (yellow)	Serious injuries that can tolerate some delay	Open fractures, minor burns, moderate bleeding
Minimal (green)	Walking wounded, non-life-threatening injuries	Superficial shrapnel wounds, minor anxiety or burns
Expectant (black)	Unsurvivable injuries in current resource setting	Devastating head trauma, full-thickness burns >85% TBSA

- *Communication with CASEVAC/Medevac teams must include triage category, injury mechanism, and interventions completed (MIST report).*
- *Decontamination protocols should be considered in quinary injuries with suspected CBRN exposure.*

FORCE Tactical Pearl

In high-volume settings like VBIED attacks or IED ambushes, apply the SALT or START triage system only if MARCH-based assessment is not feasible due to provider limitations.

Case Resolution

As the evacuation team arrives after a 55-min delay, the casualty's vital signs remain tenuous but stable. His GCS holds at 13 with intermittent confusion, and his respiratory rate remains elevated at 28/min, but without accessory muscle use or overt signs of airway collapse. The nasopharyngeal airway remains in place and patent. The team rechecks for worsening hoarseness, stridor, or inability to clear secretions—none of which are observed. Given the absence of rapidly progressing symptoms, surgical cricothyrotomy is deferred, but the medic remains on standby with the kit primed should airway patency worsens.

The chest decompression site remains dry and functional. SpO_2 is holding at 93% on ambient air, indicating moderate blast lung injury without critical hypoxia. The field medic opts against further fluid boluses, recognizing that excessive crystalloid administration could exacerbate pulmonary contusion. Instead, fluid administration is limited to maintaining a radial pulse and mentation, aligning with the principles of permissive hypotension in blast lung.

The tourniquet on the amputated limb remains dry and secure. No rebleeding or distal tissue bulging is noted. The pelvic binder remains in place due to the proximity of the blast and low BP. Shrapnel wounds on the left thigh are dry and cleanly dressed. No signs of expanding hematoma or compartment syndrome are noted.

The casualty's stump is padded and gently elevated. His body is insulated using a foil blanket, dry clothing from a teammate, and layers of palm leaves to create a heat barrier against the jungle's damp floor. These jungle-adapted measures help prevent further hypothermia, especially critical given the casualty's borderline perfusion and risk of coagulopathy.

The field team maintains continuous documentation of:

- Airway status and GCS
- Chest decompression efficacy
- Fluid volume administered
- Vital signs every 15 min
- Time and site of tourniquet placement

The casualty is psychologically reassured with calm verbal cues and brief touch, reinforcing that help has arrived. On CASEVAC arrival, the casualty is:

- Placed laterally with the stump elevated
- Transported with ongoing reassessments of airway and breathing
- Handed over with detailed notes on tourniquet time, fluids, medications, and interventions performed

In the hospital, thoracic imaging revealed localized pulmonary contusion not requiring chest tube insertion. He undergoes below-knee amputation revision and burn debridement. Due to timely decompression, airway protection, and conservative fluid use, he survived without major pulmonary or airway complications or neurological deficits and demonstrated partial lower limb function with prosthetic rehabilitation. He was subsequently redeployed in a noncombat support role.

Key Messages

- Blast injuries produce complex polytrauma involving multiple mechanisms—pressure, penetration, blunt trauma, and burns—*often overlapping in a single casualty!*
- The MARCH algorithm remains the foundation of field management, guiding providers through prioritized, lifesaving interventions in high-threat settings.
- Primary blast injuries often present with subtle signs but carry high mortality (e.g., blast lung, bowel rupture, and tympanic rupture)—*maintain a high index of suspicion, especially in enclosed space detonations.*
- Tourniquet use, hemostatic dressings, and junctional control are critical in managing massive hemorrhage—the leading preventable cause of death in blast casualties.

(continued)

- *Airway burns and blast lung should be anticipated even without obvious trauma*; field airway support and early chest decompression can be lifesaving.
- Judicious fluid resuscitation and early TXA administration are key to maintaining perfusion while avoiding complications, such as worsening pulmonary edema or coagulopathy.
- Environmental factors like terrain, weather, and delayed evacuation must inform both clinical decisions and tactical planning in Indian operational theatres.
- Early evacuation, ongoing reassessment, and structured response to mass casualty are essential for optimizing survival and minimizing long-term disability.

Conclusion

Blast injuries represent some of the most complex and high-risk scenarios in combat trauma care. In the Indian context, where terrain, threat dynamics, and evacuation delays compound medical complexity, *structured field response is nonnegotiable*. The MARCH framework serves as a vital tool, guiding combat provider to prioritize life-threatening conditions systematically while maintaining tactical awareness. *However, successful outcomes are not determined by protocol alone—they hinge on the provider's clinical judgment, adaptability under fire, and commitment to core combat trauma principles*. In resource-limited and high-stress environments, *even basic interventions, when performed with precision and timeliness, can make the difference between life and death*. When executed correctly, *this approach transforms chaos into coordinated care*—preserving life, function, and the fighting strength of the force.

Bibliography

1. Born CT, Briggs SM, Ciraulo DL, et al. Disasters and mass casualties: II. explosive, biologic, chemical, and nuclear agents. *J Am Acad Orthop Surg*. 2007;15(8):461–473. https://doi.org/10.5435/00124635-200708000-00003
2. Champion, Howard R et al. "Injuries from explosions: physics, biophysics, pathology, and required research focus." *The Journal of trauma* vol. 66,5 (2009): 1468–77; discussion 1477. https://doi.org/10.1097/TA.0b013e3181a27e7f
3. Eiseman, B. "Combat casualty management for tomorrow's battlefield: urban terrorism." *The Journal of trauma* vol. 51,5 (2001): 821–3. https://doi.org/10.1097/00005373-200111000-00001
4. Irwin, R J et al. "Cardiopulmonary physiology of primary blast injury." *The Journal of trauma* vol. 43,4 (1997): 650–5. https://doi.org/10.1097/00005373-199710000-00015
5. Kapur, G Bobby et al. "The United States twenty-year experience with bombing incidents: implications for terrorism preparedness and medical response." *The Journal of trauma* vol. 59,6 (2005): 1436–44. https://doi.org/10.1097/01.ta.0000197853.49084.3c

6. Kashuk, Jeffry L et al. "Bomb explosions in acts of terrorism: evil creativity challenges our trauma systems." *Journal of the American College of Surgeons* vol. 209,1 (2009): 134–40. https://doi.org/10.1016/j.jamcollsurg.2009.01.049
7. Tintinalli JE, Ma OJ, Yealy DM, et al. *Tintinalli's Emergency Medicine: A Comprehensive Study Guide*. 9th ed. New York: McGraw-Hill Education; 2019. ISBN: 978-1405296434.
8. Wolf SJ, Bebarta VS, Bonnett CJ, et al. Blast injuries. *Lancet*. 2009;374(9687):405–415. https://doi.org/10.1016/S0140-6736(09)60257-9.

Combat Triage and Mass Casualty Response

19

Ashwin S. Raj

Learning Objectives
By the end of this chapter, the reader will be able to:

- Understand and apply the structured triage system across all phases of Tactical Combat Casualty Care (TCCC).
- Integrate the MARCH protocol effectively to address battlefield life threats in priority order.
- Conduct rapid, resource-efficient triage even under hostile and high-casualty environments.
- Differentiate between immediate, delayed, minimal, and expectant triage categories for optimal resource utilization.
- Adapt triage decisions dynamically during Care Under Fire, Tactical Field Care, and Tactical Evacuation.
- Optimize casualty management to enhance survival during mass casualty incidents in combat settings.

Introduction

Combat operations, by their very nature, often result in multiple simultaneous casualties across dispersed or hostile terrains. Whether triggered by ambushes, improvised explosive devices (IEDs), indirect fire, or urban engagements, mass casualty (MASCAL) scenarios in the battlefield demand a departure from conventional care

A. S. Raj (✉)
Department of Emergency Medicine, NCI Jhajjar, AIIMS, New Delhi, India

N. T. Rai, S. Misra (eds.), *Frontline Operational Resuscitation and Combat Emergencies (FORCE) Manual*, https://doi.org/10.1007/978-981-92-1622-2_19

models. In such situations, *the standard of care shifts from providing maximal care to each casualty individually to achieving the greatest good for the greatest number.* This pivot requires an unwavering commitment to structured triage, tactical adaptability, and ruthless prioritization under fire.

Tactical Combat Casualty Care (TCCC) offers a well-established framework for battlefield casualty management. By embedding the phases of care—Care Under Fire (CUF), Tactical Field Care (TFC), and Tactical Evacuation Care (TACEVAC)—within the triage process, combat providers can systematically assess, intervene, and re-triage casualties based on evolving tactical and physiological realities. Simultaneously, the MARCH algorithm—Massive hemorrhage, Airway, Respiration, Circulation, Hypothermia/Head injury—guides focused lifesaving interventions in a prioritized manner.

In Indian operational environments—ranging from the remote heights of Siachen, dense insurgency zones of Chhattisgarh, to urban counter-terrorism theaters—the ability to conduct rapid triage becomes even more critical due to limited medevac options, hostile weather, and delayed access to surgical care. *Battlefield triage is not a single event; it is a continuous, dynamic process demanding constant reassessment.*

This chapter integrates the concepts of primary, secondary, and tertiary triage, linked directly with TCCC phases, into a cohesive model for managing combat MASCALs. Through structured decision-making, tactical flexibility, and disciplined application of the MARCH principles, combat providers and frontline providers can maximize survivability, sustain operational momentum, and preserve force strength in the most challenging conditions.

Case Scenario

During an anti-insurgency patrol in the dense jungles of Chhattisgarh, a 12-man team is ambushed by an IED blast followed by small arms fire (Fig. 19.1).

Upon neutralizing the immediate threat, the patrol leader calls for mass casualty triage.

You, the designated combat lifesaver, find:

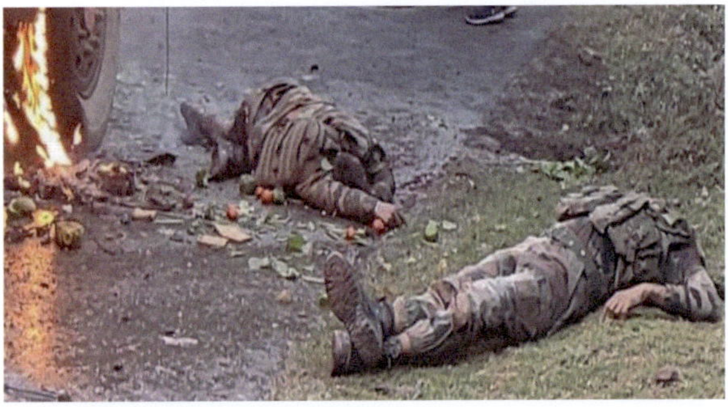

Fig. 19.1 Jungle ambush mass casualty during anti-insurgency patrol

- *Casualty 1*: 25-year-old with bilateral lower limb amputations, pale, thready radial pulse, semiconscious
- *Casualty 2*: 32-year-old with deep facial lacerations, intact airway, GCS 15, bleeding controlled
- *Casualty 3*: 28-year-old walking wounded, minor shrapnel wounds to the upper arm
- *Casualty 4*: 24-year-old unconscious, massive chest trauma, agonal breathing, absent radial pulse

There is an urgent need to perform primary triage under fire risk and organize rapid CASEVAC under limited resources.

- How do you categorize each casualty (immediate, delayed, minimal, expectant) based on field triage principles?
- What interventions, if any, should be prioritized before initiating evacuation?
- In limited CASEVAC space, which two casualties should be evacuated first?
- How should unconscious casualties be managed to prevent further deterioration en route?

Importance of Structured Triage in Combat Settings

In combat environments, chaos is the norm, not the exception. The injured are often interspersed among the dead, rescuers are under threat, resources are scarce, and time is brutally unforgiving. In such circumstances, *structured triage is not merely useful—it is essential to survival.*

Unlike civilian trauma, where immediate evacuation to hospitals is often feasible, battlefield casualties may face prolonged field care and delays in reaching surgical teams. *Structured triage allows providers to allocate limited time, manpower, and equipment rationally, ensuring that those who can be saved with available interventions are prioritized.*

In tactical mass casualty events:

- *Over-triage* (classifying minor injuries as critical) can overwhelm limited medical capacity, leading to preventable deaths among truly critical casualties.
- *Under-triage* (missing severe injuries) may condemn salvageable soldiers to death or permanent disability.

Combat triage frameworks must thus be rapid, repeatable, and ruthlessly pragmatic, balancing individual care against operational priorities. The FORCE principle emphasizes that triage must integrate seamlessly with tactical casualty evacuation (CASEVAC), mission continuation, and force preservation. *Structured triage transforms chaos into controlled response*, empowering tactical medical teams to save the maximum lives possible under adverse conditions.

Phases of Combat Triage Linked to TCCC Phases

Effective triage during combat operations is closely tied to the phases of Tactical Combat Casualty Care (TCCC). Each phase demands specific triage decisions suited to the tactical and threat environment.

1. *Care Under Fire (CUF)—Primary Triage*
   - *Environment*: Ongoing hostile threat (gunfire, explosions).
   - *Priorities*:
     - Suppress enemy fire.
     - Move casualties to cover.
     - Perform a rapid MARCH sweep focused only on:
       Controlling massive hemorrhage (tourniquet application)
   - *Triage decisions*:
     - *Dead or expectant casualties* (no movement, catastrophic wounds, no response) may be bypassed temporarily.
     - *Ambulatory casualties* (those who can walk) are directed to self-extricate and provide self-care.
       Nonambulatory but salvageable casualties (responsive, bleeding controlled) prioritized for rescue and protection.

> **FORCE Tactical Pearl**
> *In CUF, triage is brutal—focus only on immediate life threats you can control under fire.*

2. *Tactical Field Care (TFC)—Secondary Triage*
   - *Environment*: Reduced threat; secured zone or tactical pause.
   - *Priorities*:
     - Full MARCH algorithm assessment:
       Control bleeding, secure airway, decompress chest, manage circulation, prevent hypothermia, and identify head injuries.
       Begin field treatments based on available resources.
   - *Triage decisions*:
     - Use simple methods to categorize casualties:
       - *Immediate*: Life-threatening injuries needing urgent intervention (e.g., airway compromise and massive hemorrhage)
       - *Delayed*: Serious injuries but stable enough to wait (e.g., fractures and moderate burns)
       - *Minimal*: Minor injuries; walking wounded
         Expectant: Severe, non-survivable injuries when resources are limited (e.g., devastating head trauma + pulselessness).

FORCE Tactical Pearl

Triage categories may evolve—reassess casualties frequently, especially if resources or evacuation timelines change.

3. *Tactical Evacuation Care (TACEVAC)—Tertiary Triage*
   - *Environment*: Organized evacuation to definitive care facility (ambulance, helicopter, CASEVAC convoy).
   - *Priorities*:
     - Continue care initiated during TFC.
       Prepare for handover to advanced medical teams.
   - *Triage Decisions*:
     - Prioritize *immediate* and *delayed* casualties for CASEVAC.
     - *Casualties requiring urgent surgical intervention (*e.g., *airway compromise, uncontrolled hemorrhage, and penetrating chest trauma) are loaded first.*
       Document injuries and interventions clearly during handover.

Triage Categories and Battlefield Color Coding Systems

In combat and mass casualty settings, triage relies on rapid categorization to prioritize scarce resources for those most likely to survive.

Standard triage categories are color coded for quick recognition and universally understood by tactical medical teams (Table 19.1).

Practical Battlefield Triage Tagging

In most Indian military and paramilitary field settings:

- *Triage tags* (color-coded cards or tapes) may be pre-issued (Fig. 19.2a).
- *Improvised systems* (e.g., colored cloth, tape, or even labeled medical gloves) are used if official tags are unavailable (Fig. 19.2b).
- *Documentation on triage tags should minimally include*:
  - Mechanism of injury
  - Injuries noted
  - Interventions done (e.g., tourniquet time)
    Vital signs if available

Table 19.1 Triage categories and battlefield color coding systems

Triage category	Color code	Description	Examples	Field actions
Immediate (Priority I)	Red	Life-threatening injuries requiring urgent intervention to survive	Airway obstruction, uncontrolled hemorrhage, tension pneumothorax, open globe injury, blast lung	Immediate intervention and fastest evacuation
Delayed (Priority II)	Yellow	Serious but not immediately life-threatening injuries; can tolerate some delay	Closed long bone fractures, stable abdominal injuries, moderate burns	Stabilize and monitor; evacuate after "immediate"
Minimal (Priority III)	Green	Minor injuries; able to walk and perform self-care	Abrasions, minor fractures, superficial burns	Group separately for later evacuation; assist in field care if able
Expectant (Priority IV)	Black	Injuries incompatible with survival in current resource-limited environment	Devastating head trauma with GCS 3, pulseless after major thoracic trauma, multiple traumatic amputations with profound shock	Provide comfort measures if possible; focus resources elsewhere

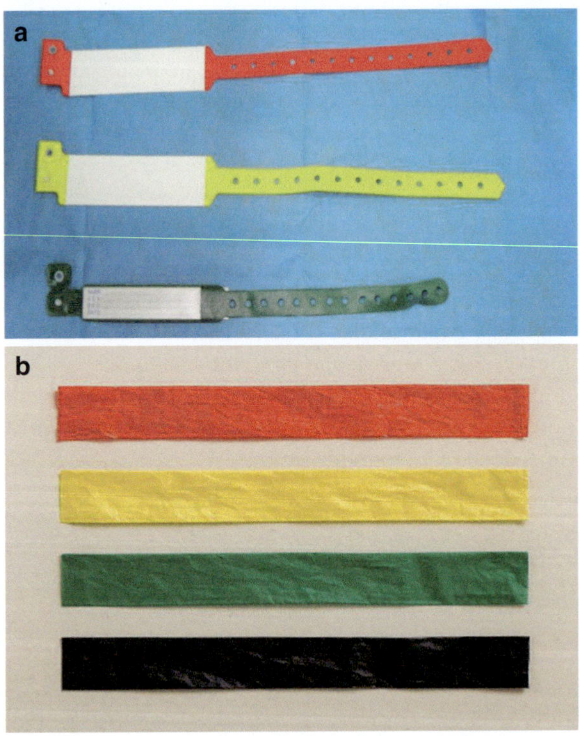

Fig. 19.2 (**a**) Standard triage bands. (**b**) Improvised triage bands made from biomedical waste polybags

FORCE Tactical Pearl

When overwhelmed, simple visual signs guide tagging:

- *Breathing difficulty → immediate*
- *Walking wounded → minimal*
- *Unconscious without major bleeding → expectant unless recoverable airway secured*

Principles of Battlefield Mass Casualty Management

Mass casualty events (MCEs) in combat, such as IED blasts, ambushes, or artillery strikes, overwhelm available medical resources. Effective management hinges on structured, scalable responses that prioritize lifesaving care over perfect care.

Key battlefield MCE management principles include the following:

1. *Establish Command and Control (C2)*
   - First responder with the highest tactical medical training assumes temporary medical incident commander (MedIC) role.
   - Clear communication chains are essential: radio or visual signals to direct providers and stretcher-bearers.
   - Designation of triage officer separate from treatment teams—ensures continuous casualty sorting without delay.
2. *Rapid Scene Assessment*
   - Estimate:
     - Number of casualties
     - Types of injuries (blast, gunshot, crush, burns)
       Available resources (medics, stretchers, evacuation platforms)
   - *Declare a mass casualty event (MCE) if casualties exceed immediate treatment capability.*
3. *Create a Casualty Collection Point (CCP)*
   - Choose safe, defensible location:
     - Sheltered from enemy fire or secondary hazards
       Accessible for evacuation vehicles (ambulance, helicopter)
   - Organize:
     - *Entry point*: For incoming casualties.
     - *Triage zone*: Color-code and sort casualties.
     - *Treatment zone*: Minimal interventions only (airway, bleeding control).
       Evacuation holding area: Prioritize loading based on triage color.
4. *Follow MARCH Priorities at Triage*
   Even in mass casualty settings:
   - *Massive Hemorrhage* control comes first (tourniquets, hemostatic dressings).
   - *Airway* support follows immediately.

- *Respiration* assessment: Expose chest injuries quickly.
- *Circulation* support: Position shock casualties flat, and prepare IV/IO access.
- *Hypothermia prevention*: Strip wet clothing, and cover casualties early.

5. *Prioritize Rapid Evacuation (CASEVAC/MEDEVAC)*
   - Immediate priority (red-tagged) casualties should move out first.
   - Group green-tagged (minimal) casualties separately to reduce congestion.
   - Expectant (black-tagged) casualties receive comfort care only if resources allow.
6. *Documentation and Handover*

   Each of the injured should carry:
   - Field triage tag
   - Brief injury/intervention record
   - Time-sensitive details (e.g., tourniquet application time)

   At evacuation, *handover must be short, clear, and critical.*

   > "Gunshot chest, needle decompressed, GCS 13, tourniquet time 0930, TXA given."

FORCE Tactical Pearl

In MCEs, efficiency trumps perfection. Most lives are saved by structured triage, minimal interventions, and rapid evacuation.

Tactical Evacuation Planning in Mass Casualty Settings

Effective evacuation planning in combat mass casualty incidents (MCIs) is crucial to maximize survival and operational continuity. *Evacuation must be dynamic, threat adaptive, and resource conscious.* Prioritization hinges on triage categorization—immediate (red) casualties requiring urgent CASEVAC/MEDEVAC within the "golden hour" take precedence. Delayed (yellow) casualties follow, with minimal (Green) casualties evacuated last or tasked to self-mobilize where feasible.

Critical elements of tactical evacuation planning include the following:

1. *CCP (Casualty Collection Point) Security*: Ensure the CCP is shielded from direct enemy fire or secondary threats. If insecure, prioritize "scoop and move" rather than detailed interventions.
2. *Evacuation Loadout Discipline*: Injured should be loaded based on triage tags and injury severity, not first-come-first-served. Heavily wounded but salvageable must ride out first.
3. *Dynamic Reassessment*: Conditions evolve; triage tags must be revalidated periodically, particularly before and during CASEVAC loading.
4. *Minimal Handling*: Especially in hypothermic, spinal, ocular, and blast injury, limit unnecessary movements that could destabilize patients further.

5. *CASEVAC Platform Optimization*: Use tactical vehicles, helicopters, or any available means; environmental adaptations (e.g., insulation in cold terrain) must be integrated.
6. *Buddy Reinforcement*: Injured capable of minimal function (green) can assist in litter carrying or security, easing the burden on medical assets.

BHISHM Cube: Modular Medical Support for Combat and Humanitarian Response

The *BHISHM Cube* (Bharat Health Initiative for Sahyog, Hita and Maitri) is a next-generation modular medical support system developed by HLL Life Care under the *Aarogya Maitri Project* of the Government of India. Designed for rapid deployment in austere and high-risk environments, the BHISHM Cube supports integrated medical care, survival, and surgical capability in both combat and disaster response settings (Fig. 19.3).

It consists of a modular system of 72 mini-cubes, configured into two "mother cubes" that together form a single BHISHM Cube. Each mini-cube is compact (15 in.), individually portable (weighing less than 20 kg), and packed with medical supplies organized according to specific injury patterns and operational priorities. The entire unit is designed for deployment via multiple modes—air, land, sea, or drone—and has been successfully airdrop tested from altitudes up to 15,000 ft. There are two primary configurations:

- *BHISHM Cube 1*: Enables the autonomous survival of a five-member team for up to 48 h, including provisions for food, potable water, shelter, power supply, and Advanced Trauma Life Support (ATLS) care.
- *BHISHM Cube 2*: Designed as a mobile field surgical suite, it contains essential instruments to support 10–15 basic life- or limb-saving surgeries per day in forward-deployed environments.

The BHISHM Cube offers a game-changing solution for delivering advanced medical care in forward combat zones and austere environments. Its compact, modular structure allows rapid deployment close to the point of injury, supporting immediate trauma resuscitation, damage control surgery, and stabilization during mass casualty situations. Capable of treating up to 200 battlefield casualties—including bullet wounds, burns, amputations, and blast-related injuries—it significantly enhances the operational efficiency of combat medical teams. With integrated power, oxygen generation, and AI-enabled inventory and coordination systems, the BHISHM Cube ensures sustained, self-contained medical support under the most challenging conditions.

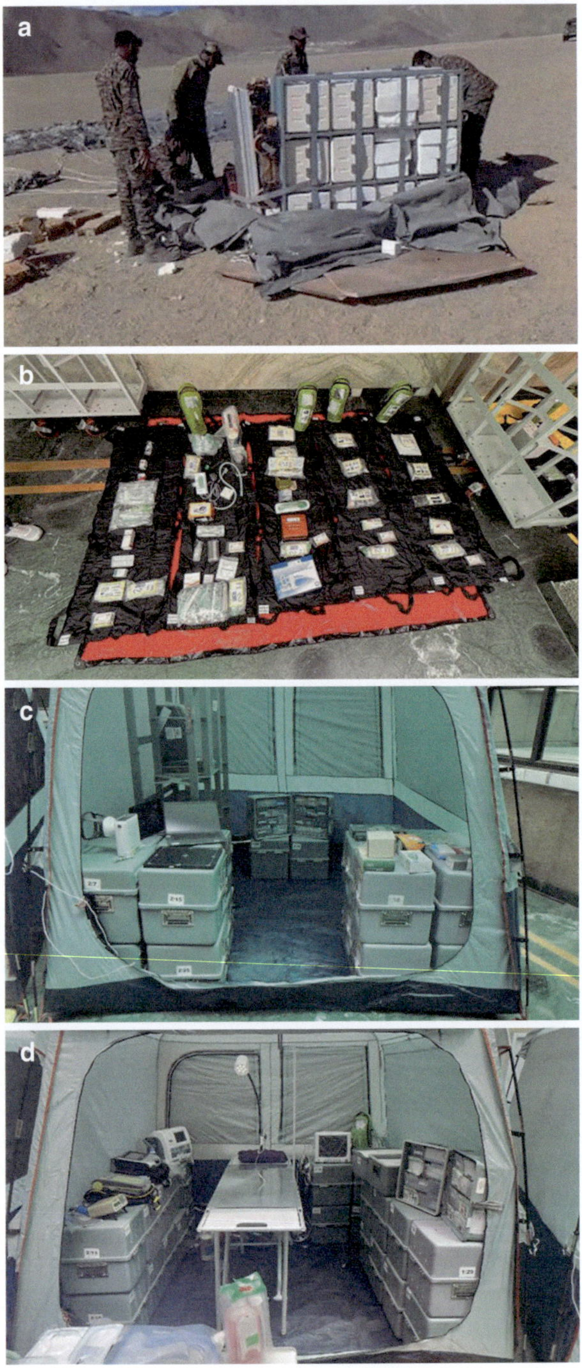

Fig. 19.3 The BHISHM Cube. (**a**) Airdrop testing of the BHISHM Cube. (**b**) Medical equipment and supplies packed within a mini-cube. (**c**) BHISHM Cube 1—configured for first-line care and survival support. (**d**) BHISHM Cube 2—deployable mobile field surgical suite

Case Resolution

Following the IED ambush and subsequent neutralization of hostile threat, you proceed to conduct primary triage using the SALT and TCCC-military triage model. The priority is to identify salvageable casualties and allocate limited evacuation assets effectively.

Triage Categorization:

- *Casualty 1*: 25-year-old with bilateral lower limb amputations, pale, semiconscious, thready radial pulse:
  - *Triage category*: *Immediate (red)*
  - *Rationale*: High threat of exsanguination and shock, but salvageable with prompt hemorrhage control and evacuation. Tourniquets should be applied to both limbs if not already in place, TXA should be administered, and IV access with fluid resuscitation initiated. Monitor GCS and vitals continuously.
- *Casualty 2*: 32-year-old with deep facial lacerations, GCS 15, airway patent, bleeding controlled:
  - *Triage category*: *Delayed (yellow)*
  - *Rationale*: Injuries are serious but not immediately life-threatening. No airway compromise or major hemorrhage. Dress wounds, provide analgesia, and reassess frequently.
- *Casualty 3*: 28-year-old walking wounded with superficial shrapnel wounds to the upper arm.
  - *Triage category*: *Minimal (green)*
  - *Rationale*: Ambulatory and stable. Provide basic first aid and reposition to help with team logistics if needed.
- *Casualty 4*: 24-year-old with massive chest trauma, unconscious, agonal breathing, and no radial pulse:
  - *Triage category*: *Expectant (black)*
  - *Rationale*: Signs of impending cardiac arrest and non-survivable injuries in the given resource-limited environment. Comfort care only. Use resources for casualties more likely to survive.

Evacuation Priority:

1. *Casualty 1* (Immediate): Requires urgent resuscitation, likely survivable with rapid surgical care
2. *Casualty 2* (Delayed): Though not critically unstable, needs specialized care for facial trauma; can deteriorate with delayed evacuation, hence second priority

Pre-evacuation Interventions:

- Apply tourniquets and hemostatic dressings to life-threatening bleeds.
- Secure IV access and administer TXA to those with risk of hemorrhagic shock.
- Use hypothermia prevention strategies (e.g., Mylar blanket and poncho liner).
- Label tourniquet time, and administer analgesia if time permits.

Unconscious Casualty Management (Casualty 4):

- If evacuation is not possible, ensure airway is patent.
- Position laterally to avoid aspiration.
- Monitor for signs of life and administer comfort measures.
- If breathing ceases and pulselessness confirmed, cease resuscitation and document.

This scenario highlights the brutal, necessary decisions in combat triage—optimizing survival for the maximum number of teammates under fire.

Key Messages

- *Combat triage focuses on maximizing survival, not individual outcomes.* Rapid and accurate categorization using immediate, delayed, minimal, and expectant priorities is essential to preserve the fighting force.
- *The MARCH algorithm must be completed before triage decisions.* Life threats like massive hemorrhage, airway compromise, and tension pneumothorax must be addressed even during mass casualty scenarios.
- *Expectant category is a hard but necessary decision.* In limited-resource environments, casualties with unsurvivable injuries must receive comfort measures, conserving efforts for salvageable lives.
- *Triage is dynamic, not static.* Casualties must be reassessed continuously, especially during prolonged field care or delayed evacuation.
- *Simple triage tools like START, SALT, and MIST tagging can be adapted to the tactical context.* Field-friendly adaptations ensure rapid decision-making even in austere settings.
- *Evacuation planning must integrate triage outcomes.* CASEVAC resources must first lift immediate (Priority I) casualties, even if it means temporarily leaving minimal (Priority III) casualties on scene.
- *Combat medical leadership matters.* Providers and first responders must coordinate triage, treatment, and evacuation simultaneously under operational constraints—*leadership under chaos saves lives.*

Conclusion

Combat triage and mass casualty management represent the sharpest test of a provider's skills, judgment, and resilience. In battlefield conditions where time is short, resources are scarce, and lives hang in the balance, structured triage allows rescuers to bring order to chaos. The principles of prioritization, rapid MARCH interventions, dynamic reassessment, and disciplined evacuation planning must be ingrained into every tactical team.

Combat triage is not about saving everyone—it is about saving the most lives possible under fire.

Through adherence to systematic triage protocols and decisive leadership, *combat providers can transform overwhelming casualty events into controlled operations*, preserving combat power and upholding the sacred duty to care for the wounded.

Bibliography

1. Army U.S. Tactical Combat Casualty Care Handbook. Version 5. Morrisville (NC): Lulu Press Inc.; 2017. 130 p. ISBN: 9781678198312.
2. Auerbach PS, Cushing TA, Harris NS. Auerbach's Wilderness Medicine. 7th ed. 2 vols. Philadelphia: Elsevier; 2016. ISBN: 9780323359429
3. Feliciano DV, Mattox KL, Moore EE. Trauma. 9th ed. New York: McGraw Hill Medical; 2020. ISBN: 978-1260143355
4. Press Information Bureau. *Aarogya Maitri: India Launches BHISHM – A Portable Hospital for Disaster Relief and Humanitarian Assistance* [Internet]. New Delhi: Ministry of Information and Broadcasting; 2024 Jan 2. Available from: https://www.pib.gov.in/PressNoteDetails.aspx?NoteId=152055&ModuleId=3
5. Ranger Training Brigade, U.S. Army Infantry School. Ranger Handbook: U.S. Army Ranger Handbook SH 21-76 (Revised February 2011). 5th June 2013. ISBN: 978-1304107619.
6. St. John Ambulance Association (India), Indian Red Cross Society. First Aid Manual 7th Edition. Available from: https://www.indianredcross.org/publications/FA-manual.pdf

FORCE Skill Stations

20

Samir Misra and Aman Arora

Learning Objectives
By the end of this chapter, the learner should be able to:

- Apply the MARCH algorithm to systematically assess and manage trauma patients in combat and austere environments.
- Adapt trauma care interventions to operational constraints, such as moving vehicles, aircraft, and confined or hostile environments.
- Recognize and prioritize life-threatening conditions, including massive hemorrhage, airway compromise, respiratory failure, shock, hypothermia, and traumatic brain injury.
- Demonstrate effective hemorrhage control techniques, including direct pressure, wound packing, and tourniquet application, along with indications for pelvic stabilization and traction splinting.
- Establish and manage vascular access (IV and intraosseous) and initiate appropriate fluid resuscitation based on clinical context.
- Perform airway assessment and management, including basic maneuvers (jaw thrust), airway adjuncts (OPA/NPA), bag-valve-mask ventilation, supraglottic devices, endotracheal intubation, and surgical airway techniques when indicated.

(continued)

S. Misra (✉)
Department of Traumatology & Surgery, King George's Medical University, Lucknow, Uttar Pradesh, India

A. Arora
Department of General Surgery, AMC Centre and College, Lucknow, Uttar Pradesh, India

N. T. Rai, S. Misra (eds.), *Frontline Operational Resuscitation and Combat Emergencies (FORCE) Manual*, https://doi.org/10.1007/978-981-92-1622-2_20

- Identify and manage life-threatening thoracic injuries, including tension pneumothorax and hemothorax and perform procedures, such as needle decompression, occlusive dressing application, and tube thoracostomy.
- Conduct focused neurological assessment (AVPU, GCS, pupillary exam) and implement early management of traumatic brain injury.
- Recognize and prevent hypothermia and implement appropriate passive and active warming strategies in field conditions.
- Apply spinal motion restriction techniques, including cervical collar application and spine board immobilization in constrained environments.
- Demonstrate situational awareness, reassessment, and decision-making under stress, including identifying the need for escalation, definitive care, and evacuation.
- Utilize improvisation techniques to deliver effective care with limited resources in austere and combat settings.

Introduction

Combat casualty care does not occur in ideal conditions—it unfolds in the back of moving trucks, inside cramped aircraft, under hostile fire, and within frigid trenches. In such realities, lifesaving decisions must be rapid, tactile, and repeatable under stress. This chapter on FORCE skill stations is designed to transform theory into field-ready muscle memory using the MARCH algorithm—Massive Hemorrhage, Airway, Respiration, Circulation, and Hypothermia/Head Injury—as a structured response framework. Unlike traditional training modules that assume a controlled environment, FORCE skill stations simulate operational chaos by embedding tactical constraints, such as limited space, noise, low visibility, unstable surfaces, and extreme climates.

Each station presents a critical skill set that directly correlates with preventable causes of battlefield mortality. Trainees learn to apply tourniquets in darkness, secure airways amidst vibrations, decompress chests mid-transport, and improvise with minimal gear. Whether applying a pelvic binder in a helicopter or performing needle cricothyrotomy in a trench, every task is executed with the anticipation of real-world friction.

The purpose is not only technical mastery but also *situational fluency—the ability to adapt, prioritize, and act decisively under fire.* These stations emphasize role-based execution, allowing buddies, medics, and commanders to function within their competencies, creating a distributed, fail-safe trauma response system.

Ultimately, FORCE skill stations reinforce the doctrine that *survival begins not at the hospital, but at the point of injury.* By replicating operational constraints, these training modules cultivate the courage, clarity, and competence required to save lives in the moments that matter most.

Tactical Considerations

In combat and austere environments, casualty care is often delivered under extreme constraints that significantly impact the safety, efficacy, and prioritization of interventions. Whether in moving vehicles, airborne platforms, or confined spaces, such as trenches, each setting presents unique challenges—including limited space, unstable platforms, compromised asepsis, and environmental hazards like cold, dust, or altitude. Effective field management requires adaptability, improvisation, and forethought to mitigate risks, such as tube dislodgement, hypothermia, or worsening injuries during transport. Table 20.1 outlines key considerations and tactical adaptations necessary for providing safe and effective care in these dynamic operational contexts.

Table 20.1 Operational considerations for casualty management in dynamic and austere settings

(a) *Moving vehicle* 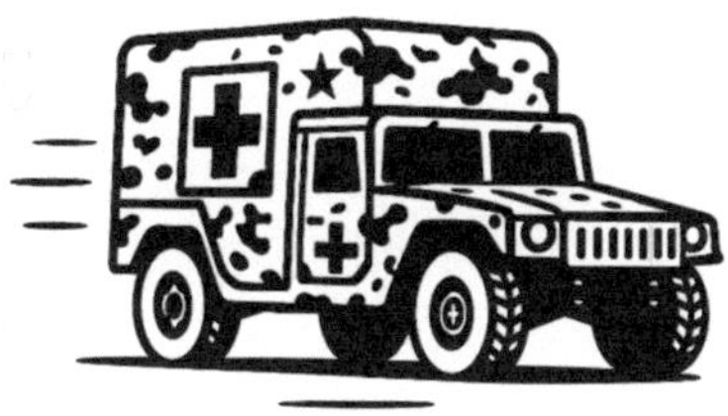	(i) Space Limited space Uncomfortable seating Limited treatment facility Unstable platform: Intubation and surgical cricothyrotomy are high risk—use supraglottic airway devices (LMA/LT) Unable to maintain asepsis due to less space (ii) Movement Jerky movement: Tubes/iv lines may dislodge—secure lines properly, ensure c-collar + lateral supports Uncontrolled patient's stable position (iii) Other considerations Hypothermia risk: Cold fluids + ventilation loss increase risk; keep patient covered and insulated Neuromonitoring: Use GCS or AVPU frequently as vitals may fluctuate en route
(b) *Flying aircraft/helicopter*	(i) Space Limited space Background noise—auscultation unreliable and communication issues Unable to maintain asepsis due to less space (ii) Movement Turbulence—tubes/iv lines may dislodge and movement constraints due to seat belts during landing/takeoff (iii) Other considerations Pressure drops at altitude—fluid flow may slow; use pressure infusion bags or gravity assist Ventilator may fail to deliver at high altitude if not configured Small untreated pneumothorax can become tension pneumothorax during flight Ambient temperature may be low at altitude: Ensure all extremities covered, fluids pre-warmed Noise prevents verbal GCS: Use AVPU and pupillary exam

(continued)

Table 20.1 (continued)

(c) *On the ground/trench/closed spaces* 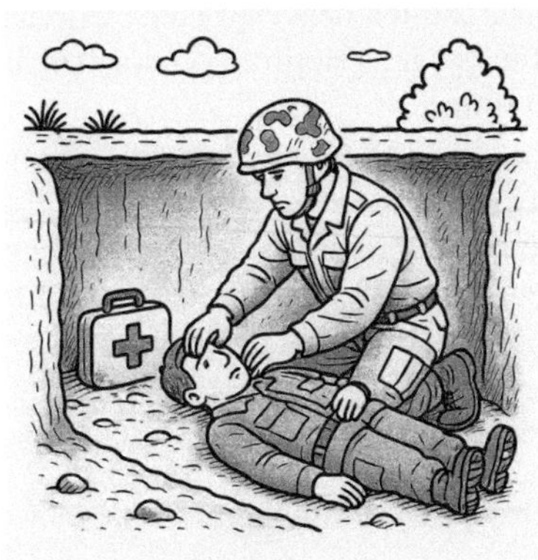	(i) Space Limited space Unable to maintain asepsis due to contaminants—debris, dust, and water Low visibility Restricted access to head and neck (ii) Movement Limited movement due to space constraints Difficult to log-roll or apply spine board: Prioritize cervical collar and lateral padding (iii) Other considerations Hypothermia from snow/rain exposure: Remove wet clothing, elevate torso, wrap completely Limited gear: Improvise with jackets, rucksacks, dry sleeping mats

Abbreviations: *LMA* laryngeal mask airway, *LT* laryngeal tube, *GCS* Glasgow Coma Scale, *AVPU* alert, verbal, pain, unresponsive

Massive Hemorrhage and Circulation

Case Scenario

A 48-year-old soldier sustains a gunshot wound to the left anterior chest with no exit wound during a forward patrol. He is conscious but hypotensive. Another soldier is recovered from a vehicle crash with an open femoral fracture and profuse bleeding from the thigh. Extraction is delayed due to terrain constraints. Immediate hemorrhage control and stabilization are crucial to prevent death from exsanguination.

Core Skill Components

I. Wound Packing

Equipment required:

Equipment	Number
Gauze pads, hemostatic dressings	As needed
Gloves, tape	As needed
Rolled gauze, combine dressing	As needed

Procedure:

1. Ensure the scene is tactically safe; approach only when under cover or enemy fire is suppressed.
2. Expose the wound completely by cutting away clothing to assess the bleeding source.

3. Identify if the bleeding is from a deep, narrow wound—especially in junctional areas like the groin, axilla, or neck—where tourniquets are not effective.
4. Apply firm direct pressure with a gloved hand or plain gauze to slow bleeding while preparing your packing material.
5. Open the hemostatic gauze (or plain gauze if unavailable), maintaining sterility as much as possible in the field.
6. Insert your finger into the wound to locate the point of maximal bleeding.
7. Begin packing the gauze into the wound cavity, pressing it firmly against the bleeding vessel or source with your finger.
8. Continue inserting gauze in a controlled, layered manner—*like stuffing a cavity*—without removing previously packed material.
9. Ensure the entire cavity is tightly and completely packed; if one roll is not enough, use additional gauze as needed.
10. Once fully packed, apply sustained direct pressure over the wound for a *minimum of 3 min* (longer if non-hemostatic gauze is used).
11. Secure the packed wound with a pressure dressing (e.g., Israeli bandage or improvised wrap) to maintain pressure during movement or evacuation.
12. Reassess frequently for continued bleeding or saturation of the dressing.
13. Document time of intervention and communicate the wound site, packing used, and bleeding status during casualty handover (Fig. 20.1).

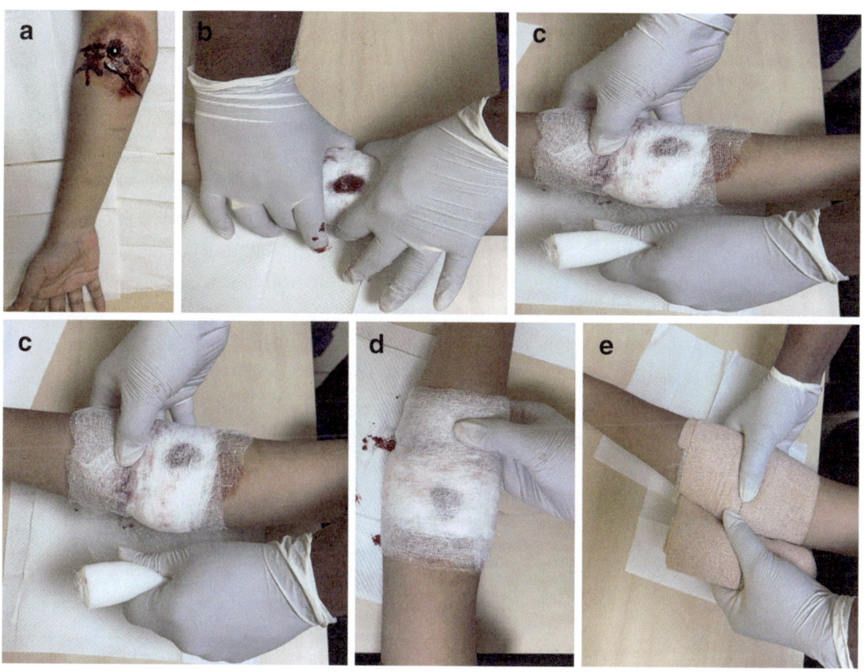

Fig. 20.1 Steps of direct pressure and packing. (**a**) Image showing arterial injury of the right upper limb around elbow. (**b**) Application of gauze over the wound with pressure. (**c**–**e**) Application of roller gauze over the wound with firm pressure. (**f**) Application of crepe bandage/Israeli bandage over the wound

II. Tourniquet Application

Equipment required:

Equipment	Number
Task trainer for tourniquet placement (alternatively, providers may apply tourniquets on one another)	1
Task trainer for wound packing	1
CAT tourniquet (or improvised tourniquet)	1
Clamps	1
Gauze pads	1
Large combine dressing packet	1
Rolled gauze, minimum of four disposable gloves box of various sizes	1

Procedure:

1. Confirm the scene is secure and safe to approach; always prioritize your safety before initiating care.
2. Identify the site of life-threatening limb bleeding—look for spurting blood, pooling, or bright red bleeding from a major vessel.
3. Choose a location 2–3 in. above the bleeding site; avoid placing the tourniquet directly over joints or on the wound itself.
4. If the wound is not visible, apply the tourniquet *high and tight* on the limb—upper thigh or upper arm—to ensure proximal control.
5. Slide the CAT tourniquet strap around the limb and pass the free end through the buckle; pull it as tight as possible and fasten it back on itself using the Velcro.
6. Twist the windlass rod until the bleeding stops and distal pulse is no longer palpable—this usually requires several full rotations.
7. Lock the windlass rod into the clip to prevent it from unwinding.
8. Secure the windlass by fastening the retaining strap completely over it; ensure the tourniquet is stable and would not loosen during casualty movement.
9. Write the time of application clearly on the tourniquet's white label or on the casualty's forehead or limb using a permanent marker.
10. Do not remove or loosen the tourniquet once applied unless directed by a higher-level provider in a controlled environment.
11. Reassess frequently to ensure bleeding remains controlled and the tourniquet remains tight during transport or movement (Fig. 20.2).

III. IV Access

Equipment required:

Equipment	Number
IV cannulae (16 G, 18 G, 20 G), IV dressing, and IV set	As needed
Alcohol soaked gauze/antiseptic wipes	As needed
IV fluids and syringes	As needed
Gloves, tape	As needed

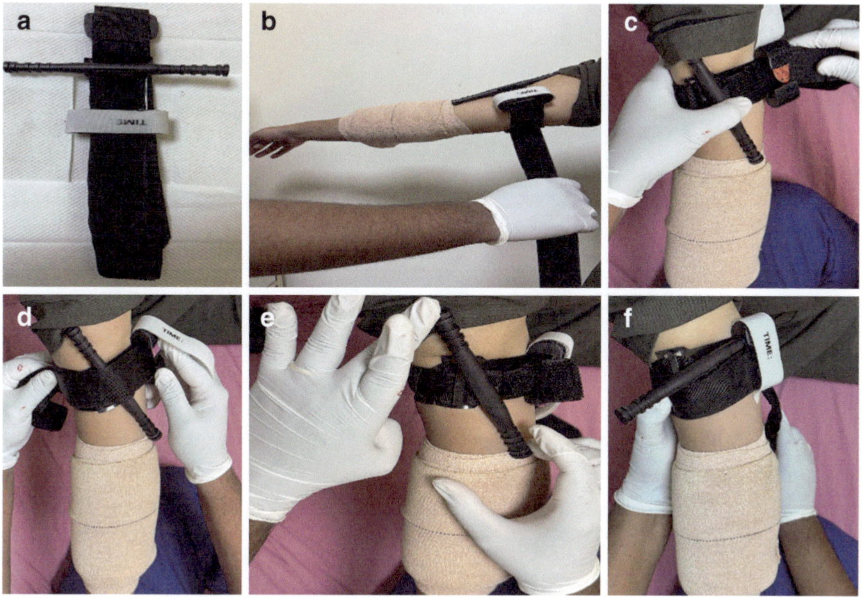

Fig. 20.2 Steps of CAT tourniquet application. (**a**) Image showing CAT tourniquet. (**b**) Pass the CAT around the arm 5–7 cm above the wound. (**c**) Pass the band through the buckle. (**d**) Fix the band tightly around the arm. (**e**) Rotate the windlass rod till the bleeding stops. (**f**) Fix the rod in the holder, attach the clip, and document the time of application

Procedure:

1. Select a suitable site for IV access, typically the antecubital fossa or forearm; avoid injured or contaminated limbs.
2. Use gloves and aseptic technique as much as the tactical situation allows; if in a high-threat setting, prioritize speed over sterility.
3. Apply a tourniquet above the selected site to engorge the vein and make it more visible or palpable.
4. Select appropriate IV cannula (Fig. 20.3). Palpate and stabilize the vein with one hand while holding the IV cannula bevel-up at a shallow angle (15–30°) in the other hand.
5. Insert the cannula into the vein until a flashback of blood appears in the chamber.
6. Advance the catheter slightly to ensure it is fully within the vein, and then slide the catheter off the needle into position.
7. Remove the needle carefully and dispose of it in a sharps container or secure location if unavailable.
8. Release the tourniquet and connect the IV line or saline lock; flush with normal saline to confirm patency.
9. Secure the catheter with tape or dressing to prevent dislodgement during movement.

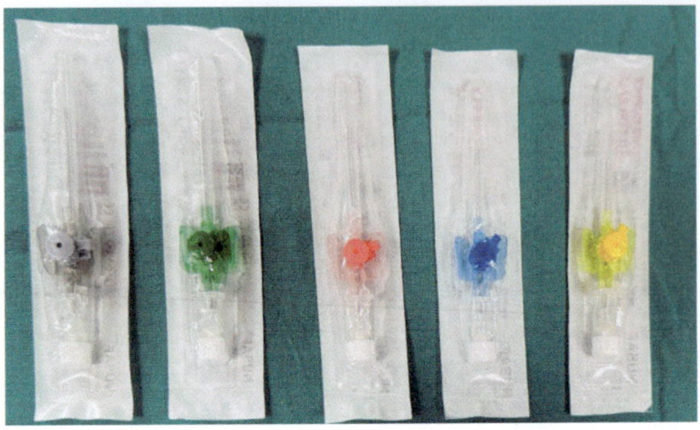

Fig. 20.3 Different sizes of IV cannula: 16 G, gray; 18 G, green; 20 G, pink; 22 G, blue

10. Label the IV site with time of insertion and type of fluid started, if applicable.
11. Begin fluid resuscitation only if indicated (e.g., signs of shock), and monitor for signs of infiltration or dislodgement.
12. Reassess frequently during evacuation or transport to ensure continued patency and secure placement.

IV. Intraosseous Access

Equipment required:

Equipment	Number
Intraosseous leg trainer or chicken or turkey legs	1 (or 4 chicken legs)
EZ-IO driver 1 EZ-IO intraosseous needles or manual IO devices	1
IO dressing to secure access	1
IV fluids: normal saline	2
10 mL syringes	2
IV pole	1
Sharps container	1
Disposable gloves	1 box of various sizes

Procedure:

1. Identify the need for intraosseous (IO) access—typically in cases of shock or cardiac arrest when peripheral IV access is difficult or delayed.
2. Choose an appropriate IO insertion site, most commonly the proximal tibia (just below the tibial tuberosity, medial side) or alternatively the humeral head (Fig. 20.4).
3. Clean the insertion site if time and resources allow; in tactical scenarios, prioritize rapid access over sterility.
4. Stabilize the limb and align the IO device perpendicular to the bone surface.
5. Insert the IO needle using a mechanical driver or manual pressure, advancing it steadily through the cortex until a sudden "give" is felt.

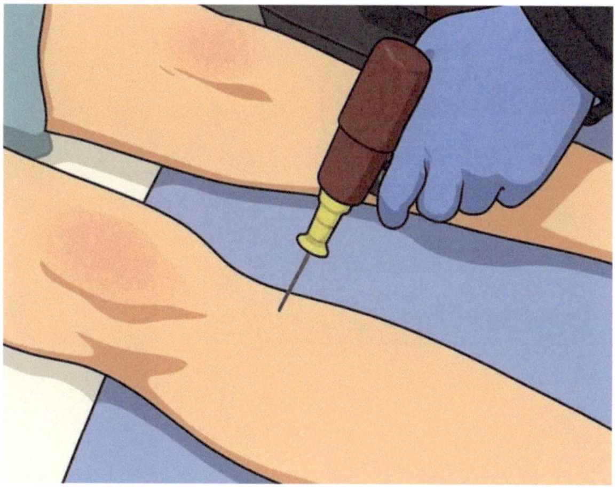

Fig. 20.4 Intraosseous (IO) access at the proximal tibia

6. Stop advancing once the needle hub is flush with the skin; avoid over-penetration.
7. Remove the stylet and immediately attach a syringe to aspirate the bone marrow; a flash of blood or marrow confirms placement.
8. If aspiration is not successful, flush with 5–10 mL of saline to confirm patency; resistance-free flow also indicates correct placement.
9. Secure the IO device with tape or a stabilization device to prevent dislodgement during movement.
10. Begin fluid resuscitation using a pressure bag or manual push, as flow through IO lines is slower than IV.
11. Label the site with time of insertion and type of fluid administered.
12. Monitor for complications, such as infiltration, swelling, or pain; reassess frequently during ongoing care or transport.

V. Pelvic Binder

Equipment required:

Equipment	Number
Pelvic stabilizing device	1
Long sheet	1
Clamps	2
Pelvic X-ray	1

Procedure:

1. Identify signs suggestive of a pelvic fracture: mechanism of injury (e.g., high-speed impact, blast, and fall), pelvic instability, leg-length discrepancy, or hypotension without obvious external bleeding.

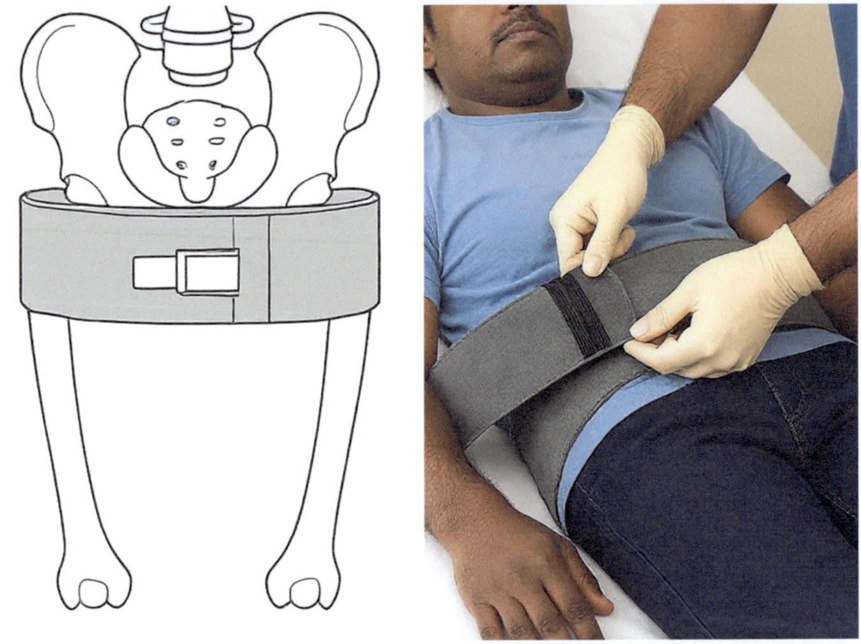

Fig. 20.5 Application of pelvic binder at the level of greater trochanters

2. Explain to team members that a pelvic binder is being applied to control potential internal hemorrhage and stabilize the pelvis.
3. Expose the pelvis and remove any bulky clothing to ensure correct placement and avoid misapplication.
4. *Locate the greater trochanters of both femurs*—this is the correct anatomical landmark for binder placement, not the iliac crest or waist (Fig. 20.5).
5. Slide the binder or sheet under the patient's pelvis, centering it over the greater trochanters.
6. Pull the binder or sheet tightly and symmetrically across the pelvis to achieve compression; in case of a sheet, twist and secure it with clamps or knots to maintain tension.
7. Confirm that the binder is positioned correctly—*low across the hips*, not over the abdomen or lower spine.
8. Avoid repositioning once applied, as excessive movement can worsen hemorrhage.
9. Document the time of application and reassess periodically for signs of improved perfusion or complications, such as pressure injury.
10. Keep the casualty immobilized and prepared for definitive imaging and surgical care; do not remove the binder in the field.

VI. Femoral Traction Splint

Equipment required:

Equipment	Number
Thomas splint/traction device/improvised traction	1
Roller gauze	1
Skin traction set	1
Counterweights (saline bottle or improvised)	2
Femur X-ray	1

Procedure:

1. Identify indications for femoral traction splinting, typically a suspected or confirmed midshaft femur fracture with associated limb shortening, rotation, swelling, or severe pain.
2. Explain the procedure to team members and casualty if conscious, emphasizing pain control and the goal of stabilizing the fracture and reducing bleeding.
3. Expose the entire limb and check for additional injuries, open wounds, or contraindications (e.g., pelvic fracture and lower leg amputation).
4. Assess distal neurovascular status—check pulses, capillary refill, sensation, and motor function before applying the splint.
5. Gently support the injured leg while preparing the traction device (Thomas splint or equivalent), adjusting its length to fit the patient from ischial tuberosity to just beyond the foot.
6. Place the ischial ring or proximal support of the splint against the groin, ensuring it sits firmly without compressing genitalia.
7. Apply the ankle hitch or distal strap to the casualty's foot, securing it tightly and attaching it to the traction mechanism.
8. Begin applying traction by gradually pulling the foot in line with the leg, aiming to restore limb length and reduce muscle spasm.
9. Secure intermediate straps around the thigh and lower leg to immobilize the limb within the splint (Fig. 20.6).
10. Reassess and adjust the amount of traction until the leg appears aligned, pain is reduced, and distal pulses remain intact.
11. Recheck neurovascular status after traction is applied and at regular intervals during transport.
12. Document the time of application, traction amount if measurable, and reassessment findings for handover.

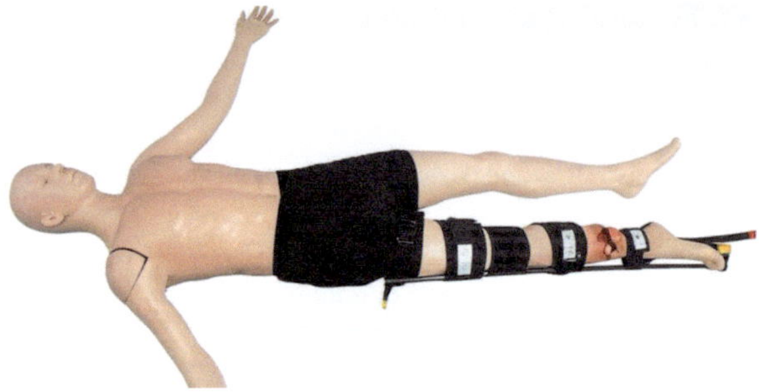

Fig. 20.6 Application of femoral traction splint

Airway

Key Messages

- *Recognize shock early* via pulse, mental status, and capillary refill. Differentiate between compensated versus uncompensated shock.
- *Control bleeding first*—airway comes second if patient is exsanguinating. Use direct pressure, tourniquet, and pelvic and long bone stabilization devices appropriately.
- Begin resuscitation. Replace losses with judicious isotonic crystalloids and blood products if feasible.
- Ensure access for resuscitation. *Use IO early if IV access fails or delay is expected.*
- *Pelvic fractures are "internal bleeders"*—treat them with urgency.
- Activate massive transfusion protocol with significant hemorrhage.
- *Log time of tourniquet and IO insertion* visibly on the casualty card.
- Secure lines properly before transport—especially in tactical evacuation.

Case Scenario

A soldier is pulled out from a burning tank with facial burns, soot in the oropharynx, and deteriorating consciousness. He is tachypneic, hypoxic, and agitated. A definitive airway is urgently required. Evacuation is 45 min away. The responder must choose and execute the most appropriate airway intervention, considering movement, lighting, and equipment constraints.

Core Skill Components

Equipment required:

Equipment	Number
Intubation manikin	1
Oropharyngeal airway (OPA) of various sizes	1 each
Nasopharyngeal airway (NPA) of various sizes	1 each

Equipment	Number
Endotracheal tubes 3.0, 4.0, 6.0, 7.0, 7.5, 8.0	1 each
Direct laryngoscope with blades of various sizes	1
Video laryngoscope (if available)	1 each
Adult high-flow oxygen mask, pulse oximeter	1-1
Bag mask	1 adult
Eye protection, masks, gloves, and gowns (to reinforce universal precautions)	1
End tidal CO_2 colorimetric detector	1
Towel or pad to place under the patient	1 each
Disposable syringe	1
7.5 ET connector	3
Cricothyrotomy manikin	1
Surgical and needle cricothyrotomy trays—scalpel (10, 11, 15), Kelly clamp, or tracheal spreader	1
Tracheostomy tubes, LMA, LTA, Guedels	1-1-1-1
Eye protection	1
Masks, gowns, and gloves	1 set
End tidal CO_2 colorimetric detector	1
ET tube connector and bag mask	1
Jet insufflation equipment and/or oxygen tubing	1
Syringe	1
Three-way stopcock	1

Basic Airway Management

I. Jaw-Thrust Maneuver

Procedure:

1. Position yourself at the head of the patient, facing their feet, ideally in a supine position.
2. Place both of your hands on either side of the patient's head, with your elbows resting on the surface to provide stability.
3. Use your index and middle fingers to grasp the angles of the patient's mandible (lower jaw), just behind the corners of the jawline.
4. Simultaneously, use your thumbs to gently press down on the patient's cheeks or lower lip to open the mouth slightly if needed.
5. Apply firm, upward, and forward pressure with your fingers to lift the mandible anteriorly, displacing the jaw away from the posterior pharyngeal wall (Fig. 20.7).
6. This motion pulls the tongue forward and helps relieve obstruction caused by the tongue falling back in an unconscious patient.
7. Maintain this position while assessing for air movement or while a partner provides ventilation with a bag-valve mask.
8. Avoid tilting the head or neck during this maneuver, *especially if a cervical spine injury is suspected.*
9. Reassess airway patency continuously, and be prepared to insert an airway adjunct (OPA/NPA) or escalate to advanced airway if needed.

Fig. 20.7 Jaw-thrust maneuver

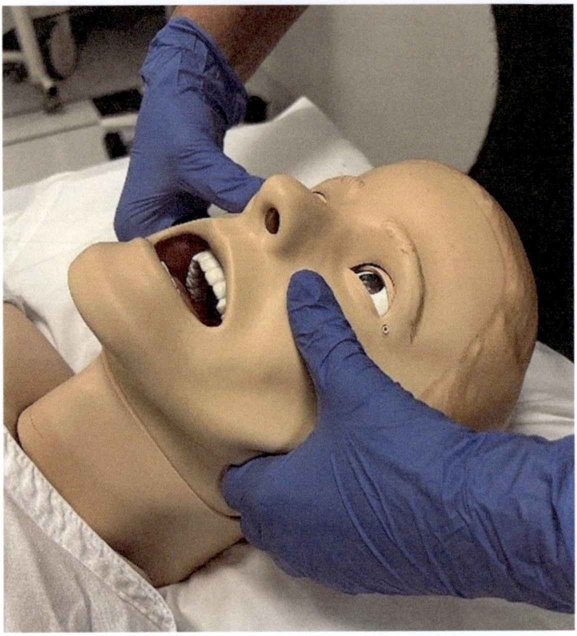

II. Oropharyngeal airway (OPA) and Nasopharyngeal airway (NPA) Insertion

Procedure:

1. *Assess the patient for airway compromise*—check for snoring, gurgling, or absence of effective air movement.
2. If the patient is unresponsive with no gag reflex, prepare to insert an oropharyngeal airway (OPA); if the patient is semiconscious or has an intact gag reflex, choose a nasopharyngeal airway (NPA) instead (Fig. 20.8).
3. For NPA, choose the correct size by *measuring from the tip of the nose to the earlobe* (Fig. 20.9a).
4. Lubricate the NPA with water-based gel to reduce friction.
5. Insert the NPA into the right nostril (preferably), bevel facing the nasal septum, advancing it gently along the floor of the nose; if resistance is encountered, try the left nostril.
6. For OPA, select the correct size by *measuring from the corner of the mouth to the angle of the mandible* (Fig. 20.9b).
7. Open the mouth using a cross-finger technique and insert the OPA upside down and then rotate 180° as it advances into the oropharynx; alternatively, insert following the curve of the tongue using a tongue depressor.
8. Once the airway adjunct is in place, reassess airway patency and check for chest rise during ventilation.

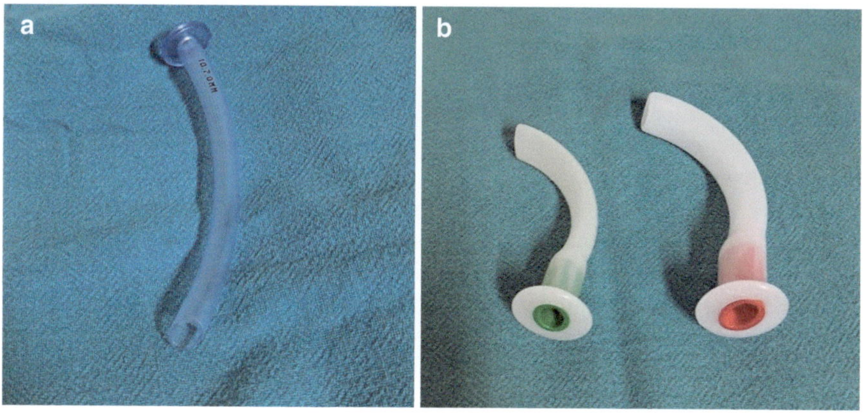

Fig. 20.8 (**a**) Nasopharyngeal airway. (**b**) Oropharyngeal airway

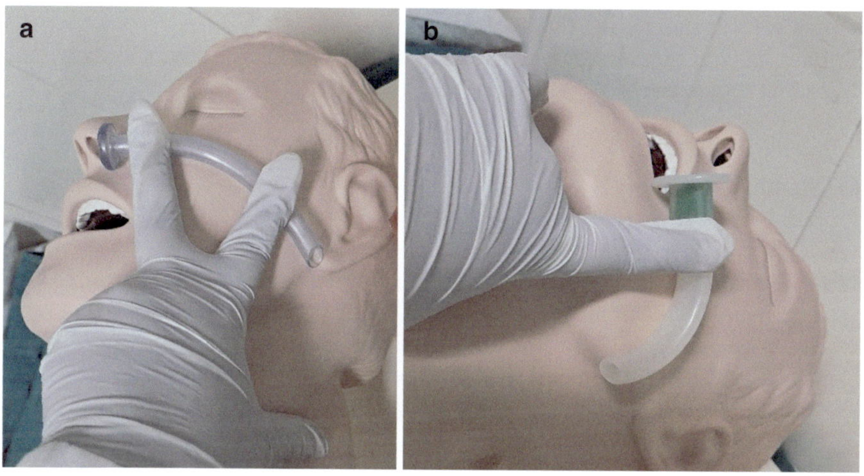

Fig. 20.9 Measurement of appropriate size of airway adjunct: (**a**) Nasopharyngeal airway. (**b**) Oropharyngeal airway

9. If using a bag-valve mask (BVM), ensure a proper seal and deliver ventilations synchronized with spontaneous effort or at a rate of 10–12 breaths per minute if apneic.
10. Continuously monitor for dislodgement, gagging, or obstruction, and remove the airway adjunct if it causes vomiting or airway irritation.
11. Document the type, size, and time of insertion of the airway adjunct, and monitor airway status regularly.

III. Bag-Valve Mask (BVM) Ventilation

Procedure:

1. Assess the patient's breathing—if they are apneic and breathing inadequately or have a low respiratory rate with poor effort, prepare to assist ventilation using a bag-valve mask (BVM).
2. Position the patient supine and ensure the airway is open using the head tilt–chin lift or jaw-thrust maneuver (if cervical spine injury is suspected).
3. Select the correct mask size to cover the nose and mouth without gaps; connect the BVM to an oxygen source if available, ideally at 15 L/min (Fig. 20.10).
4. Create a tight seal using the E-C clamp technique: Use the thumb and index finger to form a "C" around the mask, and the other three fingers to lift the mandible, forming the "E" for a proper jaw seal.
5. Squeeze the bag slowly over 1 s to deliver a visible chest rise; avoid excessive force or rate to prevent gastric insufflation.
6. Ventilate at a rate of 10–12 breaths per minute for adults, or one breath every 5–6 s, while monitoring for chest rise and fall.
7. Reassess the airway continuously for obstruction, mask seal adequacy, and patient response.

IV. Manual Suctioning

Procedure:

1. If the airway is compromised by blood, vomitus, or secretions, prepare to perform manual suctioning before or during ventilation.
2. Use a wide-bore suction catheter (e.g., Yankauer tip) connected to a manual or battery-powered suction unit (Fig. 20.11).
3. Turn the patient's head to the side if spinal injury is not suspected, or use a jaw-thrust maneuver to open the airway.

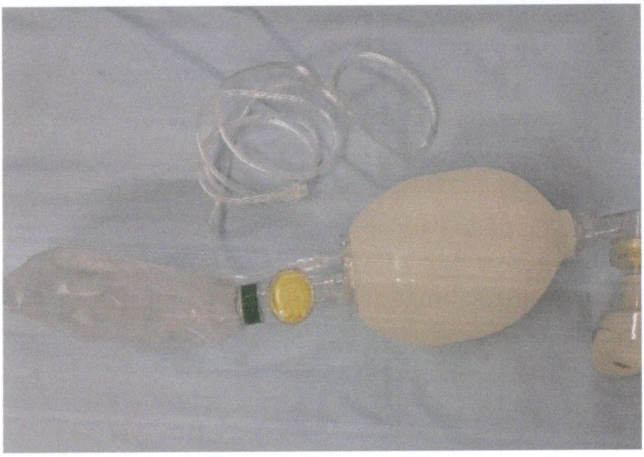

Fig. 20.10 A bag-valve mask device

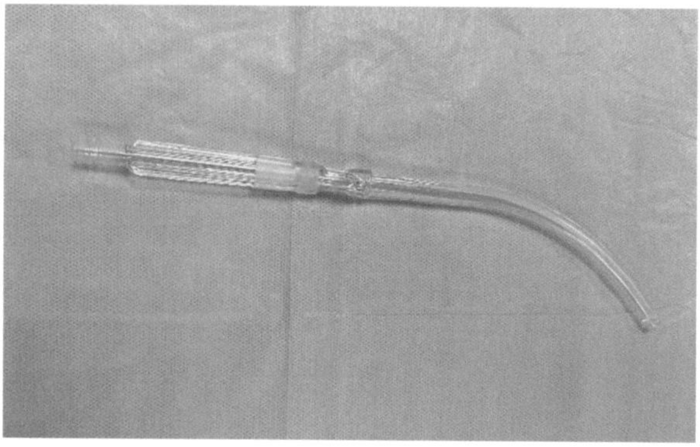

Fig. 20.11 Yankauer tip suction—wide bore suction catheter

4. Insert the suction catheter into the mouth only as far as you can visualize, without blindly probing.
5. Apply suction only while withdrawing the catheter in a circular motion, limiting each pass to no more than 10–15 s to prevent hypoxia.
6. Repeat suctioning as necessary, especially if gurgling or bubbling sounds return or ventilation becomes difficult.
7. Monitor oxygen saturation and respiratory effort throughout the process, and be prepared to reinsert an airway adjunct or reassess BVM effectiveness after suctioning.

Advanced Airway Management

I. Laryngeal Mask Airway

Laryngeal mask airway is a device that is inserted into the oral cavity, so that it slides and rest over the larynx (Fig. 20.12). It is a temporary device and must be replaced by a definitive airway (ET tube/surgical airway).

Procedure:

1. Clear the oropharynx.
2. Pre-oxygenate
3. Choose the appropriate size of LMA.
4. With the deflated cuff, apply a small amount of lubricant to the posterior surface of the distal mask and cuff.
5. Insert the LMA into the mouth, manually guiding it along the hard and soft palates and into the throat by pushing with the index or long finger in the v-shaped notch where the tube attaches to the mask. Push the tube, so the lubricated posterior surface of the mask follows the curve of the hard and soft palates.
6. The mask should enter the hypopharynx along the posterior wall, to avoid deflecting and possibly causing a tube obstruction by the epiglottis. At the proper distance of insertion, inflate the cuff with the correct volume of air

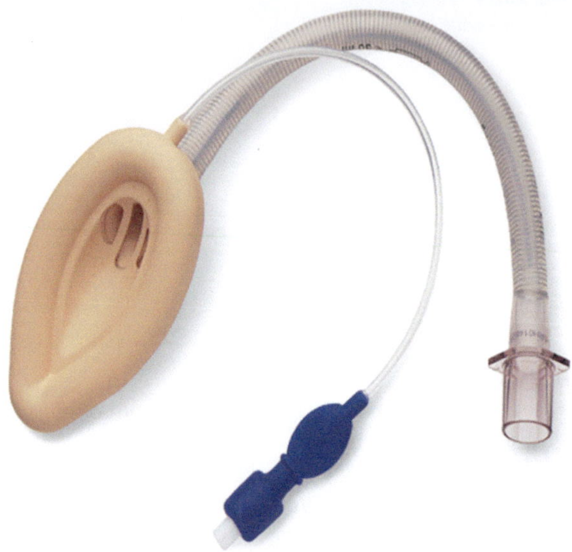

Fig. 20.12 Laryngeal mask airway

7. Check placement of the LMA by applying bag ventilation.
8. Confirm proper position by auscultation, chest movement, and ideally verification of CO_2 by capnography.

II. Laryngeal Tube

Laryngeal tube (LT) is quite similar to LMA device. The principle is to insert a tube through the oral cavity, which has two openings, with the assumption that one of the openings is going to ventilate the lungs, and selecting the same for ventilation (Fig. 20.13).

Procedure:

1. Clear the oropharynx.
2. Pre-oxygenate.
3. The LT device should be the correct size, sterile, and have no visible damage.
4. Pass the LT device to slide into the oral cavity to pass into the pharynx.
5. Without excessive force, advance the LT until the base of the connector is aligned with the patient's teeth or gums.
6. Inflate the cuffs.
7. While gently bagging the patient to assess ventilation, simultaneously withdraw the airway until ventilation is easy and free flowing (large tidal volume with minimal airway pressure).
8. Reference marks are provided at the proximal end of the LTA; when aligned with the upper teeth, these marks indicate the depth of insertion.
9. Confirm proper position by auscultation, chest movement, and ideally verification of CO_2 by capnography.
10. Secure LTA to patient using tape or other accepted means. A bite block can also be used, if desired.

Fig. 20.13 Laryngeal tube device

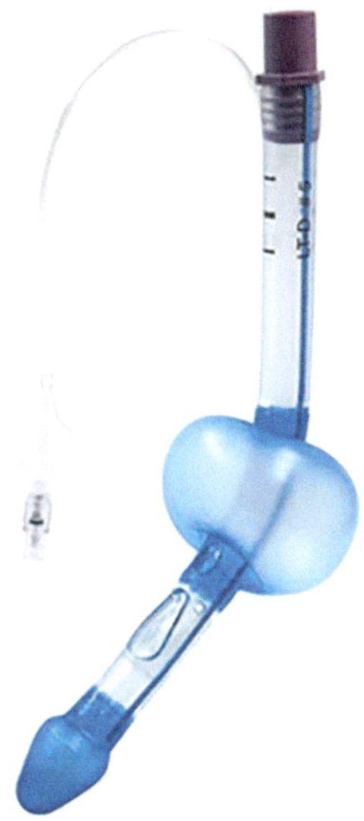

III. Endotracheal Intubation

Procedure:

1. Ensure the environment is tactically secure and assess whether intubation is immediately necessary (e.g., airway burns, GCS $\leq$ 8, apnea, and agonal respirations).
2. Pre-oxygenate the casualty with a bag-valve mask (BVM) using high-flow oxygen, if available, for at least 30–60 s or until SpO_2 improves, recognizing that time may be limited.
3. Position the casualty in a supine position with *the sniffing position if no spinal injury is suspected; if spine trauma is a concern, maintain manual in-line stabilization (MILS).*
4. Select and prepare equipment:
   (i) Endotracheal tube (ETT), appropriate size (usually 7.0–8.0 mm for adults), with stylet preloaded and curved
   (ii) Laryngoscope (Macintosh blade for DL or video laryngoscope screen for VL)
   (iii) Suction device ready and functional
   (iv) Syringe (10 mL) to inflate the cuff
   (v) Bag-valve mask with $EtCO_2$ detector or capnography (if available)
5. Apply tactical lighting (headlamp or angled torch) and have an assistant support the head if terrain is unstable or space is tight.
6. Open the airway using jaw thrust if spinal injury is suspected; insert an OPA to maintain patency during pre-oxygenation.

Fig. 20.14 Endotracheal intubation

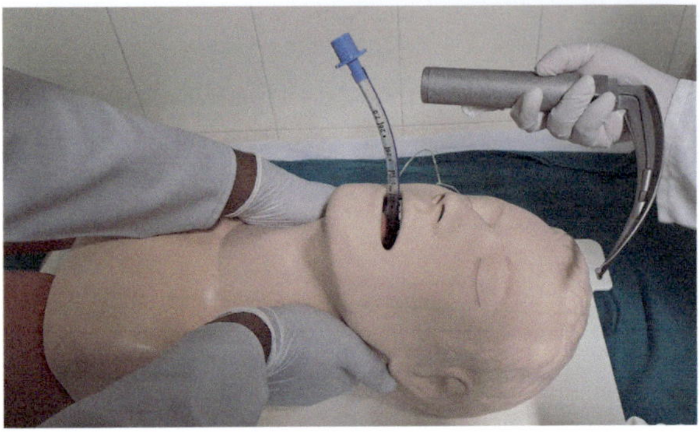

7. Hold the laryngoscope in the left hand, open the mouth, and insert the blade into the right side of the mouth, sweeping the tongue to the left (Fig. 20.14).
8. Advance the blade until the tip reaches the vallecula (Macintosh) or lifts the epiglottis (straight blade); in VL, watch the screen and align anatomy.
9. Lift the blade up and away at a 45° angle, not levering on the teeth, until the vocal cords come into view.
10. With your right hand, insert the lubricated, stylet-curved ETT through the cords until the cuff passes 2–3 cm beyond the glottis.
11. Remove the stylet carefully while holding the tube securely.
12. Inflate the cuff with air (5–10 mL) using a syringe.
13. Confirm placement:
    (a) Look for chest rise.
    (b) Auscultate both the lungs and epigastrium if possible.
    (c) Use $EtCO_2$ detector (color change to yellow or waveform if available).
    (d) Observe for improved oxygenation, reduced work of breathing, and absence of gastric sounds.
14. Secure the tube with tape or a commercial tube holder, ensuring it is firmly fixed in anticipation of casualty movement.
15. Document depth at teeth or lips (usually 21–23 cm for adults).
16. Reassess tube placement frequently, especially during movement or extraction, and be prepared to ventilate with BVM.

Surgical Airway

I. Needle Cricothyrotomy
Procedure:

1. Identify the cricothyroid membrane. Begin at the base of the neck by locating the cricoid cartilage, a firm, circular structure just above the top of the trachea. Move your finger cranially (upward) until you feel a soft, step-off depression between the cricoid cartilage and the lower border of the thyroid cartilage—this is the cricothyroid membrane (Fig. 20.15).

2. Stabilize the trachea with the thumb and forefinger of the nondominant hand to prevent lateral movement of the trachea during the procedure.
3. Inject a local anesthetic along the anticipated skin incision site (if the patient is capable of feeling pain.)
4. Puncture the skin in the midline with the cannula attached to a syringe, directly over the cricothyroid membrane. Direct the cannula at a 45° angle caudally while applying negative pressure to the syringe.
5. Carefully insert the cannula through the lower half of the cricothyroid membrane, aspirating as the needle is advanced. The addition of 2–3 cc of saline to the syringe will aid in detecting air.
6. Note the aspiration of air, which signifies entry into the tracheal lumen.
7. Remove the syringe and withdraw the needle while gently advancing the cannula downward into position, taking care not to perforate the posterior wall of the trachea.
8. Attach the jet insufflation equipment to the cannula, or attach the oxygen tubing or 3 mL syringe (7.5) endotracheal tube connector combination over the catheter needle hub, and secure the catheter to the patient's neck.
9. *Adequate* PaO_2 *can be maintained for only around 30–45 min*, and CO_2 accumulation can occur more rapidly.
10. Continue to observe lung inflation and auscultate the chest for adequate ventilation. To avoid barotrauma, which can lead to pneumothorax, pay special attention to lung deflation. If lung deflation is not observed, in the absence of serious chest injury, it may be possible to support expiration by using gentle pressure on the chest.

II. Surgical Cricothyrotomy

Procedure:

1. Place the patient in a supine position with the neck in a neutral position. Have an assistant restrict the patient's cervical motion.
2. Palpate the thyroid notch, cricothyroid cartilage, and sternal notch for orientation.
3. Surgically prepare and anesthetize the area locally, if the patient is conscious.
4. Stabilize the thyroid cartilage with the nondominant hand, and maintain stabilization until the trachea is intubated.
5. Make a 2–3 cm vertical skin incision over the cricothyroid membrane and, using the dominant hand from a cranial direction, spread the skin edges to reduce bleeding. Reidentify the cricothyroid membrane and then incise through the base of the membrane transversely and dilate the site using mosquito artery forceps (Fig. 20.16).

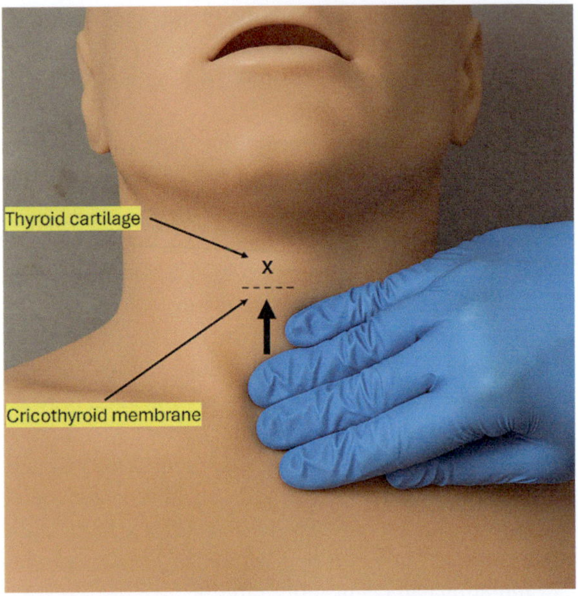

Fig. 20.15 Identifying cricothyroid membrane by palpating from the base of the neck

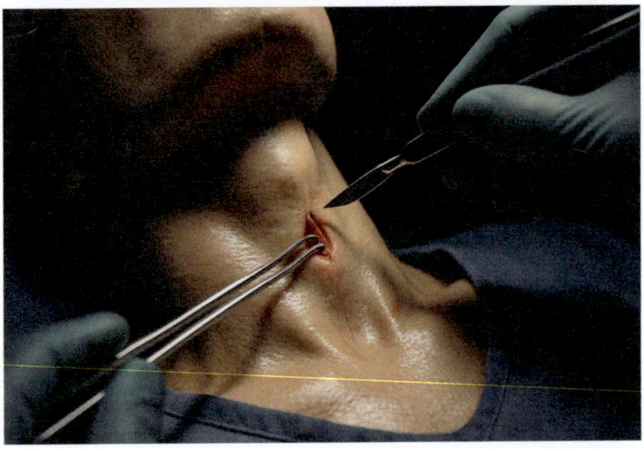

Fig. 20.16 Surgical cricothyrotomy

6. Insert a properly sized, cuffed endotracheal tube or tracheostomy tube (usually a size 5–6) through the cricothyroid membrane incision, directing the tube distally into the trachea. If an endotracheal tube is used, advance only until the cuff is no longer visible to avoid mainstem intubation. Inflate the cuff and ventilate.
7. Observe lung inflation and auscultate the chest for adequate ventilation. Confirm the presence of CO_2 and obtain a chest X-ray. Secure the endotracheal or tracheostomy tube to the patient, to prevent dislodgement.

Key Messages

- Airway takes precedence only after massive hemorrhage is controlled.
- Burns, trauma, and decreased mental status are red flags for early airway intervention.
- *Choose the simplest effective airway* in a high-risk or low-resource environment.
- Confirm tube position with *at least two methods.*
- Do not attempt multiple intubation attempts in unstable or moving settings.
- Surgical airways are last resort but must be practiced regularly.

Respiration

Case Scenario

Two soldiers are rescued after sustaining chest injuries in combat. One has a penetrating bullet injury to the right hemithorax at the sixth intercostal space midclavicular line. The other sustained blunt trauma from a collapsed wall and is short of breath with crepitus on palpation. Evacuation is delayed, and signs of tension pneumothorax emerge en route.

Core Skill Components

I. Three-Sided Occlusive Dressing

Equipment required:

Equipment	Number
Airtight material/chest seal	As needed
Dry gauze	As needed
Gloves, tape	As needed

Procedure:

1. Expose the chest and identify the wound—*typically a penetrating injury with a sucking sound or bubbling at the wound site during respiration.*
2. Immediately apply a gloved hand or airtight material (plastic wrap, chest seal, or glove) over the wound to temporarily seal it while preparing the dressing.
3. Clean and dry the area surrounding the wound as much as the tactical situation allows to help adhesive stick, but do not delay application if bleeding or air leak is active.
4. Cut or select a piece of nonporous, airtight material (e.g., chest seal, plastic wrapper, foil, or glove) *at least 5–6 cm larger than the wound in all directions.*

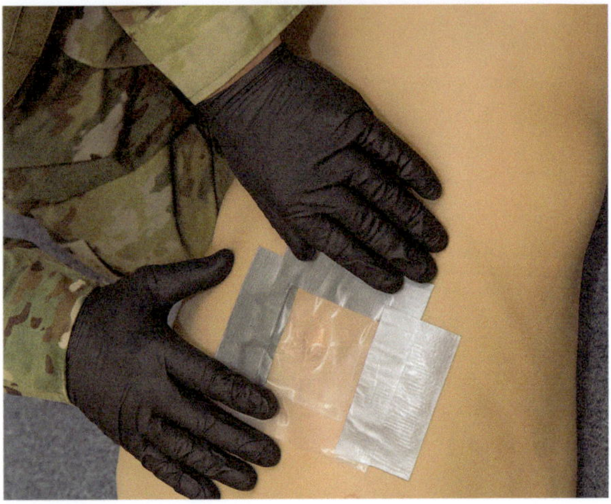

Fig. 20.17 Three-sided occlusive dressing

5. Place the material directly over the wound, ensuring full coverage of all wound edges.
6. Tape down *three sides* of the dressing—*typically the top, right, and left edges*—leaving the bottom edge open to act as a flutter valve (Fig. 20.17).
7. The open edge allows air to escape during exhalation while preventing air from entering the pleural space during inhalation, reducing the risk of tension pneumothorax.
8. Instruct the casualty (if conscious) to exhale fully while the dressing is sealed, to evacuate trapped air before final placement.
9. Continuously monitor the casualty for signs of deterioration—increasing respiratory distress or decreased breath sounds may indicate progression to tension pneumothorax.
10. If tension develops, *lift or remove the occlusive dressing temporarily ("burping" it) or perform needle decompression.*
11. Document the time of application and monitor closely during transport or movement.

II. Needle Decompression

Equipment required:

Equipment	Number
Thoracic manikin	1
3-way stopcock	1
14–16 G IV needle over catheter	1
Syringe	1

Procedure:

1. Identify signs of tension pneumothorax: *respiratory distress, absent or diminished breath sounds on one side, distended neck veins, tracheal deviation (late sign), hypotension, and cyanosis.*
2. Confirm the need for immediate needle decompression—this is a lifesaving intervention and should not be delayed if clinical suspicion is high.
3. Expose the chest and choose the appropriate anatomical site: *either the fifth intercostal space at the anterior axillary line (preferred) or the second intercostal space at the midclavicular line on the affected side* (Fig. 20.18).
4. Clean the area if time and situation permit, prioritizing speed over sterility in tactical conditions.
5. Prepare a 14–16 gauge cannula/catheter, preferably at least 8 cm in length, attached to a syringe partially filled with saline or air.
6. Insert the needle perpendicular to the chest wall at the chosen site, *just above the upper border of the rib to avoid the neurovascular bundle.*
7. Advance the needle until a sudden release of air or a "pop" is felt—this confirms entry into the pleural space; you may also see bubbling in the syringe.
8. Remove the needle, leaving the catheter in place; listen for air escape and observe for clinical improvement (e.g., improved breathing and SpO_2 rise).
9. Secure the catheter to the chest wall with tape to prevent dislodgement during movement or transport.
10. *Monitor for reaccumulation of tension*—reassess breath sounds and patient condition frequently; repeat decompression may be necessary.
11. Document time, site, and side of decompression, and communicate it clearly during casualty handover.

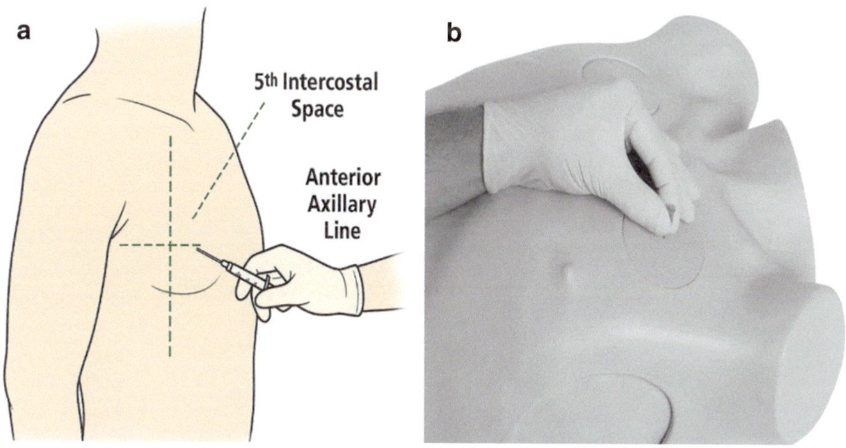

Fig. 20.18 Needle decompression. (**a**) Fifth intercostal space at the anterior axillary line. (**b**) Second intercostal space at the midclavicular line

III. Tube Thoracostomy

Equipment required (Fig. 20.19):

Equipment	Number
Thoracic manikin	1
Surgical drapes and sterile gown and gloves	As needed
Surgical instruments:	
Scalpel handles: sizes 3, 4 Scalpel blades: sizes 10, 11 or 15 Tissue forceps Large clamps (e.g., Kelly) Suture scissor Needle holder	1 each 1 each 2 2 1 1
Suture, heavy nonabsorbable (0, 1, or 2) 20 mL syringe Lidocaine Skin preparation solution Gauze pads Chest tube, 28 and 32 Chest tube drain set	4 1 1 bottle 1 10 2 each 1
Occlusive dressing	1 in. strips, large
4 in. tape	1 roll

Procedure:

1. Identify the need for thoracostomy—typically in cases of penetrating or blunt chest trauma with suspected tension pneumothorax, hemothorax, or persistent air leak unrelieved by needle decompression.
2. Choose the correct anatomical site: *the fifth intercostal space at the anterior or mid-axillary line, on the affected side.*
3. Position the patient with the arm raised above the head to expose the lateral chest wall, if spinal injury is not suspected.
4. Don gloves and eye protection; clean the area as much as the tactical situation allows, but do not delay if the patient is in extremis.
5. *Make a 4–5 cm horizontal incision* over the fifth intercostal space, *just above the upper border of the sixth rib to avoid the neurovascular bundle.*

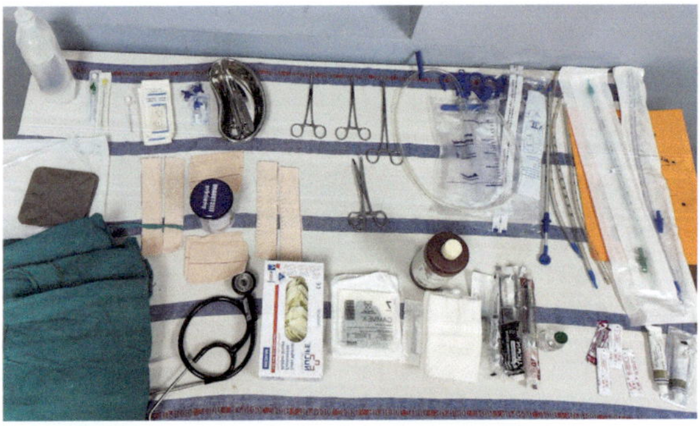

Fig. 20.19 Equipment required for tube thoracostomy

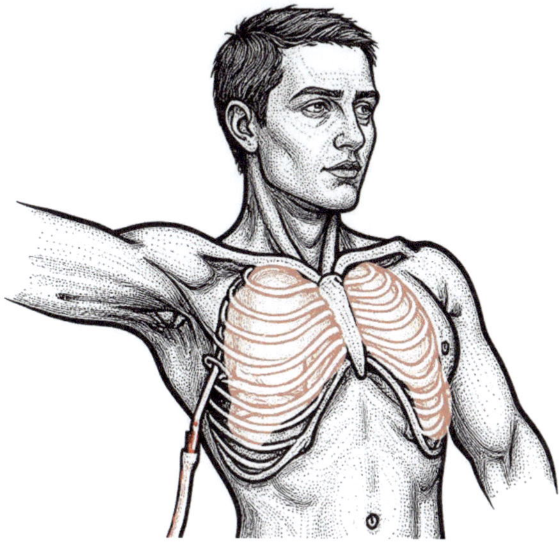

Fig. 20.20 Tube thoracostomy for a pneumothorax

6. Use blunt dissection with a curved clamp (e.g., Kelly or mosquito forceps) through the intercostal muscles until the pleural space is entered.
7. Insert a gloved finger into the pleural space to confirm entry, break any adhesions, and verify lung re-expansion and absence of solid organ injury—*this is the finger thoracostomy.*
8. If placing a chest tube, insert a 28–32 Fr thoracostomy tube through the same tract, directing it posteriorly and superiorly for pneumothorax (Fig. 20.20) or posteriorly and inferiorly for hemothorax.
9. Advance the tube until the last side hole is inside the thoracic cavity; do not force against resistance.
10. Connect the tube to a Heimlich valve, improvised water seal, or drainage system depending on resources available.
11. Suture the tube in place using heavy silk and apply an occlusive dressing to seal the wound.
12. Reassess breath sounds, SpO_2, and chest movement; check for air leak or continued blood drainage.
13. Document the procedure details: side, site, time, output, and improvement, and include this in casualty handover.

Key Messages

- Tension pneumothorax is the most rapidly correctable cause of preventable combat death.
- *If in doubt, decompress with needle or finger.* Delay can be fatal.
- The majority of life-threatening injuries to the chest can be treated with a tube thoracostomy.
- Chest tubes should be secured firmly; *poorly secured tubes risk dislodgement in transit.*
- Always reassess for recurrence of pneumothorax or hemorrhage.
- Improvisation is key—*glove + tape can seal a sucking chest wound.*

Hypothermia/Head Injury

Case Scenario

A 47-year-old soldier is rescued unconscious after falling from a cliff during mountain patrol. His clothes are soaked in icy water, and the ambient temperature is below freezing. Another casualty from a blast shows confused behavior and unequal pupils. Evacuation is delayed for 2 h due to terrain and enemy fire.

Core Skill Components

Equipment required:

Equipment	Number
Space blanket/thermal (Mylar) blanket	1
Sleeping bag or insulated roll	1
Waterproof ground insulation mat or foam pad	1
Dry blankets or clothes (for base insulation layer)	1
Plastic sheet/vapor barrier material	1
Towels or absorbent cloths	As needed
Warm packs/chemical heat packs	As needed
Cap, hood, or head covering	1
Trauma shears (to remove wet clothing)	1
Penlight (for pupillary exam)	1
GCS/AVPU reference chart	1
Stopwatch/timer	1
Cervical collars (adjustable and/or multiple sizes)	2
Measuring guide for collar sizing	1
Training mannequin (preferably with adjustable neck position)	1
Rigid spine board (full-length)	1
Head immobilizer blocks with straps or foam supports	1
Cross-body securing straps or Velcro belts	1 set

(continued)

Equipment	Number
Forehead and chin securing straps or medical tape	1
Log roll checklist/step-by-step diagram	1
Three-person team (for log-roll demonstration)	1
Gloves (non-sterile)	As needed
Documentation sheet	As needed

I. Hypothermia Management: Improvised Wrap with Internal Vapor Barrier
Procedure:

1. Move the casualty to a sheltered or covered area if possible to prevent further heat loss.
2. Gently remove all wet clothing and cutting garments away if needed to avoid excessive movement or pain.
3. Dry the patient thoroughly using towels, absorbent materials, or any available clean fabric, focusing on the chest, back, and groin.
4. Lay a thermal or foil blanket, sleeping bag, or insulating surface on the ground to prevent heat loss through conduction.
5. *Wrap the patient in dry layers*—start with base layers (like dry clothes or blankets), followed by a thermal or space blanket, and then cover with any available windproof or waterproof layer (Fig. 20.21).

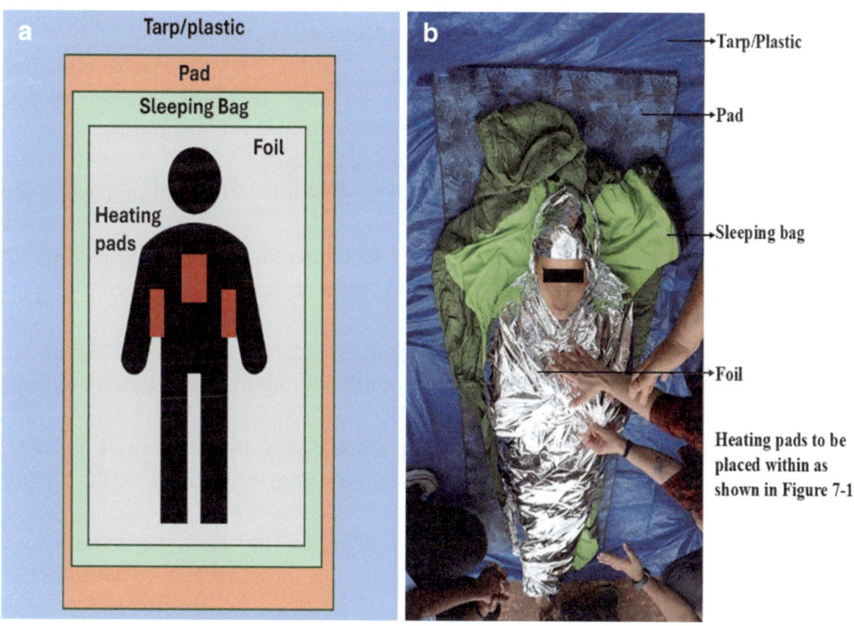

Fig. 20.21 Burrito wrap technique—improvised wrap with internal heating pads and vapor barrier

6. Ensure the head is covered with a cap or hood and place warm packs near the neck, armpits, and groin if available and the patient is not unconscious.
7. Elevate the casualty's legs slightly if not contraindicated to support circulation.
8. *Avoid active rewarming if the patient is unconscious or severely hypothermic to prevent afterdrop*; focus instead on passive insulation.
9. Continuously monitor for changes in mental status, respiratory rate, and pulse, and reassess the wrap to ensure it remains dry and sealed against wind or cold.

II. TBI and Neurological Assessment

Procedure:

1. Assess the patient's level of consciousness using the AVPU scale (Alert, responds to Voice, responds to Pain, Unresponsive) as a rapid screening tool.
2. Follow up with a detailed Glasgow Coma Scale (GCS) assessment: Check eye opening (1–4), verbal response (1–5), and motor response (1–6), recording a total score out of 15.
3. Perform a bilateral pupillary check using a penlight—evaluate for size, equality, and reactivity to light; *asymmetry or fixed dilated pupils may suggest raised intracranial pressure.*
4. Assess limb movement and motor function, noting any asymmetry, posturing (decorticate/decerebrate), or flaccidity that may indicate neurological compromise.
5. Monitor for signs of rising intracranial pressure (ICP), including *Cushing's triad: bradycardia, hypertension (widened pulse pressure), and irregular respirations.*
6. Maintain neutral head positioning to promote cerebral venous drainage—*avoid flexion, hyperextension, or lateral rotation of the neck.*
7. Elevate the head of the bed or upper body to about 30°, if spinal injury is ruled out, to reduce ICP.
8. Take airway precautions: Ensure patency while avoiding aggressive suctioning or hyperventilation; provide oxygen if available and support ventilation if GCS ≤ 8.
9. Watch for seizure activity, including tonic-clonic movements, eye deviation, jaw clenching, or brief posturing; also monitor for subtle signs like lip smacking or limb twitching.
10. If a seizure occurs, protect the airway, maintain lateral positioning if possible, prevent injury, and administer benzodiazepines (e.g., midazolam or diazepam) if equipped.
11. Reassess neurological status regularly and document any changes; deterioration may indicate expanding hematoma, worsening cerebral edema, or herniation.

III. Spinal Immobilization

(a) *Cervical Collar Application*

Procedure:

1. Assess the need for cervical spine immobilization—typically in cases of trauma with altered mental status, neck pain, distracting injuries, or mechanism suggestive of spinal risk (e.g., fall, blast, and MVC).
2. Explain the procedure to the patient if conscious and instruct them to minimize head movement.
3. Position yourself at the head of the patient and maintain manual in-line stabilization of the cervical spine throughout the procedure.
4. Select the appropriate size cervical collar by measuring from the top of the shoulder (trapezius) to the angle of the jaw; most commercial collars have adjustable sizing guides (Fig. 20.22).

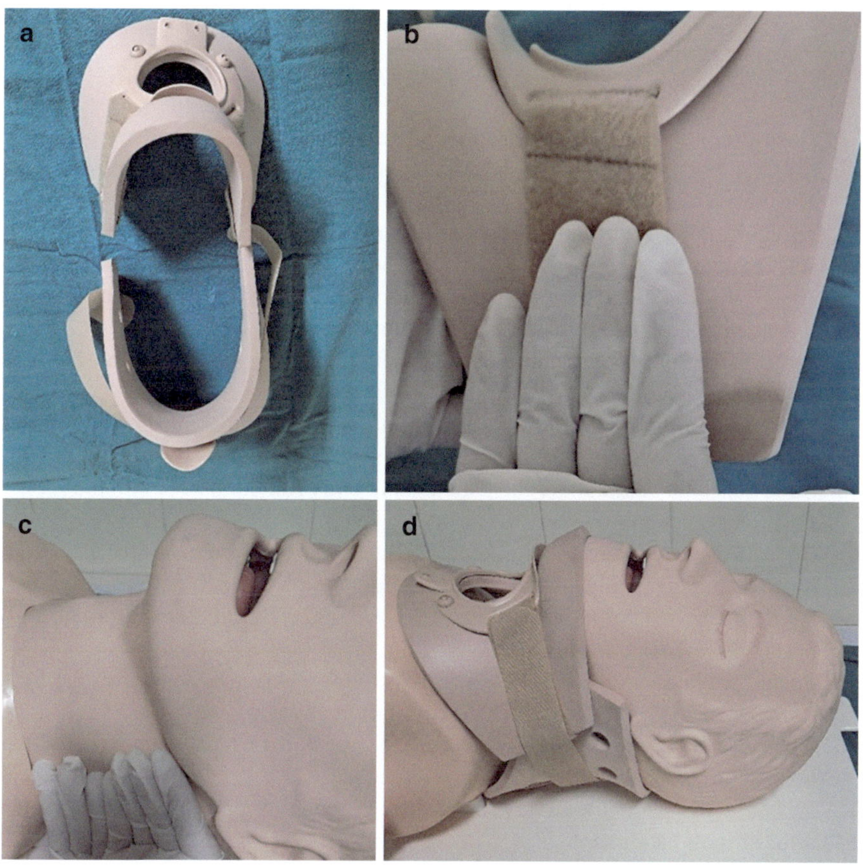

Fig. 20.22 Cervical collar application. (**a**) Hard cervical collar. (**b**) Choosing appropriate size of hard cervical collar. (**c**) Measurement of appropriate size of hard cervical collar on a manikin. (**d**) Hard cervical collar applied on a manikin

5. Pre-size and prepare the collar by adjusting it to fit the patient's neck height, locking it into position before application.
6. Slide the back portion of the collar behind the patient's neck, ensuring it centers evenly beneath the occiput.
7. Bring the front of the collar up under the chin, cupping the jawline gently while ensuring the chin is supported but not overly flexed.
8. Fasten the Velcro or side straps securely on both sides, *ensuring a snug fit without excessive tightness or gaping.*
9. Reassess to ensure proper alignment, comfort, and maintenance of a neutral position; *confirm that the collar does not obstruct the airway or interfere with breathing.*
10. Release manual stabilization only once the collar is secured and additional spinal immobilization (e.g., spine board and head blocks) is in place if required.
11. Document the time of application, collar type/size, and any neurological findings before and after application.

(b) *Spine Board Immobilization*

Procedure:

1. Determine the need for spinal immobilization based on mechanism of injury, altered mental status, neck or back pain, neurologic deficits, or inability to reliably assess the spine.
2. Explain the procedure to the patient if conscious, and instruct them to remain still throughout.
3. *Assign roles to at least three providers:* one at the head to maintain manual in-line stabilization and two others at the shoulders, hips, and legs.
4. Position the spine board adjacent to the patient, ideally on the side to which the patient will be rolled.
5. With the person at the head giving commands, perform a coordinated log roll by rotating the patient as a unit onto their side, keeping the spine in alignment.
6. Slide the spine board under the patient and gently roll them back into the supine position on the board (Fig. 20.23).
7. Reposition the patient to align their body centrally on the board, ensuring the head, shoulders, spine, and legs are all midline.
8. Apply a cervical collar if not already done and place head blocks or foam supports on either side of the head.
9. Secure the head with straps or tape across the forehead and chin, ensuring neutral alignment without neck flexion or rotation.
10. Use cross-body straps or belts to secure the chest, pelvis, and legs firmly to the board to prevent shifting during movement.
11. Reassess the patient's airway, breathing, circulation, and neurological status after immobilization.
12. Document the time of immobilization, findings before and after, and any changes during transport.

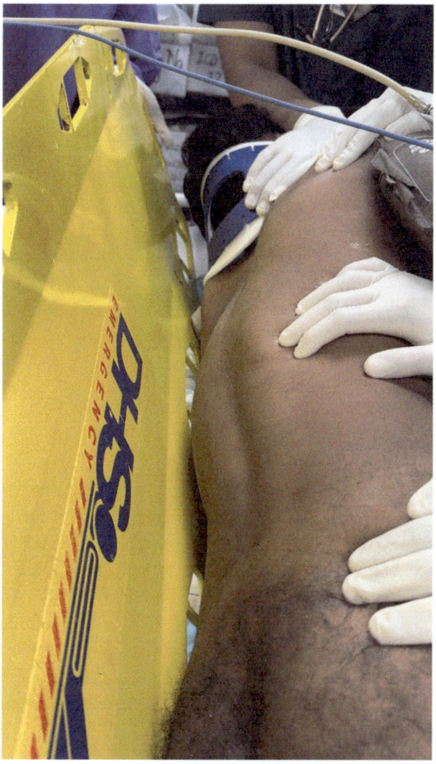

Fig. 20.23 Spine board immobilization

Key Messages

- Even warm environments pose hypothermia risk after fluid loss or wet exposure.
- Hypothermia worsens coagulopathy and increases mortality—*cold kills.*
- *Warm from core outward, not extremities first,* to prevent afterdrop.
- Prevention of secondary brain injury is the priority—oxygenation, perfusion, and warmth.
- *Head injury signs may be subtle*—monitor mental status and pupils repeatedly.
- Do not hyperventilate patients with suspected raised ICP unless absolutely indicated.
- Avoid moving spinal injury patients unless airway or scene safety dictates.

Conclusion

The FORCE Skill Stations chapter translates battlefield theory into tactile competence, enabling providers to perform under the most austere and chaotic conditions. Structured around the MARCH algorithm, each station is crafted to reinforce lifesaving skills in environments where seconds count and resources falter. From controlling hemorrhage with improvised tourniquets to managing airways inside a vibrating vehicle, this chapter embeds procedural fluency, tactical judgment, and adaptive improvisation into every drill. Skill acquisition is not merely about mastering checklists—it is about internalizing action patterns that can be executed under fire, in cold, or in silence. The modular, scenario-based structure also ensures applicability across combat, disaster, and civilian field settings. By emphasizing realism, resilience, and role-based proficiency, the FORCE Skill Stations prepare each provider—not just to react, but to lead, stabilize, and save. In the end, FORCE is not about procedures—it is about presence, preparedness, and performance when everything else is uncertain.

Bibliography

1. American College of Surgeons Committee on Trauma. ATLS: Advanced Trauma Life Support. 10th ed. Chicago: American College of Surgeons; 2018. ISBN: 978-0996826235
2. Army U.S. Tactical Combat Casualty Care Handbook. Version 5. Morrisville (NC): Lulu Press Inc.; 2017. 130 p. ISBN: 9781678198312.
3. Auerbach PS, Cushing TA, Harris NS. Auerbach's Wilderness Medicine. 7th ed. 2 vols. Philadelphia: Elsevier; 2016. ISBN: 9780323359429
4. Butler, Frank K et al. "Tactical Combat Casualty Care and Wilderness Medicine: Advancing Trauma Care in Austere Environments." *Emergency medicine clinics of North America* vol. 35,2 (2017): 391–407. https://doi.org/10.1016/j.emc.2016.12.005
5. Butler, Frank K Jr et al. "Tactical combat casualty care 2007: evolving concepts and battlefield experience." *Military medicine* vol. 172,11 Suppl (2007): 1–19. https://doi.org/10.7205/milmed.172.supplement_1.1
6. Butler, Frank K Jr. "Fluid Resuscitation in Tactical Combat Casualty Care: Yesterday and Today." *Wilderness & environmental medicine* vol. 28,2S (2017): S74–S81. https://doi.org/10.1016/j.wem.2016.12.007
7. Feliciano DV, Mattox KL, Moore EE. *Trauma*. 9th ed. New York: McGraw Hill Medical; 2020. ISBN: 978-1260143355
8. Giebner, Stephen D. "The Transition to the Committee on Tactical Combat Casualty Care." *Wilderness & environmental medicine* vol. 28,2S (2017): S18–S24. https://doi.org/10.1016/j.wem.2016.11.005
9. Giebner, Stephen. "TCCC Updates: Tactical Combat Casualty Care Curriculum Annual Update 2014." *Journal of special operations medicine: a peer reviewed journal for SOF medical professionals* vol. 14,4 (2014): 144–145. https://doi.org/10.55460/W2P1-7IUE
10. Tintinalli JE, Ma OJ, Yealy DM, et al. *Tintinalli's Emergency Medicine: A Comprehensive Study Guide*. 9th ed. New York: McGraw-Hill Education; 2019. ISBN: 978-1405296434.

MIX
Papier aus verantwortungsvollen Quellen
Paper from responsible sources
FSC® C105338

If you have any concerns about our products,
you can contact us on
ProductSafety@springernature.com

In case Publisher is established outside the EU,
the EU authorized representative is:
Springer Nature Customer Service Center GmbH
Europaplatz 3, 69115 Heidelberg, Germany

Printed by Libri Plureos GmbH
in Hamburg, Germany